Clinical Cases
and OSCEs
in Surgery

Clinical Cases and OSCEs in Surgery

The definitive guide to passing examinations

THIRD EDITION

Manoj Ramachandran

BSc(Hons) MBBS(Hons) MRCS(Eng) FRCS(Tr&Orth)

Consultant Orthopaedic and Trauma Surgeon (Paediatric and Young Adult)
Lead for Paediatric Orthopaedics and Director of Informatics, Surgery and Cancer,
The Royal London and Barts and The London Children's Hospitals, Barts Health NHS
Trust, London

Honorary Reader and Director of Clinical Strategy, School of Engineering and Material
Sciences, Queen Mary, University of London

Marc A Gladman

MBBS DRCOG DFFP PhD MRCOG MRCS(Eng) FRCS(Gen Surg) FRACS

Professor of Colorectal Surgery, Sydney Medical School, University of Sydney, Australia

Head, Academic Colorectal Unit and Consultant Colorectal Surgeon, Concord Hospital,
Sydney, Australia

Director, Enteric Neuroscience and Gastrointestinal Research Group, ANZAC Research
Institute, University of Sydney, Australia

Photographer: Pramod Achan

MBBS FRCS(Eng) FRCS(Tr&Orth)

Consultant Orthopaedic Surgeon, The Royal London
and St Bartholomew's Hospitals, Barts and The
London NHS Trust, London, UK

Contribution from: Roshana Mehdian

MBCHB BMSC (Hons) MRCS(Eng) PGCMedEd

Trauma and Orthopaedic Registrar, South West
London Deanery, London, UK

ELSEVIER

Edinburgh   London   New York   Oxford   Philadelphia   St Louis   Sydney   Toronto   2018

ELSEVIER

First edition 2003
Second edition 2011
Third edition 2018

Notices

Knowledge and best practice in this field are constantly changing. As new research and experience broaden our understanding, changes in research methods, professional practices or medical treatment may become necessary.

Practitioners and researchers must always rely on their own experience and knowledge in evaluating and using any information, methods, compounds or experiments described herein. In using such information or methods they should be mindful of their own safety and the safety of others, including parties for whom they have a professional responsibility.

With respect to any drug or pharmaceutical products identified, readers are advised to check the most current information provided (i) on procedures featured or (ii) by the manufacturer of each product to be administered, to verify the recommended dose or formula, the method and duration of administration and contraindications. It is the responsibility of practitioners, relying on their own experience and knowledge of their patients, to make diagnoses, to determine dosages and the best treatment for each individual patient and to take all appropriate safety precautions.

To the fullest extent of the law, neither the Publisher nor the authors, contributors or editors assume any liability for any injury and/or damage to persons or property as a matter of products liability, negligence or otherwise, or from any use or operation of any methods, products, instructions or ideas contained in the material herein.

The Publisher

ISBN 978-0-7020-6629-0

Printed in China

Last digit is the print number: 9   8   7   6   5   4   3   2   1

Senior Content Strategist: Laurence Hunter
Senior Content Development Specialist: Ailsa Laing
Project Manager: Deepthi Unni
Designer: Miles Hitchen
Marketing Manager: Deb Watkins

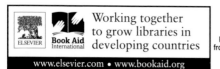

Working together
to grow libraries in
developing countries

ELSEVIER   Book Aid International

www.elsevier.com • www.bookaid.org

The publisher's policy is to use paper manufactured from sustainable forests

PREFACE

Increasingly, the art of surgical examination is being lost from the repertoire of clinical skills of undergraduate and postgraduate students of surgery. Unlike many other branches of medicine in the 21st century, many surgical diagnoses depend on clinical assessment. Consequently, the maintenance and fine-tuning of clinical skills remain imperative to good surgical practice. The primary aim of this book is to demystify and simplify the clinical assessment of surgical cases. This third edition – the definitive guide to passing examinations – is aimed squarely at candidates preparing for surgical examinations, be it at undergraduate, postgraduate or exit examination level. We have included lessons learned from our own personal experience of sitting and conducting surgical examinations and have provided Top Tips, acronyms and up-to-date summaries of current practice wherever possible. As a new addition, we have included photographs of surgical signs to assist with exam preparation, whilst retaining images of key manoeuvres during specific surgical examination routines.

As with previous editions, the cases in the book are carefully framed to allow interpretation for not only short cases but also OSCEs, reflecting recent changes to College exams. For each case, an example of the opening instruction is given, followed by a discussion of the steps required to complete the examination. To assist with your exam preparation, this book is organised as follows:

By subspecialty: Cases are listed in clusters that reflect the subspecialties of surgery to assist with revision and exam preparation.

Common to rare: Certain cases tend to appear more commonly than others in examinations.

This book attempts to list cases in decreasing order of frequency of likely appearance in the examination within each subsection; this is denoted by the star rating given to each case, three stars being the most frequently encountered.

Instruction: This is the same for short cases and OSCEs and defines the flow of the case which follows.

Top tips: These are included to emphasise specific areas (often favourites of examiners), which cause confusion or are described differently by different surgeons and teachers.

Finish your examination here: This instruction is added to demonstrate where the marking sheets for an OSCE, or the expectations of a short-case examiner, are likely to conclude. Going beyond this is unlikely to score any further marks and you are more likely to impress by answering some supplemental questions accurately.

Questions and advanced questions: These are designed to fit in with both short-case and OSCE formats, and also cover supplemental questions asked following 'history' scenarios.

Procedures and props: We have included examples of common procedures and props that come up in the skill-based examination format, such as reduction of fractures and description of intramedullary nails and external fixators.

We hope that this book will help you prepare with confidence for any surgical examination you may have to face in the future.

Manoj Ramachandran, London, 2018

Marc A Gladman, Sydney, 2018

ABOUT THE AUTHORS

Manoj Ramachandran is Consultant Orthopaedic and Trauma Surgeon, Lead for Paediatric Orthopaedics and Director of Informatics, Surgery and Cancer at The Royal London & Barts and The London Children's Hospitals, London and Honorary Reader at Queen Mary, University of London. He qualified from King's College School of Medicine, University of London with a double honours degree and *proxime accessit* to the University of London Gold Medal. He undertook basic surgical training on the Oxford and Hammersmith rotations and specialist orthopaedic training on the Royal National Orthopaedic Hospital rotation, Stanmore, Middlesex, with fellowships in Sydney, Los Angeles and London. He has a strong interest in education, digital health, medical technology and entrepreneurship. For more on Manoj's projects and achievements, please visit his personal website at manoj.strikingly.com.

Marc A Gladman is Professor of Colorectal Surgery at the Sydney Medical School, University of Sydney and Head of the Academic Colorectal Unit and Consultant Colorectal Surgeon, Concord Hospital, Sydney. He is also Director of the Enteric Neuroscience & Gastrointestinal Research Group, ANZAC Research Institute, University of Sydney, Australia. Having qualified from King's College School of Medicine, University of London, he undertook training in Obstetrics & Gynaecology, General Surgery and Colorectal Surgery in London before moving to Sydney. He is committed to undergraduate and postgraduate education and career development, using technology-enhanced techniques. During the last twenty years he has been extensively involved in surgical examinations at multiple centres in the UK and Australia and has designed, directed and delivered numerous examination revision courses, including the online resource, masterclass.surgery.

ACKNOWLEDGEMENTS

Acknowledgements for the third edition

The authors would like to thank the entire team at Elsevier, specifically, **Mr Laurence Hunter** for his continued support and belief in the project, and **Ms Ailsa Laing** for her expert guidance through the stages of publication. Special thanks also go to **Mr Lee Parker**, Consultant Orthopaedic Surgeon, for his help with his vital contribution to the foot cases in the musculoskeletal section, to **Mr Ian Whiteley** and **Dr Jake Sloane** for their help collecting clinical images and to **Roshana Mehdian**, Specialty Trainee in Trauma and Orthopaedics for her valuable and significant contributions throughout the book.

Acknowledgements for the second edition

The authors express their sincere gratitude to **Mr Pramod Achan**, Consultant Orthopaedic Surgeon, The Royal London and St Bartholomew's Hospitals, Barts and The London NHS Trust, London for his role as photographer of the high-quality images that have beautifully complemented the updated text of the new edition of this book. We would also like to thank **Dr Elizabeth Owen** for her excellent body-art painting on our student models and **Ms Noemi Montes** for her vital help with the photographic editing.

The authors would also like to thank **Tom Crompton**, Specialist Registrar in Orthopaedics and Trauma, South East Thames rotation, London for his significant contribution to the Communication Skills cases.

The authors are grateful to the following current medical students (and one postgraduate surgeon) at Barts and The London School of Medicine and Dentistry, University of London for volunteering to act as photographic models: **Katie Chan, Harry Craven, Marc Gladman, Archchana Radhakrishnan, Catherine Rees, Emily Shepherd** and **Natalie Soobadoo**.

Acknowledgements for the first edition

The authors are grateful to the following individuals for their advice:

Rachel Bell, Joanna Broomfield, Timothy Cheadle, Paul Dilworth, Barry Ferris, Richard Harrison, Charlie Knowles, Gordon Kooiman, Emma Jackson, Will Jackson, Tim McCormick, Ian McDermott, Navin Ramachandran, Sally Richardson, Marc Swan, Hazel Warburton and **Dan Weaver.**

INTRODUCTION

It is important to appreciate that clinical examination is essentially the same irrespective of whether the examination employs short cases or OSCEs. Whilst the conduct is slightly different between the two formats, the surgical knowledge and skills assessed are identical. Increasingly, OSCEs are being used for examinations, including the Intercollegiate MRCS, since they ensure consistency (and thus reliability) of assessment between candidates.

Irrespective of the format of the examination, the importance of technique cannot be overstated. Put simply, clinical examinations demand a demonstration of your skill, knowledge and ability to examiners. Successful negotiation, and the all-important 'pass', is largely dependent on two factors: (1) preparation/revision leading up to the exam, requiring repeated rehearsal and practice of clinical skills; and (2) performance in front of the examiners with deliberate and explicit demonstration of clinical information using a systematic approach.

SHORT CASES

Format

At the beginning of the examination, candidates wait in a specific central area to be collected by the examiners, who often work in pairs. One asks the questions and the other listens and often makes notes. The examiners lead you round the patients, who are organised in clusters (or 'bays'), and choose which patients you meet and in which order.

Often a prop, an X-ray or another data interpretation-style question can be introduced, but these are usually supplemental to the major theme, which is the physical examination of a sign or system. The vast majority of the time will be spent examining the patient and answering questions on the case, e.g. treatment options.

The examiners choose how many patients you see per bay, which can vary between just one patient to six or seven. The time limitation is usually imposed on the whole bay, which may be 10–15 minutes. Within that time it is up to the examiner how many patients the candidates see and how deep (and difficult) the supplemental questions become. In Final MB short cases, there is usually only one bay where all the cases are examined, which might be part of a ward or a day-surgery unit.

The *pros* of short cases are that they:

- Allow good candidates to progress rapidly to harder cases or more complex supplemental questions
- Give flexibility for examiners to choose different patients who are waiting in the bay, which is less boring for both examiner and patients
- Allow rapid assessment of clinical skills across areas, e.g. in superficial lesions, cases vary from skin lesions to lumps and bumps to thyroid nodules, etc.
- Incorporate data interpretation questions, such as chest X-rays, as appropriate
- Test clinical skills across a broad spectrum.

The *cons* of short cases include that:

- They allow little control of choice of patients an individual examiner picks (except the presence of the co-examiner)
- They can emphasize 'favourite' clinical signs, which may not reflect clinical relevance
- It is difficult to control the marking scheme to ensure transparency and fairness
- They are almost entirely subjective
- It is difficult for the candidate to feel confident about doing well (or badly), as the questions tend to get increasingly difficult.

OBJECTIVE STRUCTURED CLINICAL EXAMINATION (OSCE)

Format

OSCEs comprise a series of stations in a circuit that cover different aspects of the syllabus, around which the candidates rotate. At each station the candidate is required to undertake a clearly defined task, such as taking a focused history or performing a clinical examination, interpreting an X-ray or performing a simulated practical procedure. The time spent at each station is fixed (often 7–10 minutes) and is the same for every candidate, irrespective of how well (or badly!) the candidate is performing at the station. Often a bell rings between stations to let the examiners know to move on to the next candidate. One minute is allowed between stations for circulation from one station to the next. This also allows the examiners to complete the mark sheet for each candidate and for the patient or simulated patient to prepare for the next candidate. Each OSCE usually contains between 10 and 20 stations. The whole examination therefore lasts at least 2 hours, but can be longer. The marking sheet used by examiners is pre-set and only allows them to score on specific criteria that are standard for every other examiner as well.

The *pros* of OSCEs are that:

- The marking scheme is explicit and therefore seen as being 'fairer'
- They reduce inter-examiner variability, and usually mean assessment by a larger number of examiners in total because each scenario is examined by a different clinician
- They allow the possibility of assessment by other doctors (e.g. specialist registrars, medical educators) or other healthcare professionals
- There tends to be much greater emphasis on patient-centred examining, including communication skills and rapport, i.e. testing a greater range of skills (not just clinical examination)
- They allow for much more extensive use of simulated patients – see below.

The *cons* of OSCEs include that they:

- Are repetitive for examiners and patients – seen as being 'boring' and may lead to error
- Provide little or no scope for examiners to push very strong candidates
- Make it easier to score an average mark, and more difficult to pull out a clear fail or an exceptional candidate
- May present patients as having a certain set of characteristic symptoms or signs, which may not mirror their personal clinical situation
- Usually under-represent unusual cases as they focus on 'common' scenarios.

Simulated patients

Simulated patients are actors. There is a growing industry of simulated patients across medicine. Actors were originally used in teaching and assessment in general practice, and the success of this has led to a huge expansion into other specialties over the last few years. Actors can, of course, be trained and

will play a clinical scenario very effectively. Clearly there are drawbacks and their use is confined to history taking and, in particular, examination of communication skills. Dummies and mannequins (such as for trauma, breast examination, scrotal and digital rectal examination cases) are also being used much more commonly for the clinical parts of examinations.

The *pros* of using simulated patients are that they:

- Allow accurate portrayal of 'typical' patients, e.g. response to grief, being given a diagnosis or information on the treatment of a relative
- Are the most effective way of testing communication skills
- Contribute to discussion of each candidate's performance and even the mark awarded.

The *cons* of using simulated patients are that:

- They reduce the number of clinical scenarios, and tend to increase history taking and communications stations
- In the same way as practicing basic resuscitation on a dummy, it is different in a real-life situation
- It can be difficult to believe if the same actor is used for more than one scenario with the same candidate.

Range of testing

OSCEs don't *just* test clinical examination technique but can also test knowledge/skills in other areas that can be classified into five different headings:

1. Clinical examinations
2. History taking
3. Knowledge (e.g. surgical anatomy/pathology/critical care) and data analysis
4. Communication skills technique
5. Practical skills

So how do you know which of these is being tested in a given station?

Clinical examinations

Who will be at the station (other than examiners)?

- A patient with an identifiable pathology (inguinal hernia, thyroid lump, etc.)
- Occasionally a mannequin.

What will be available to you?

- Everything required to complete the examination adequately, e.g. in a thyroid scenario, a glass of water is provided; in a vascular bay a hand-held Doppler probe is provided.

What instructions are given to the candidate?

- Normally 'examine …', or 'have a look at …', and you will be directed to the side of the patient's examination couch, or to the area where the patient is sitting.

What kind of questions will be used?

- These will often close in on the pathological problem, especially if the candidate is getting side-tracked with something which is not on the marking sheet for the scenario.

What kind of supplemental questions should you expect?

- Supplemental questions might be asked (as included in the chapters of this book) to ascertain background knowledge and understanding of potential treatments.

History taking

Who will be at the station (other than examiners)?

- A simulated patient or a real patient.

What will be available to you?

- Possibly paper on which to make notes as you take the history.

What instructions are given to the candidate?

- You may be asked to gain some information about the symptoms a patient is describing and to formulate a differential diagnosis
- Be aware of the time; you are not going to be able to complete a whole history but should focus on answering the *exact* question posed, without going into a whole stream of closed questioning. The time limit for the station will usually be provided.

What kinds of questions will be used?

- During the scenario none, but if you are interrupted you should infer that you may be getting side-tracked and the examiners are providing a 'subtle hint' to get you back on track.

What kind of supplemental questions should you expect?

- Again, supplemental questions may relate to further parts of the assessment of the patient's symptoms.

Knowledge and data analysis

Who will be at the station (other than examiners)?

- Nobody.

What will be available to you?

- Here a 'prop' will be used, which might be arterial blood gas results, blood laboratory results, joint aspiration results, histopathology results or possibly an X-ray, CT scan or barium series.

What instructions are given to the candidate?

- Explicit instructions will be provided either written at the station or directly from the examiners or a combination of both.

What kind of questions will be used?

- Often very specific (and quite closed) questioning will be used to ensure you understand the clinical significance of any abnormality you pick up.

What kind of supplemental questions should you expect?

- Usually these will relate to the clinical situation which has been diagnosed, and are unlikely to relate specifically to history or examination technique.

Communication skills

Who will be at the station (other than examiners)?

- Simulated patient.

What will be available to you?

- Probably a sheet detailing the communications exercise (which is usually given to you in advance to allow you to prepare).

What kind of questions will be used?

- None; the scenario is a test of your rapport and communication with the patient, not with the examiners.

What kind of supplemental questions should you expect?

- None, for the same reason.

Practical skills

Who will be at the station (other than the examiners)?

- Nobody.

What will be available to you?

- A prop or mannequin.

What instructions are given to the candidate?

- An instruction to demonstrate a specific technique, such as advanced trauma life

support, or suturing, or reduction of a Colles' fracture on the examiner's arm.

What kind of questions will be used?

- Usually you talk through as you are proceeding with the case; the only role the examiners have is to ensure that you can adequately perform the specific skill.

What kind of supplemental questions should you expect?

- Possibly none.

SCORING SYSTEMS

We set ourselves one objective in writing this book – to help you to pass any surgical examination – and the first stage is to understand under what basis you will be assessed and how you will score marks.

SCORING IN SHORT CASE ASSESSMENTS

As mentioned above, this is largely subjective, but marks here are awarded for:

- Introducing yourself to the patient and establishing rapport
- Taking care to expose the patient appropriately (as described in each individual chapter)
- Examining the relevant parts of the body – including starting with the hands
- Accurately identifying the pathological problems (if there are any)
- Coming up with possible further examinations or tests that could be done

- Thinking of a list of differential diagnoses, or a definite diagnosis, and a list of investigations that would tip you towards a particular cause
- Following the train of thought of the examiner, picking up on suggestions and letting yourself be 'taught' technique at the bedside.

Consequently, it is *imperative* that you do not drop marks by omitting to demonstrate deliberately each of these points to the examiners.

SCORING IN OSCE ASSESSMENTS

This is an objective test, and there is a specific marking sheet, which usually contains separate headings, such as clinical knowledge and application; clinical and technical skills; communication and professionalism. Under each of these headings, marks are then awarded for various tasks that are being assessed, e.g in the case of a thyroid examination: (1) introduction to patient; (2) adequate exposure; (3) observing the neck from the front; and (4) observing the swallow test and protrusion of tongue.

It is possible to come up with a marking scheme for each case in this book by picking out the

detail of the examination and making a list of the things you would need to do in order to demonstrate competence. In the same way as in the short cases, there comes a point where you should finish your examination and tell the examiner how you would proceed. This is clearly listed under each case in the book. The examiner indicates if you should continue, and this would imply there are more marks yet to be awarded.

At the end of each case your marks are allotted, then totalled at the end of the entire examination to come up with a score which translates into a pass/fail.

FAILING THE CLINICAL EXAMINATION

Failing a clinical exam is most likely if you are not professional and respectful to the patient, e.g. not introducing yourself, not exposing adequately and/or not asking permission before examining. The examiners are usually there to help you pass the exam and may provide hints if you start to head in completely the wrong direction. Ignoring these hints, and not listening carefully enough to the question, may also lead to a failed case. Gross lack of knowledge or understanding is the third possibility.

A common misconception in OSCEs is to assume that you can pass simply by showing concern for the patient and establish rapport – making the patient 'like you'. Whilst it is imperative to do this, it isn't sufficient to pass the exam, and you are also expected to ask questions or examine intelligently and come up with the right answers to most of the questions at all levels. It is important to appreciate that you won't fail the whole examination because of poor performance (failure) at one OSCE station, so it is crucial to approach each new station afresh, leaving the performance of the previous (good or bad) behind you.

In the OSCE, reducing as many variables as possible from the assessment reduces the chance that a candidate who should have passed will actually fail (i.e. the false-negative rate). Variables that are reduced (or eliminated) in this format include the following:

- **Intra-examiner variability** – where an examiner (by chance) chooses a 'harder' set of cases for a given candidate compared with the one he examines immediately before or afterwards
- **Inter-examiner variability** – where different examiners have wildly different expectations of the appropriate amount of knowledge required to pass
- **Testing one single modality** – where, instead of just being tested on clinical examination, a range of skills (as above) is examined.

A 'pass' mark for the OSCE may therefore be more fairly ascertained than in short cases.

A GENERAL APPROACH TO CLINICAL EXAMINATIONS: TECHNIQUE

Attention to sound technique that is systematic, thorough and slick is crucial in securing maximum marks in clinical examinations. Repeated rehearsal, including under simulated exam conditions, is very important leading up to the exam. Through a process of 'mental rehearsal' it is possible to walk through each of the important steps/points of every clinical scenario long before you stand before the examiners. For each individual clinical case, a series of specific points will be relevant and will be detailed in the remainder of this book. However, it is essential to commence every clinical case with the same general approach that is applicable to *all* cases, even though it may start to sound very repetitive. Failure to do this will result in you losing valuable marks. One such general approach to be employed at every station would include:

1. Read/listen to the instructions *carefully* and then read them *again* (if written)
2. Introduce yourself
3. Ascertain the patient's name/confirm patient's identity

4. Explain what you have been asked to do to the patient
5. Obtain the patient's consent to the required task
6. Clean your hands before (and after) patient contact with alcohol-based hand gel
7. Follow the instructions provided throughout the entire case.

There is always debate about whether to describe clinical examination findings during the course of the exam or to remain silent and summarise and report to the examiner(s) at the end. In some situations, the instructions provided will clarify whether candidates should describe what they are doing as they proceed. However, if explicit instruction is not given to do so, dialogue is not necessary as the examiner will be observing you perform the task and you will have the opportunity to report your findings at the appropriate time at the end of the case. For most candidates, it comes down to personal choice and comfort, and what you have rehearsed.

It cannot be emphasised enough that it is absolutely imperative that you follow the instructions *precisely*, as marks will only be awarded in relation to these in each short case/OSCE station. For instance, if you are instructed to conduct a physical examination of the shoulder, you should *not* take a history or undertake a general examination. All too often, failure to adhere to the specific instructions, in addition to poor preparation and (mental) rehearsal for each of the commonly encountered clinical scenarios, leads to poor performance in the exam. We recommend that you employ the same general approach to each case (for example, as outlined above) and then append a specific approach tailored to the individual case being examined; the clinical cases throughout the rest of this book will provide assistance with this. In this way, candidates can prepare, rehearse and deliver a systematic, comprehensive and slick performance that will lead to exam success.

CONTENTS

SECTION 3   MUSCULOSKELETAL AND NEUROLOGY

SECTION 4   CIRCULATION AND LYMPHATIC SYSTEMS

SECTION 5   COMMUNICATION SKILLS WITH THOMAS CROMPTON AND ROSHANA MEHDIAN

CASE 1   LUMPS AND ULCERS – HISTORY   ***

INSTRUCTION

'Ask this gentleman a few questions about his lump/ulcer.'

APPROACH

It is common to be asked to take a focused history from a patient presenting with relatively common problems, such as a lump or ulcer. Listen carefully to the instruction. After introducing yourself and establishing the patient's name and age, go straight to questions about the lump or ulcer. You may continue on to further relevant surgical questions such as fitness for anaesthesia. The examiner will usually stop you once you have extracted the necessary information. You may not always be asked to continue to examine the patient.

TOP TIP

☑ If the examiner tells you the patient's name, then do not embarrass yourself by asking his name again – this only shows that you have not been listening to the examiner!

VITAL POINTS

Ask the following questions about the lump/ulcer:

Onset

- When did you first notice it?
- What made you notice it?
- Were there any predisposing events (e.g. trauma, insect bite)?

Continued symptoms

- How does it bother you, i.e. what symptoms does it cause? (Ask particularly about pain)
- Has it changed since you first noticed it? (colour, shape and size changes are important in malignant melanoma)
- Have you noticed any other lumps?
- Has it ever disappeared or healed?

Treatments and cause

- What treatments have you had in the past for this?
- What do you think is the cause of the lump/ulcer?

You will usually find that as you extract the relevant information, the examiner will move you on to the examination relatively quickly.

TOP TIP

☑ When asked to take a history, keep eye contact with the patient throughout your questioning.

☑ Don't stare awkwardly at the lump!

CASE 2   LUMPS AND ULCERS – EXAMINATION   ***

INSTRUCTION

'Examine the lump on this patient's chest.' (Fig. 1.1)

APPROACH

Most clinical examinations in surgery include the description of a lump. The examiners may even expect an on-the-spot diagnosis. The description given here of the examination technique is complete and exhaustive, but be prepared to give a diagnosis and to describe the specific features which have led you to this conclusion.

VITAL POINTS

Inspect

- Site – most accurately measured with respect to a fixed landmark, such as a bony prominence

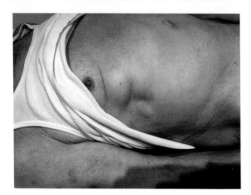

Figure 1.1 A lump.

- Size – measure the dimension in centimetres (if the lump is large enough, be seen to use a measuring tape/ruler, but do not use a tape on a small lump as it can appear awkward)
- Shape
- Skin changes
- Symmetry
- Scars
- Colour

Ask the patient if the lump is tender before proceeding with palpation.

Palpate

- Surface – smooth/irregular
- Edge – well/poorly defined
- Consistency – soft/firm/hard
- Temperature – using the dorsal surface of the examining fingers or hand
- Tenderness
- Transilluminability – using a pen torch on one side of the lump and looking through an opaque tube, such as an empty Smarties tube (this is difficult and cumbersome to perform in a well-lit room and we therefore recommend not taking an empty Smarties tube into the exam, especially if the lump is a hydrocoele!)
- Pulsatility – place a finger on opposite sides of the lump
  - Expansile pulsation – fingers pushed apart
  - Transmitted pulsation – fingers pushed in the same direction (usually upwards)
- Compressibility/reducibility – press firmly on the lump and release

- Compressible – lump disappears on pressure but reappears on release, e.g. arteriovenous malformations
- Reducible – lump disappears on pressure but reappears only when another opposite force is applied, such as coughing in hernia examination
- Fluctuation (for small lumps) – rest two fingers of one hand on opposite sides of the lump and press the middle of the lump with the index finger of your other hand – if the fingers are moved apart, the lump is fluctuant. (Repeat the test at right angles to the first in order to confirm your findings.) This is also known as Paget's sign (see Case 109)
- Fluid thrill – for large lumps – ask the patient to place the edge of his/her hand on the centre of the lump and then flick one side of it, feeling the other side for a percussion wave (most commonly performed in ascites; see Case 57)
- Fixation – decide which plane the lump is in by determining which structures it is attached to, e.g.:
  - Skin/subcutaneous – if you can move the skin over the lump it is subcutaneous. If not, it is within the skin.
  - Muscle – move the lump in two planes perpendicular to each other, ask the patient to tense the relevant muscle and reassess the motion in the two planes.

Percuss

- Dull/resonant (the former indicating fluid, latter indicating an air-filled mass).

Auscultate

- Bruits or bowel sounds may be heard.

Finish your examination here

Completion

Say that you would like to:

- Examine the draining lymph nodes
- Assess the neurovascular status of the area/limb
- Look for similar lumps elsewhere
- Perform a general examination (as necessary).

☑ When assessing consistency, imagine:

- Soft, comparable with the consistency of the flesh of your nostrils (i.e. the ala)
- Firm, comparable with your nasal septum
- Hard, comparable with the bridge of your nose.

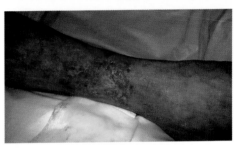

Figure 1.2 An ulcer.

Mnemonic

We use the following mnemonic to remind us what to do with a lump. It is very useful as an aide-mémoire for completeness, but note that it does not provide you with the correct order for examination:

Should **T**he **C**hildren **E**ver **F**ind **L**umps **R**eadily

S – size/site/shape/surface/skin changes/ symmetry/scars

T – temperature/tenderness/transilluminability

C – colour/consistency/compressibility

E – edge/expansility and pulsatility

F – fluctuation/fluid thrill/fixation

L – lymph nodes/lumps elsewhere

R – resonance/relations to surrounding structures and their state, e.g. neurovascular status.

A note on ulcers (Fig. 1.2)

Ulcers should be examined in a similar way to a lump, but important additional points to look for on examination can be remembered in the form of the mnemonic **BEDD**:

Base. Look for the presence of granulation tissue, slough (i.e. dead tissue) or evidence of malignant change

Edge. Five types of edges to be aware of are:
a. Sloping – a healing ulcer (usually venous or traumatic)
b. Punched-out – ischaemic or neuropathic (rarely syphilis)
c. Undermined – pressure necrosis or tuberculosis
d. Rolled – basal cell carcinoma
e. Everted – squamous cell carcinoma

Describe which structure is visualised at the base of the ulcer, e.g. is the ulcer down to fascia, muscle or bone?

Discharge. Is the discharge serous (clear), sanguineous (blood-stained), serosanguineous (mixed) or purulent (infected)?

Individual ulcers, e.g. arterial, venous, neuropathic, are considered in the appropriate sections.

CASE 3 | LIPOMA ★★★

INSTRUCTION

'Examine this lesion on this gentleman's arm.' (Fig. 1.3)

APPROACH

Examine as for any lump (see Case 1).

VITAL POINTS

Lipomas can occur anywhere in the body where there are fat cells, although they most commonly occur in the subcutaneous layer of the skin, particularly in the neck and trunk.

Inspect

- Discoid or hemispherical swelling
- May appear lobulated
- Look carefully for scars (may be a recurrent lipoma).

Palpate

- Lobulated surface
- May be soft or firm depending on the nature of the fat within the lipoma and the temperature at which it liquefies
- If soft and large in size, may show fluctuation

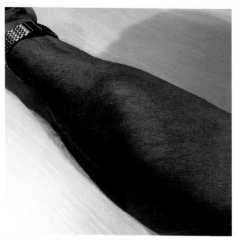

Figure 1.3   A lipoma.

- 'Slip sign' – describes the manner in which a lipoma tends to slip away from the examining finger on gentle pressure
- Skin freely mobile over the lipoma (compared with a sebaceous cyst where it isn't)
- Try to elicit which layer the lipoma is in, e.g. whether subcutaneous or intramuscular (in the latter case, the lipoma disappears on contraction of the relevant muscle).

Completion

Say that you would like to ask the patient:

- How the lipoma affects his life, e.g. cosmetic symptoms, pain
- Whether he has noticed similar lumps elsewhere.

? QUESTIONS

(a) What is a lipoma?

A lipoma is a benign tumour consisting of mature fat cells. Multiple, painful lipomas are known as adiposis dolorosa or Dercum's disease, and are associated with peripheral neuropathy.

(b) Do lipomas undergo malignant change?

- It is thought that malignant change does not occur
- Liposarcomas arise de novo and usually occur in an older age group in deeper tissues of the lower limbs.

(c) How would you treat a lipoma?

- Non-surgical: reassure and 'watch and wait'
- Surgical: if the patient wants it removed, e.g. pain, cosmesis. Some surgeons remove lipomas using suction lipolysis via a small, remote incision. Usually this is performed under local anaesthetic. However, nuchal lipomas have extremely fibrous septa and are difficult to excise, any lipoma close to a joint may communicate with the joint and it may not be possible to excise it under local anaesthetic.

? ADVANCED QUESTIONS

(a) Do you know of any variants of lipomas or syndromes associated with lipomas?

- Angiolipomas, which have a prominent vascular component
- Hibernomas, which consist of brown fat cells similar to those seen in hibernating animals
- Bannayan–Zonana syndrome – rare autosomal-dominant hamartomatous disorder, characterised by multiple lipomas, macrocephaly and haemangiomas.

(b) How are liposarcomas classified?

- Liposarcomas can be classified pathologically into three main groups:
  a. Well-differentiated
  b. Myxoid and round cell (poorly differentiated myxoid) liposarcoma
  c. Pleomorphic liposarcoma.

Francis X. Dercum (1856–1931). North American neurologist, born in Philadelphia.

FURTHER READING

Dalal KM, Antonescu CR, Singer S: Diagnosis and management of lipomatous tumors. *J Surg Oncol* 97(4):298–313, 2008.

Dei Tos AP: Liposarcoma: new entities and evolving concepts. *Ann Diagn Pathol* 4(4):252–266, 2000.

www.cancerhelp.org.uk/help/default.asp?page=18503 – information for patients on lipoma removal.

CASE 4   SEBACEOUS CYST   ***

INSTRUCTION

'Examine this gentleman's lump.' (Fig. 1.4)

APPROACH

Examine as for any lump (see Case 1).

VITAL POINTS

Inspect

- Smooth hemispherical swelling
- Usually solitary
- Found most commonly on the face, trunk, neck and scalp
- Punctum present at apex of cyst in 50%.

Palpate

- Smooth surface
- Firm to soft on palpation
- Punctum may exhibit plastic deformation on palpation
- All sebaceous cysts are attached to the skin, therefore the cyst does not move independently from the skin.

Completion

Say that you would like to ask the patient:
- How the cyst affects his life, e.g. cosmetic symptoms

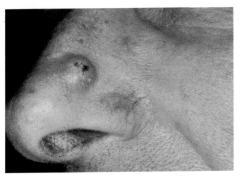

Figure 1.4   Epidermal Cyst. Patient Education. October 15, 2015. ExitCare® Patient Information ©2015 ExitCare, LLC.

- Whether he has noticed similar lumps elsewhere.

? QUESTIONS

(a) What are the complications of a sebaceous cyst?

- Infection – frequent complication, there may be an associated discharge
- Ulceration
- Calcification (trichilemmal cysts; see below) – this may cause the cyst to feel hard on palpation
- Sebaceous horn formation (hardening of a slow discharge of sebum from a wide punctum)
- Malignant change.

(b) How would you treat a sebaceous cyst?

- Non-surgical: may be left alone if small and asymptomatic
- Surgical: to prevent recurrence, complete excision of cyst and its contents is required, which involves removal of an elliptical portion of skin containing the punctum.

? ADVANCED QUESTIONS

(a) What are the different histological subtypes of sebaceous cysts?

Two types of cysts are recognised according to their histological features:

- Epidermal cyst – thought to arise from the infundibular portions of hair follicles
- Trichilemmal cysts – thought to arise from hair follicle epithelium and so are most common on the scalp, and are frequently multiple; these cysts have an autosomal-dominant mode of inheritance.

(b) What is a Cock's peculiar tumour?

Proliferating trichilemmal cysts are usually solitary, occur on the scalp in 90% of cases and can grow to a large size and ulcerate. Clinically and histologically, they may resemble a squamous cell carcinoma; such cases are known as a Cock's peculiar tumour. Very rarely, malignant transformation can occur.

(c) What is Gardner's syndrome?

Multiple epidermal cysts may be part of Gardner's syndrome, which is also associated with:

- Adenomatous polyposis of the large bowel
- Multiple osteomata of the skull
- Desmoid tumours.

Note that Gardner's syndrome is now part of the spectrum of familial polyposis coli syndromes, which includes familial adenomatous polyposis.

> *Edward Cock (1805–1892).* English surgeon at Guy's Hospital, who was the nephew of Sir Astley Cooper and performed the first pharyngectomy in England.
>
> *Eldon J. Gardner (1909–1989).* American geneticist and Professor of Zoology, Utah State University.

FURTHER READING

Dastgeer GM: Sebaceous cyst excision with minimal surgery. *Am Fam Physician* 43(6):1956–1960, 1991.

www.intelihealth.com/IH/ihtIH/WSIHW000/9339/9779.html – information for patients on sebaceous cysts.

CASE 5 GANGLION ***

INSTRUCTION

'Examine this lady's hand.' (Fig. 1.5)

APPROACH

Expose to elbows and ask the patient to place the hands palm upwards on a pillow (if available).

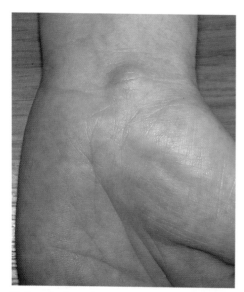

Figure 1.5 A ganglion.

VITAL POINTS

Ganglia can occur anywhere in the body, although they are commonly found around the wrist, on the dorsum of the hand and on the dorsum of the ankle. In fact, the most common soft-tissue mass found in the hand is a ganglion.

Inspect

- Usually single
- Hemispherical swelling
- Look carefully for scars (may be recurrent).

Palpate

- Smooth surface
- May be multiloculated
- May be soft and fluctuant (especially if large) or firm (if small with tense, viscous contents)
- Associated with a synovial-lined structure such as a tendon or joint
- Weakly transilluminable due to its viscous fluid contents.

Completion

Say that you would like to ask the patient:

- How the ganglion affects her life, e.g. cosmetic symptoms

- Whether she has noticed similar lumps elsewhere
- Which hand is dominant (considering treatment options)
- Her occupation (also to consider treatment options).

? QUESTIONS

(a) What is a ganglion?

A ganglion is a cystic swelling related to a synovial-lined cavity, either a joint or a tendon sheath. The origin of ganglia is controversial – they are seen as a pocket of synovium communicating with the joint or tendon sheath, or as a myxomatous degeneration of fibrous tissue.

(b) What is the differential diagnosis?

- Bursae
- Cystic protrusions from the synovial cavity of arthritic joints
- Benign giant cell tumours of the flexor sheath (indistinguishable from flexor sheath ganglia)
- Rarely, malignant swellings, e.g. synovial sarcoma.

(c) How would you treat a ganglion?

- Non-surgical: 'watch and wait', or aspiration followed by 3 weeks of immobilisation (successful in 30–50% of patients). (The old method of striking the ganglion with the family Bible is now out of favour!)
- Surgical: complete excision to include the neck of the ganglion at its site of origin.

(d) What complications are associated with surgical treatment of a ganglion?

- Wound complications, e.g. scar, haematoma, infection
- Recurrence – can be as high as 50%, but can be lower if care is taken to excise the neck completely
- Damage to adjacent neurovascular structures.

FURTHER READING

Thornburg LE: Ganglions of the hand and wrist. *J Am Acad Orthop Surg* 7(4):231–238, 1999.

www.med.und.nodak.edu/users/jwhiting/ganglia.html – information for patients.

CASE 6 | NECK EXAMINATION – GENERAL ***

INSTRUCTION

'Examine this gentleman's neck.'

APPROACH

- Note that the patient is usually sitting in a chair and may have a glass of water next to him
- If there is a glass of water, be prepared to examine the thyroid gland in full
- Expose the whole neck down to both clavicles – this may necessitate undoing the top buttons of a shirt or even taking off a polo-neck jumper
- Ask the patient to remove any jewellery.

TOP TIP

☑ The examiners may try to catch you out by placing the patient on a chair with its back against the wall. Your first move is to ask the patient to stand up and move the chair away from the wall, allowing you to access and examine the patient's neck from behind.

VITAL POINTS

Inspect (from the front)

- Site of the lump, e.g. midline, supraclavicular fossa
- Other features on inspection of the lump, e.g. size, skin changes, scars (see Case 1).

Protrusion of the tongue

- Ask the patient to open the mouth and protrude the tongue as far as possible
- If the lump moves on protrusion of the tongue, it is likely to be a thyroglossal cyst (this is because the cyst is usually related to the base of the tongue by a patent or fibrous track, which runs through the central portion of the hyoid bone) – proceed with examination of a thyroglossal cyst (see Case 31)
- A thyroid lump does not move on protrusion of the tongue.

Swallowing

- Place the glass of water in the patient's hands
- Ask them to take a sip of water, hold it in the mouth and swallow when asked
- During the swallow, inspect the lump – if it moves on swallowing, it is likely to originate from the thyroid gland.

Palpate (from the back)

- The neck is best (and first) palpated from behind the patient
- Be as gentle as possible, as you are unable to watch the patient's face for pain
- Use the fingertips of both hands to elicit the physical signs
- Begin by showing the examiner that you know the borders of the two main triangles of the neck and tell him which triangle the lump is in (Fig. 1.6)
  - The *anterior triangle* of the neck is bordered by the anterior border of sternocleidomastoid, the midline and the ramus of the mandible
  - The *posterior triangle* of the neck is bordered by the anterior border of trapezius, the clavicle and the posterior border of sternocleidomastoid
- Next, determine whether the lump is solid or cystic. You should now be ready to consider the differential diagnosis (Table 1.1 and Fig. 1.7).

TOP TIP

☑ Multiple lumps palpable within the neck are invariably lymph nodes.

Continuing the examination

If at this stage you think that the lump is thyroid in origin, you should proceed to examine the thyroid gland in full (Fig. 1.8 and see Case 8).

If you have offered a differential diagnosis you should be prepared to offer additional evidence for your suggestions – see individual cases.

If you have not found a lump at this stage you should examine the neck thoroughly using the down-and-up technique as in Table 1.2.

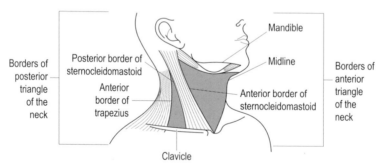

Figure 1.6 Posterior and anterior triangles of the neck.

Table 1.1 Differential diagnosis of neck lumps

Position	Solid	Cystic
Midline	Thyroid swelling (Case 8)	Thyroglossal cyst (Case 31)
Anterior triangle	Lymphadenopathy (Case 7)	Branchial cyst (Case 29)
	Chemodectoma (Case 38)	Cold abscess (secondary to tuberculosis)
Posterior triangle	Lymphadenopathy	Pharyngeal pouch (Case 36)
		Cystic hygroma (Case 37)
Within sternocleidomastoid	Sternocleidomastoid tumour	

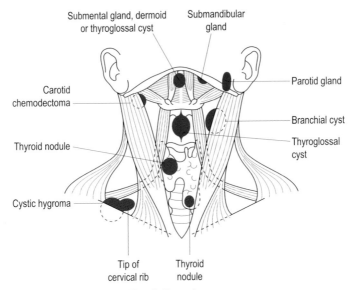

Figure 1.7   Locations of the most common swellings in the neck.

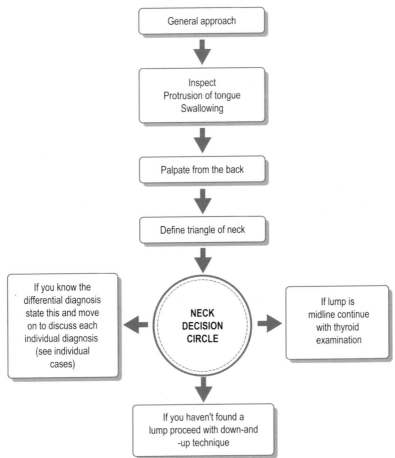

Figure 1.8   'Neck decision circle' approach to examination of the neck.

Table 1.2 The down-and-up technique

Stage	Procedure
1	Palpate from the chin backwards to below the ears
2	Move your hands behind the ears and palpate *down* the anterior border of sternocleidomastoid to the clavicle
3	Move laterally along the clavicle and then *up* the posterior border of sternocleidomastoid
4	Finish by palpating the back of the scalp for occipital nodes

Examination of cervical lymph nodes

The cervical lymph nodes are best examined using the 'down-and-up' technique:

- Use gentle rotating movements of the fingertips – this allows you to palpate even the smallest nodes
- If the patient tries to help you by raising the chin, ask them to refrain – this makes the examination easier by relaxing the anterior neck muscles
- Begin by moving from the chin backwards, palpating the submental, submandibular and parotid glands and pre-auricular nodes
- Move your fingers behind the ears and feel the mastoid (post-auricular) nodes
- Go down the anterior border of the sternocleidomastoids, feeling the anterior triangular nodes, including the jugulodigastric (tonsillar) node

- Move laterally along the clavicular region, feeling for both supraclavicular and infraclavicular nodes
- Move up the posterior border of the sternocleidomastoids, feeling the posterior triangular nodes
- Finish by palpating the occipital nodes at the back of the neck.

Palpate (from the front)

- Confirm your findings if necessary by feeling the lump from the front, watching the patient's face carefully for signs of discomfort.

Percussion and auscultation

See individual cases.

Finish your examination here

Note

Sternomastoid tumour is an ischaemic contracture of a segment of the muscle seen to appear in the first 1–2 weeks after birth (following a complicated or breech birth) and normally disappearing over the first 4–6 months of life. Babies may present with a torticollis. With early diagnosis, treatment is non-surgical with active stimulation and passive stretching and occasionally using *Botulinum* toxin injections; with late diagnosis, it may require surgery.

CASE 7   CERVICAL LYMPHADENOPATHY   ***

INSTRUCTION

'Examine this gentleman's neck.'

APPROACH

Approach as you would a neck examination (see Case 6). Note that cervical lymph nodes are the commonest neck lumps found in the clinical cases.

Inspection, protrusion of the tongue, swallowing, palpation

See Case 6.

Additional points on inspection

- Site of the lump, e.g. midline, supraclavicular fossa

- Other features on inspection of any lump, e.g. size, skin changes, scars (see Case 1).

Additional points on palpation (from the back)

- Use the 'down-and-up' routine as detailed in Case 6 to examine thoroughly for cervical lymphadenopathy
- Keep the lymph node levels (I–VII) in mind (Fig. 1.9) as you examine:
  - I – submental and submandibular
  - II – base of skull to level of hyoid
  - III – between level of hyoid and cricoid cartilage
  - IV – level of cricoid cartilage to clavicle
  - V – posterior triangle
  - VI – hyoid to suprasternal notch between carotids
  - VII – retromanubrium/sternal to innominate
- Remember also that the lymph nodes should be examined as for any other lump (see Case 1) and particularly note:

- Consistency – tends to be firm but may be rubbery
- Number – solitary, multiple or matted to each other
- Fixation – skin tethering in tuberculous nodes or malignancy.

Finish your examination here

Completion

Say that you would like to:

- Examine the face and scalp carefully for a primary site of infection or neoplasia
- Perform a full examination of the ear, nose and throat (say that you would request a formal full ENT examination), including the salivary glands and the thyroid gland
- Examine the rest of the lymphoreticular system, including palpation of the abdomen for hepatomegaly and splenomegaly
- Look for a primary site of infection or neoplasia above the umbilicus, e.g. chest examination

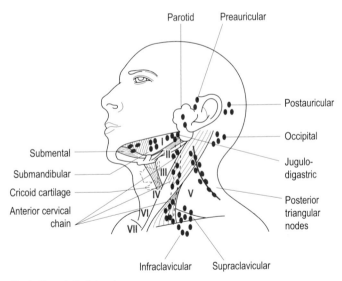

Cervical Lymph Node Levels
I. Submental and submandibular
II. Base of skull to level of hyoid
III. Between level of hyoid and cricoid cartilage
IV. Level of cricoid cartilage to clavicle
V. Posterior triangle
VI. Hyoid to suprasternal notch between carotids
VII. Retromanubrium/sternal to inominate

Figure 1.9 Typical grouping of lymph nodes.

- In a female patient, a breast examination would also be indicated, as breast malignancy can metastasise to the neck.

? QUESTIONS

(a) What questions would you like to ask this gentleman?

Directed to the possible causes (see (b) below):

- Symptoms from the lump itself, e.g. the duration, pain (e.g. in lymphomas pain is experienced on alcohol ingestion, although this is not specific to lymphomas), other lumps elsewhere
- General symptoms, e.g. night sweats, loss of appetite, loss of weight
- Local symptoms, e.g. intraoral diseases such as tooth decay
- Systemic disease, e.g. serious medical illnesses, previous surgical operations (thinking of neoplasia)
- Social history – ethnic origin (patients from high-risk areas for TB, including the Indian subcontinent), foreign travel, contact with animals (cat-scratch fever), risk factors for HIV infection.

(b) What causes of cervical lymphadenopathy do you know of?

Think of the acronym **LIST** when considering this answer:

Lymphoma and leukaemia
Infection (see below)
Sarcoidosis
Tumours (primary/secondary).

Infectious causes can, as always, be further subclassified:

- Bacterial
  - Tonsillitis, dental abscess (β-haemolytic *Streptococcus*)
  - Tuberculosis
- Viral
  - Cytomegalovirus
  - Infectious mononucleosis (Epstein–Barr virus)
  - HIV
- Protozoal
- Toxoplasmosis.

(c) How would you investigate this gentleman?

- Blood tests:
  - Haematological: full blood count, erythrocyte sedimentation rate

- Biochemical: thyroid function tests, angiotensin-converting enzyme levels, which may be raised in sarcoidosis
- Serological: Monospot or Paul–Bunnell test looking for atypical mononuclear cells in infectious mononucleosis
- Radiological:
  - Ultrasound
  - CT scan
  - MRI scan
- Histological
  - Fine-needle aspiration cytology (FNAC):
    - False-positive rate 0–3%, false-negative rate 1–10%
    - Errors reduced by experience of clinician and cytologist
  - Excision biopsy (see below).

? ADVANCED QUESTIONS

(a) What results might you expect from the FNAC and how would you proceed?

- If malignant:
  - Is it squamous cell carcinoma? – Do not perform solitary lymph node excision biopsy (spoils the field for subsequent block dissection of the neck and may reduce survival), refer to ENT surgeon for full assessment to include panendoscopy to find a primary tumour. Random biopsies from multiple sites may be needed, along with sputum cytology and chest X-ray
  - Is it adenocarcinoma? Continue to open lymph node excision biopsy and look for primary from breast or intra-abdominal viscera such as pancreas or stomach
  - Is it lymphoma? Continue to open lymph node excision biopsy, as a whole node is required for detailed histology and marker studies
- If inflammatory:
  - Is it tuberculosis? Do not perform open lymph node excision biopsy (may result in chronic sinus formation) – treat as for tuberculosis
  - Is it another infectious or inflammatory disorder? Continue to open lymph node excision biopsy and treat according to underlying cause.

(b) What are the patterns of lymphatic drainage from the head and neck? (Fig. 1.9)

- Anterior floor of mouth, anterior two-thirds of tongue, lips, cheek, mucosa to level I

- Nasopharynx to levels II, III, IV parotid nodes
- Oral cavity/pharynx to levels III, IV, V, often bilateral
- Thyroid; piriform sinus; cervical oesophagus to supraclavicular region.

(c) What surgical options are available in the management of cervical lymphadenopathy?

- Open lymph node excision biopsy:
  - Best performed under general anaesthesia
  - Beware biopsy in the posterior triangle due to risk of damaging the spinal accessory nerve, which is quite superficial – damage leads to shoulder and arm pain, paralysis of trapezius and winging of the scapula
  - In addition patients should be warned of damage to the facial nerve if the surgical approach includes dissection around the parotid gland
- Block dissection of the neck:
  - Comprehensive vs. selective
  - Comprehensive involves excision of all lymphatic tissue from levels I to V (squamous cell carcinoma: SCC):
    - Radical – includes removal of sternomastoid, jugular vein and accessory nerve
    - Modified radical – involves preservation of one or more of these structures

- Incisions used include the 'wineglass', the standard y and the McFee incision
- Selective dissection
  - For clinically/radiologically negative neck (i.e. no detectable nodes)
  - Dissection depends on site of tumour
  - The draining group/adjacent nodes are removed – e.g. level I, II and III for floor-of-mouth SCC

J. R. Paul (1893–1971). North American physician and pathologist.

W. W. Bunnell (1902–1966). North American physician.

Thomas Hodgkin (1798–1866). English physician, St Thomas's Hospital and Curator of the Pathology Museum at Guy's Hospital.

M. A. Epstein (born 1921). English physician and Professor of Pathology, Bristol.

Yvonne Barr (born 1932). English physician.

FURTHER READING

Peters TR, Edwards KM: Cervical lymphadenopathy and adenitis. *Pediatr Rev* 21(12):399–405, 2000.

Tracy TF Jr, Muratore CS: Management of common head and neck masses. *Semin Pediatr Surg* 16:3–13, 2007.

CASE 8   THYROID EXAMINATION   ***

INSTRUCTION

'Examine this lady's thyroid gland.'

APPROACH

- See general approach to examination of the neck (Case 6)
- As you start the examination, you should be looking for clues of thyroid dysfunction, such as:
  - Agitation at rest (hyperthyroidism)
  - Warm and sweaty hands (hyperthyroidism).

The objectives of thyroid examination are to:

1. Confirm that the abnormality lies within the thyroid gland (as opposed to other neck structures)

2. Determine whether there is diffuse enlargement of the thyroid (smooth or nodular) or a solitary nodule
3. Examine structures around the thyroid
4. Assess the thyroid status of the patient.

TOP TIP

☑ Examination of the thyroid should be directed at achieving these objectives and is easiest performed in three parts:

- Part 1: The thyroid gland itself
  - Begin the examination in front of the patient, then move to the back, before finally returning to the front, ready for Part 2
- Part 2: Structures around the thyroid
  - Assess trachea and oesophagus; recurrent laryngeal nerve
- Part 3: The thyroid status

PART 1: THE THYROID GLAND ITSELF

Examine (from the front)

INSPECTION, PROTRUSION OF THE TONGUE, SWALLOWING

See Case 6.

ADDITIONAL POINTS ON INSPECTION

- Obvious midline lump (see notes (below) for definition of goitre)
- Scars – horizontal skin crease incision is most common following previous thyroid surgery
- Raised jugular venous pulse – due to neck vein obstruction from mass effect.

Examine (from behind)

PALPATION

See Fig. 1.10.

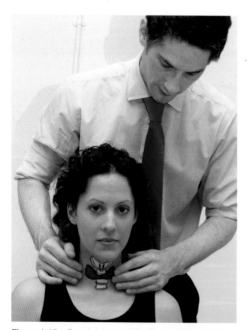

Figure 1.10 Examination position for palpation of the thyroid gland from behind.

ADDITIONAL POINTS ON PALPATION

- Ask the patient to protrude the tongue again – checking for a thyroglossal cyst – while gently palpating the thyroid gland from behind
- Repeat the swallow test, asking the patient to take another sip of water, hold it in the mouth and swallow when you indicate. Feel the thyroid gland rise, proving the mass arises from the thyroid
- Describe the features of the lump (see Case 1) – gently push on one edge of the lump so that you can palpate the other edge with ease (be gentle!) (Fig. 1.11) – feel particularly for:
  - Size
  - Tenderness
  - Mobility
  - Consistency
- Most importantly, try to work out whether there is:
  - Diffuse enlargement of the thyroid – smooth (simple goitre) or nodular (multinodular goitre)
  - A solitary nodule/lesion of the thyroid
- Move on to examining the cervical lymph nodes, performing the 'down-and-up' technique (Fig. 1.12 and see Case 6).

Examine (from the front)

PERCUSSION AND AUSCULTATION

- Listen over the thyroid for a systolic bruit – this is caused by a hypervascular thyroid – which is almost pathognomonic of Graves' disease

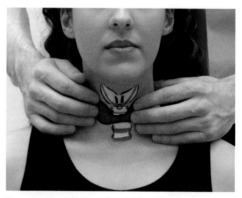

Figure 1.11 Palpation of each lobe of the thyroid gland.

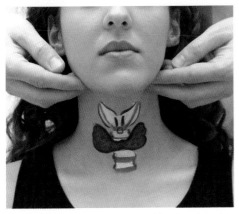

Figure 1.12 Palpation of the cervical lymph nodes using the 'down-and-up' technique.

- Percuss over the sternum from the notch downwards, listening for a change in percussion note if there is retrosternal extension.

Diffuse enlargement – smooth or nodular

- Multinodular goitre (see Case 10)
- Toxic (i.e. hyperthyroid) – Graves' disease (see Case 11)
- Simple colloid goitre (see Case 11)
- Thyroiditis, e.g. subacute (granulomatous) – de Quervain's; autoimmune (Hashimoto's); or Reidel's (invasive fibrous). In these cases, the thyroid may be tender
- Neoplastic goitre, benign/malignant.

Solitary nodule (see Case 9)

- Thyroid cysts – usually benign, although up to 10% of mixed solid/cystic lesions can be malignant
- Neoplasms: benign (follicular adenoma); malignant – primary (papillary, follicular, medullary, anaplastic SCC and malignant lymphoma) or secondary (metastatic from breast/kidney)
- Dominant nodule of a multinodular goitre masquerading as an 'apparently' solitary nodule.

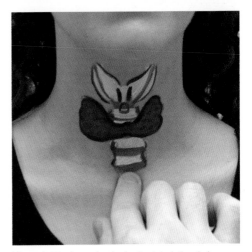

Figure 1.13 Assessing for tracheal deviation during thyroid examination.

PART 2: STRUCTURES AROUND THE THYROID

- Gently palpate the trachea for deviation by placing one finger over the trachea. It should lie equidistant between the heads of the clavicles (Fig. 1.13)
- Ask the patient if she has had any problems swallowing or has noticed any change in her voice – this completes the examination of the structures around the thyroid gland
- You could ask the patient to repeat a sentence that you read out in order to listen for the hoarse voice characteristic of a previously damaged or infiltrated recurrent laryngeal nerve.

PART 3: THYROID STATUS

This includes examination of the hands and eyes, and occasionally other areas to examine for further evidence of thyroid dysfunction. You will not usually be asked to continue to perform this part of the examination if the patient has normal thyroid status (i.e. is euthyroid).

Move on to the hands

There are seven signs to look for in the hands:

1. Increased sweating (due to hyperthyroidism)
2. Palmar erythema (due to hyperthyroidism)
3. Thyroid acropachy (a feature of Graves' disease; see Case 11) – also known as pseudoclubbing

4. Onycholysis (Plummer's nails; see Case 10)
5. Areas of vitiligo (white patches of skin ± hyperpigmented borders, seen in association with autoimmune disorders such as Graves' disease)
6. Pulse – tachycardia or atrial fibrillation in hyperthyroidism, bradycardia in hypothyroidism
7. Fine tremor – best demonstrated by placing a sheet of paper on the outstretched hands with palms facing downwards.

Proceed to the eyes

There are also seven signs to look for in the eyes, the latter six being associated with Graves' disease (see Case 11):

1. Loss of hair on outer-third of eyebrows (hypothyroidism)
2. Lid retraction – raised upper eyelid, but the whiteness of the sclera is not visible around the iris – also known as Dalrymple's sign (Fig. 1.14)
3. Lid lag. Ask the patient to look up at an examining finger and to follow it when you move your finger (Fig. 1.15). Move the examining finger *rapidly* down, while watching the patient's eyes. The globe will follow the finger, but the lid will lag behind when the sign is positive
4. Ophthalmoplegia. Fully assess eye movements, enquiring for the presence of diplopia (Fig. 1.16). The superior recti and inferior oblique muscles are most commonly affected, leading to diplopia when looking

'up and out'. In more advanced cases, it becomes impossible for the patient to complete this movement

5. Exophthalmos – both eyelids move away from the centre of the iris so that the whiteness of the sclera is visible below or all round the iris
6. Chemosis – the venous and lymphatic drainage is disturbed by the protrusion of the

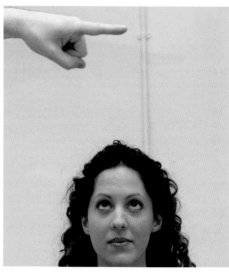

Figure 1.15 Assessing for lid lag during thyroid examination.

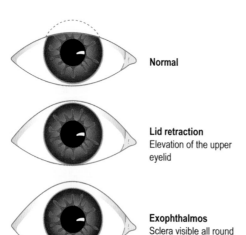

Normal

Lid retraction
Elevation of the upper eyelid

Exophthalmos
Sclera visible all round the iris

Figure 1.14 Eye signs in Graves' disease.

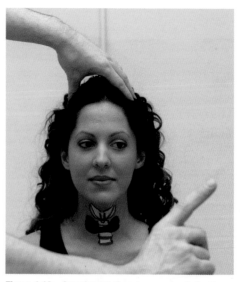

Figure 1.16 Assessment of ocular movements for the presence of ophthalmoplegia.

eye and the appearance is oedematous and wrinkled

7. Proptosis – the eye has protruded so far forward that it is visible beyond the level of the supraorbital ridge when looking over the head of the patient from behind the finger (Fig. 1.17).

In the normal eye, the upper eyelid is halfway between the pupil and the superior limbus, while the lower eyelid is at the level of the inferior limbus.

Proceed to complete a full systemic examination

- It may only be necessary to say that you would like to complete a full systemic examination, although you should be prepared to do it if the examiner wishes
- The relevant systems to be examined include the cardiorespiratory system and the lower limbs:

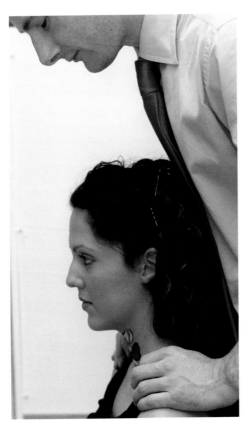

Figure 1.17   Examining for evidence of proptosis.

- Look for signs of heart failure
- Inspect the shins for pretibial myxoedema (seen in Graves' disease; see Case 11)
- Test for proximal myopathy by assessing the strength of the muscles of the upper arm (seen in Graves' disease)
- Test the reflexes – supinator jerks are inverted and ankle jerks are slow-relaxing in hypothyroidism.

Finish your examination here

Completion

Say that you would like to:
- Ask the patient how the thyroid mass is affecting her life
- Continue to assess the patient's thyroid status by asking her a few questions (see Case 12).

J. Dalrymple (1804–1852). English ophthalmologist.

F. de Quervain (1868–1940). Swiss surgeon who described subacute thyroiditis with self-limiting inflammation of the gland, pathologically characterised by giant cells and granuloma, which is probably as a result of viral infection. Some 50% of patients may experience mild hyperthyroidism.

Hakura Hashimoto (1881–1934). Japanese surgeon who described an autoimmune thyroiditis often associated with mild hypothyroidism. The pathology is thought to be due to apoptosis induced by lymphocytes bearing Fas ligands combining with thyrocytes bearing Fas.

Notes

1. The term 'goitre' is non-specific and describes any swelling of the thyroid gland. It does not imply any pathology. It is derived from the Latin for throat (*guttur*). Goitres become visible when they are three times the normal size, weighing over 50 g. Goitres can be graded according to the World Health Organization's (WHO) grading scheme:
   Grade 0: No palpable or visible goitre
   Grade 1: Palpable goitre
   Grade 2: Goitre visible with neck in normal position
   Grade 3: Large goitre visible from a distance.
2. Patients with large retrosternal goitres develop signs of compression on raising their arms above their heads, leading to

suffusion of the face, giddiness or syncope. This is Pemberton's sign – do not elicit in the examination, as the patient may faint.

3. There are some other physical signs of the eye which are of historic interest that are included here for sake of completeness:
   - Stellwag's sign: *C. Stellwag von Carion (1823–1904), Austrian ophthalmologist –* infrequent blinking in hyperthyroidism
   - Joffroy's sign: *A. Joffroy (1844–1908), French neuropsychiatrist –* absence of

wrinkling of the forehead when the patient bends her head and looks up
   - Möbius' sign: *P. J. Möbius (1853–1907), German neurologist –* difficulty in convergence elicited in a patient with ophthalmoplegia.

4. The term vitiligo is derived from the Latin *vitellus* for 'spotted calf'.

CASE 9   SOLITARY THYROID NODULE   ***

INSTRUCTION

See Cases 6 and 8 for the general examination of the neck and thyroid gland.

SPECIFIC POINTS ON EXAMINATION OF THE NECK

- Palpable nodule which moves on swallowing but not on protrusion of tongue
- Determine the characteristics of the nodule 'lump' (see Case 1)
- Palpate for associated cervical lymphadenopathy.

? QUESTIONS

(a) What is the arterial supply to the thyroid gland?

- See Fig. 1.18.

(b) What are the causes of a solitary thyroid nodule?

- Prominent nodule in a multinodular goitre
- Cyst (e.g. from haemorrhage into a nodule)
- Thyroid adenoma
- Carcinoma/lymphoma
- Thyroiditis (see Case 8).

(c) What do you know about solitary thyroid nodules?

- More common in females (F : M ratio = 4 : 1)
- Occur most commonly in the fourth and fifth decades
- 10% in middle-aged are malignant *but* 50% are malignant in the young and the elderly
- Fine-needle aspiration cytology (FNAC) is the most important investigation – if benign,

leave alone and if malignant, surgery is required.

(d) How would you investigate and treat a solitary thyroid nodule?

- All patients should undergo triple assessment:
  - Clinical examination
  - Radiological assessment, previously ultrasonographic but increasingly CT
  - Pathological, most commonly cytological following FNAC.

Note

Contrary to what is still contained in some older textbooks, technetium or iodine radioisotope scanning is *only* of value in clinical practice when assessing *solitary* nodules in *thyrotoxic* patients. In this setting, it is used to determine whether the nodule is 'functional' and the 'cause' of thyrotoxicosis, as this clearly has implications for further treatment. It has *no* value in the differentiation of benign and malignant nodules due to poor sensitivity and specificity.

- The treatment is then dependent on the findings (Fig. 1.19).

(e) What do you know about thyroid adenomas?

- Almost all are follicular adenomas
- Usually 2–4 cm and encapsulated at presentation
- Indistinguishable from carcinomas on FNAC, as the presence of a capsule cannot be demonstrated
- Surgical excision (lobectomy) is needed to confirm diagnosis.

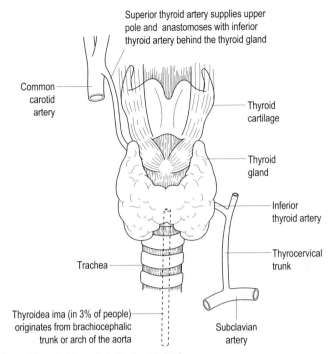

Figure 1.18 Anatomy of the arterial supply to the thyroid gland.

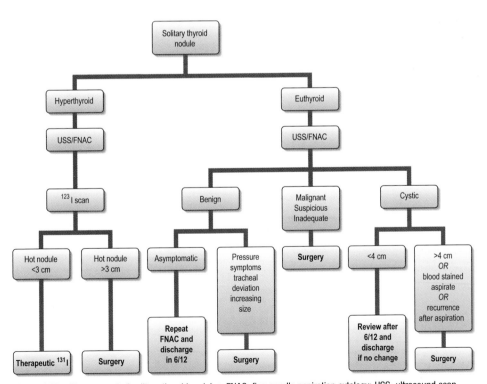

Figure 1.19 Management of solitary thyroid nodules. FNAC, fine-needle aspiration cytology; USS, ultrasound scan.

? ADVANCED QUESTIONS

(a) What do you know about thyroid malignancy?

- The incidence is low: approx. 4 per 100 000 per year
- Histological varieties are:
  - Papillary – 70%
  - Follicular – 15%
  - Medullary – 8%
  - Anaplastic – 5%
  - Lymphoma – 2%
- Papillary and follicular varieties are collectively known as differentiated thyroid cancer
- **P**apillary
  - Begins with **P** for paediatric – commonest in children and young adults
  - Ends with **y** for yellow = lymph – lymphatic spread to lymph nodes
  - Multicentric
  - 90% of children have nodal metastases at surgery
- **F**ollicular
  - Begins with **F** for fifty – mean age is 50 years at presentation
  - Ends with **r** for red = blood – spread via bloodstream
  - FNA cannot distinguish cancer from follicular adenoma
  - Note that 80% of follicular lesions on FNA are adenomas
- Staging of thyroid cancer:
  - AJCC/IUCC system – tumour nodes metastasis (TNM) staging
  - AMES (age, metastasis, extent, size) or AGES (age, grade, extent, size)
- Treatment of differentiated thyroid cancer:
  - Thyroidectomy is the treatment of choice, although the precise extent of the procedure depends on the type and size of the cancer, the number of lesions and need for radioactive iodine ablation and contraindications to total thyroidectomy, and remains controversial
  - Total thyroidectomy is advocated for lesions >1 cm. This approach addresses multifocal tumour, decreases local and distant recurrence, facilitates treatment with ^{131}I and allows postoperative monitoring with thyroglobulin concentration measurement
  - A unilateral total lobectomy and isthmusectomy is usually adequate for microlesions (<1 cm) so long as unifocal, well differentiated and intrathyroidal
- Some cancer will be diagnosed following lobectomy for a solitary nodule, especially follicular tumours that cannot be identified on FNAC. In such cases, where frankly invasive cancer has been demonstrated, completion total thyroidectomy is required
- Lymph node dissection can involve a central dissection (CLND) (level VI nodes) or lateral compartment dissection (LLND – levels II–V) (Fig. 1.9). CLND is generally recommended when there is clinically apparent lymph node involvement. LLND is only performed in biopsy-proven (on FNAC) metastatic lateral cervical lymphadenopathy
- Postoperative treatment includes:
  - ^{131}I scan to exclude residual thyroid tissue/metastases. Total uptake should be <1%. If it is greater, then therapeutic doses of ^{131}I are administered until all residual uptake is ablated.
  - Lifelong thyroxine for replacement and to suppress thyroid-stimulating hormone levels <0.1 IU, as this favourably influences the behaviour of any metastatic tumour
- Medullary
  - Arises from the parafollicular C cells (derived from ultimobranchial bodies) which produce calcitonin, a polypeptide which decreases blood calcium
  - 90% are sporadic cases
  - 10% are familial and may be associated with multiple endocrine neoplasia type 2a and 2b (see below)
  - Familial cases are associated with mutations of the ret proto-oncogene – if mutation is present, 100% risk of developing medullary carcinoma and therefore prophylactic thyroidectomy is indicated in childhood
  - Treatment is radical surgery (total thyroidectomy and bilateral CLND ± ipsilateral LLND for biopsy-proven lateral nodes) with follow-up using sequential serum calcitonin (and/or carcinoembryonic antigen) measurements
- **A**naplastic
  - Begins with **A** = aged – occur in the elderly
  - Resection of the thyroid is rarely possible
  - Treatment with radiotherapy and chemotherapy gives best survival of 1 year

- Lymphoma
  - Tru-Cut biopsy is often needed for diagnosis
  - Treated with radiotherapy and chemotherapy.

(b) What do you know about thyroid cysts?

- True cysts with a completely smooth wall are very rare
- Most are composite lesions with colloid degeneration, necrosis or haemorrhage in benign or malignant tumours
- Only benign if *completely* abolished by aspiration
- Note that cytology can be false-negative in a third of malignant cysts.

Notes

Multiple endocrine neoplasia type 1 (Wermer syndrome):

- Autosomal dominant
- Pancreatic islet cell tumour

- Pituitary adenoma
- Primary hyperparathyroidism

Multiple endocrine neoplasia type 2a (Sipple syndrome):

- Autosomal dominant
- Phaeochromocytoma
- Medullary carcinoma of the thyroid
- Primary hyperparathyroidism

Multiple endocrine neoplasia type 2b:

- Same as IIa but no parathyroid involvement.

John H. Sipple (born 1930). North American Professor of Medicine, New York.

P. Wermer (1898–1975). Contemporary North American physician, Columbia University, Presbyterian Hospital, New York

FURTHER READING

Sadler GP: The thyroid gland. In: Lennard TWJ, editor: *Endocrine Surgery*, London, 2006, Elsevier Saunders, pp 43–77.

CASE 10 | **MULTINODULAR GOITRE** ***

INSTRUCTION

'Examine this patient's neck.' (Fig. 1.20)

See Cases 6 and 8 for general examination of the neck and thyroid gland.

SPECIFIC POINTS ON EXAMINATION OF THE NECK

With a large multinodular goitre it should be relatively easy to palpate the thyroid as the patient swallows some water:

- Describe the features of the lump:
  - Multinodular
  - May be large in size
  - There may be one nodule which is more prominent than the others
- Check the position of the trachea, which may be deviated by a large multinodular goitre, and percuss for retrosternal extension.

OTHER POINTS ON SYSTEMIC EXAMINATION

- Feel the pulse – atrial fibrillation is seen in 40% of patients with multinodular goitre.

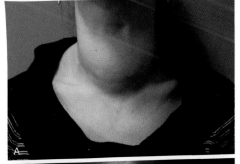
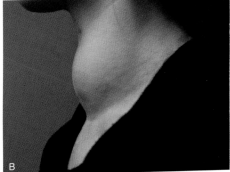

Figure 1.20 Goitre (from Young C, Gladman M. *Examination Surgery*. Chatswood, NSW, Australia: Churchill Livingstone, 2013, with permission).

? QUESTIONS

(a) What are the features of a multinodular goitre?

- Progression of simple diffuse goitre to nodular enlargement
- Female preponderance
- Positive family history
- Malignant change occurs in 5% of untreated multinodular goitres
- Overactivity in parts of a multinodular goitre may lead to mild hyperthyroidism (Plummer's syndrome)
- No ophthalmic features are seen (these are characteristic of Graves' disease; see Case 11).

(b) How would you manage a multinodular goitre?

- After triple assessment, most patients do not need any intervention
- The patient usually presents because of:
  - Cosmetic reasons, or after noticing a lump in the neck
  - Discomfort
  - Tracheal compression – causing shortness of breath
  - Oesophageal compression – causing dysphagia
  - Worries about malignancy
  - Onset of hyperthyroidism
- Investigate if:
  - Prominent nodule
  - Features suspicious of malignancy, such as cervical lymphadenopathy or recurrent laryngeal nerve palsy
- Investigate using:
  - Thyroid function tests – hyperthyroid?
  - Ultrasound/CT – dimensions of goitre and nodules, look for dominant nodules/cysts for FNAC
  - Chest X-ray – a retrosternal goitre may compress the trachea.

(c) How would you treat a multinodular goitre?

- Non-surgical:
  - Remove goitrogens, e.g. remove cabbage/Brussels sprouts from diet
  - Thyroxine 0.1–0.3 mg/day – causes regression in 50–70% of patients, probably because multinodular goitres

increase in size as a result of raised thyroid-stimulating hormone levels
  - If thyrotoxicosis, treat as in Graves' disease (see Case 11)
  - Aspiration of cysts with cytology to exclude malignancy (Fig. 1.19)
  - Radioiodine – for elderly patients, particularly those unfit for surgery
- Surgical:
  - Total thyroidectomy has replaced subtotal thyroidectomy as the procedure of choice due to 50% risk of recurrence in the long term and the risk of pathological change in the thyroid remnant (malignancy/ increasing in size, further nodularity) necessitating further re-do surgery, which carries a much greater risk of damage to recurrent laryngeal nerves and parathyroids.

(d) What are the indications for surgery?

The five **M**s:

- **M**echanical – obstructive symptoms
- **M**alignancy
- **M**arred beauty – cosmetic reasons
- **M**edical treatment failure – thyrotoxicosis
- **M**ediastinal (retrosternal) extension – unable to perform FNAC or monitor change clinically.

? ADVANCED QUESTION

(a) How can you tell the difference between toxic multinodular goitre and Graves' disease?

See Table 1.3.

H. S. Plummer (1874–1936). North American physician. Also described:

- Plummer nails: concave or ragged edge to the nail bed seen in early onycholysis occurring in thyrotoxicosis (most prominent in fourth and fifth fingers)
- Plummer sign: inability of patient to sit in a chair as a result of thyrotoxic myopathy
- Plummer treatment: the use of iodine to treat thyrotoxicosis
- Plummer–Vinson syndrome: iron-deficiency anaemia associated with dysphagia and post-cricoid oesophageal webs in middle-aged women. (Note that this is the North American variation – this syndrome is known as the Paterson–Brown-Kelly syndrome in the UK and the Waldenström–Kjellberg syndrome in Scandinavia!)

Table 1.3

Toxic multinodular goitre	Graves' disease
Older age group	Younger age group
Nodular enlargement	Diffuse enlargement
Eye signs not present	Eye signs present
Atrial fibrillation present in 40% of patients	Atrial fibrillation uncommon
No associated autoimmune diseases	Autoimmune diseases commonly associated

FURTHER READING

Hisham AN, Azlina AF, Aina EN, et al: Total thyroidectomy: the procedure of choice for multinodular goitre. *Eur J Surg* 6:403–405, 2001.

Huysmans D, Hermus A, Edelbroek M, et al: Radioiodine for nontoxic multinodular goitre. *Thyroid* 7(2):235–239, 1997.

CASE 11　DIFFUSE THYROID ENLARGEMENT ***

INSTRUCTION

'Examine this lady's neck'

See Cases 6 and 8 for the general examination of the neck and thyroid gland.

SPECIFIC POINTS ON EXAMINATION OF THE NECK

- Describe the features of the lump:
  - Diffuse enlargement (not nodular)
  - May be large in size
  - Usually non-tender in the examination
- Gently palpate the trachea for deviation (from a large goitre), and ask the patient if she has had any problems swallowing (from a large goitre) or noticed any change in her voice
- Remember to percuss over the sternum for a retrosternal extension of a large goitre.

? QUESTIONS

(a) What are the causes of a diffusely enlarged thyroid gland?

- Simple colloid goitre
- Graves' disease
- Thyroiditis (Hashimoto's, de Quervain's or Riedel's; see Case 8).

(b) What do you know about simple colloid goitres?

- Commonest form of thyroid abnormality
- Secondary to hyperplasia of the gland to meet physiological demand for thyroxine
- Secondary to defective production of thyroid hormone
- Causes are as follows:
  - Iodine deficiency (commonest cause worldwide)
  - Increased physiological demand – puberty, pregnancy and lactation (commonest cause in the UK)
  - Goitrogens (less common) – uncooked cabbage, lithium and antithyroid drugs
  - Defects of thyroid hormone production (rare).

(c) What are the features of Graves' disease?

- Commoner in females (9 : 1)
- Results from polyclonal immunoglobulins against thyroid-stimulating hormone receptor which bind and stimulate the receptor – these antibodies are found in 90% of patients
- Hyperthyroidism with goitre
- Thyroid eye disease (Fig. 1.21 and see Case 8)
- Thyroid acropachy
- Pretibial myxoedema
- Normochromic normocytic anaemia, raised erythrocyte sedimentation rate and hypercalcaemia can also occur

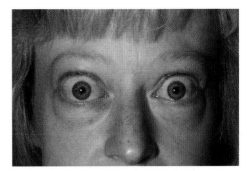

Figure 1.21 Eye changes in Graves' disease (from Quick CRG, Reed JB, Harper SJF et al. *Essential Surgery*, 5th edn. Edinburgh: Elsevier, with permission).

- Associated with other autoimmune conditions, such as type 1 diabetes and pernicious anaemia.

(d) How do you treat Graves' disease?

- Medical:
  - Antithyroid drugs, e.g. carbimazole, methimazole, propylthiouracil (to treat thyroid storm and during first trimester of pregnancy) – to inhibit thyroid peroxidase
  - Beta-blockers, e.g. propanolol – to reduce the effects of excess circulating thyroxine on the cardiac system
- Radioiodine:
  - Treatment of choice (only absolute contraindications are pregnancy and lactation)
  - Single oral dose of ^{131}I causes direct radiation damage to the replication mechanisms of thyroid follicular cells
  - Risks include early hyperthyroidism, late hypothyroidism and late hyperparathyroidism
- Surgery:
  - Particularly useful for: patients who fail medical therapy or have major reactions to medication; patients who refuse radiation therapy or relapse after an adequate course; pregnant patients or those wishing to become pregnant within 4 years; patients under the age of 40 years and those with nodular or large goitres; patients with thyroid eye disease
  - Increasingly, total thyroidectomy has replaced subtotal thyroidectomy, which carries an 8% risk of persistence or recurrence and a 50% chance of requiring thyroid hormone supplementation (the historical perceived benefit).

(e) What are the complications of thyroidectomy?

Complications of thyroidectomy can be divided into those that are general to any operation (e.g. risks of anaesthesia) and those that are specific to thyroidectomy alone. They can also be divided into *immediate* (within 24 h), *early* (within 30 days) and *late* (after 30 days) – they (mostly) begin with the letter **H**:

- Immediate:
  - **H**aemorrhage, leading to airway obstruction from secondary laryngeal oedema; patients who have recently had a thyroid operation should have a pair of suture cutters by their bed – if this complication occurs, the sutures should immediately be removed and an anaesthetist called
  - **H**yperthyroidism – severe, and known as thyroid storm
- Early:
  - **(H)**infection – a rather weak H!
  - **H**ypoparathyroidism, leading to **H**ypocalcaemia
  - **H**oarseness from damage to the recurrent laryngeal nerve
  - **H**igh-pitch tone loss/vocal fatigue from damage to the external branch of the superior laryngeal nerve
- Late:
  - **H**yperthyroidism – recurrent
  - **H**ypothyroidism
  - **H**ypertrophic scarring.

? ADVANCED QUESTIONS

(a) What is the pathology of thyroid eye disease?

- Exophthalmos is secondary to retro-orbital inflammation and lymphocytic infiltration, leading to oedema and an increase in retrobulbar orbital contents
- Lid lag is secondary to sympathetic overstimulation and restrictive myopathy of levator palpebrae superioris.

(b) How do you classify the severity of thyroid eye disease?

Use Werner's mnemonic **NO SPECS** (Table 1.4).

R. J. Graves (1797–1853). Irish physician, Dublin.

Table 1.4 NO SPECS classification of thyroid eye disease

Class 0	N	No signs or symptoms
Class 1	O	Only signs of upper-lid retraction and stare, with or without lid lag and exophthalmos
Class 2	S	Soft-tissue involvement
Class 3	P	Proptosis
Class 4	E	Exophthalmos
Class 5	C	Corneal involvement
Class 6	S	Sight loss due to optic nerve involvement

FURTHER READING

Weetman AP: Graves' disease. *N Engl J Med* 343(17):236–248, 2000.

CASE 12   THYROID HISTORY   ***

INSTRUCTION

'This lady is complaining of a swelling in her neck. Ask her a few questions about her thyroid gland.'

APPROACH

It is important to ascertain the symptoms arising from the swelling, the thyroid status, other associated symptoms and any relevant medical history.

Symptoms arising from the swelling

- Mass
  - Duration and change in size – note particularly if the swelling has suddenly increased in size (this can occur if there is haemorrhage into a necrotic nodule, subacute thyroiditis or a rapidly growing carcinoma)
- Cosmetic symptoms
- Airway
  - Dyspnoea (tracheal compression)
- Digestive tract
  - Discomfort during swallowing/dysphagia – oesophageal compression

- Voice
  - Hoarseness – due to recurrent laryngeal nerve paralysis secondary to malignant infiltration
- Pain – not common, but can occur in thyroiditis or anaplastic carcinoma.

Thyroid status

Table 1.5 shows the symptoms of hyper- and hypothyroidism.

Other associated symptoms

- Ask about eye symptoms, e.g. protruding or staring eyes, difficulty closing eyelids, double vision (secondary to ophthalmoplegia) and pain in the eye (secondary to corneal ulceration).

Relevant medical history

- Previous operations on the thyroid gland
- Previous or current medication, e.g. antithyroid drugs, thyroxine, iodine-containing medications
- Radioiodine therapy for previous Graves' disease (eye signs may persist)
- Move on to assessing fitness for surgery if relevant and time permits.

Table 1.5 Hyper- and hypothyroidism

	Hyperthyroidism	Hypothyroidism
General	Increased appetite but loss of weight	Decreased appetite and gain in weight, lethargy
Thermoregulatory	Preference for cold	Preference for hot weather
Dermatological	Increased sweating	Dry skin, 'peaches and cream' complexion, loss of hair – especially outer third of eyebrows
Musculoskeletal	Proximal myopathy (autoimmune) with wasting and weakness	Muscle fatigue
Gastrointestinal	Change in bowel habit, particularly diarrhoea and frequent defecation	Constipation
Cardiovascular	Tachycardia, atrial fibrillation	Bradycardia
Gynaecological	Oligomenorrhoea, amenorrhoea	Menorrhagia
Psychiatric	Nervousness, easy irritability, emotional lability, insomnia, psychosis	Slow thought, speech and action, depression, dementia
Neurological	Fine tremor	Symptoms of carpal tunnel syndrome (see Case 80)

CASE 13   HYPERTROPHIC AND KELOID SCARS   ✱✱✱

INSTRUCTION

'Examine this gentleman's scar.' (Fig. 1.22)

APPROACH

Your description is likely to be based solely on inspection.

VITAL POINTS

- The scar can be on any part of the body where there has been an incision in the skin
- Describe the scar – point out that the scar area is more prominent than the surrounding skin (Fig. 1.22) and add details as in Table 1.6.

Finish your examination here

Completion

Say that you would like to ask the patient:

- How the scar affects his life, e.g. cosmetic symptoms.

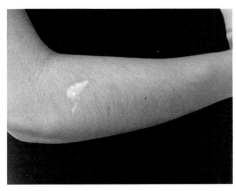

Figure 1.22   Hypertrophic scarring.

❓ QUESTIONS

(a) What do you know about the epidemiology of hypertrophic and keloid scars?

See Table 1.7.

(b) What types of wounds are prone to hypertrophic and keloid scar formation?

Wounds associated with:

- Infection
- Trauma
- Burns
- Tension, especially over the sternum, such as after coronary artery bypass grafting
- Wounds on certain areas of the body (Table 1.6).

(c) Is there a difference in the clinical course of hypertrophic and keloid scars?

Hypertrophic scars tend to appear soon after injury and usually regress spontaneously, while keloid scars appear months after injury and continue to grow.

(d) How do you treat these scars?

Recurrence can be as high as 55% with surgical revision alone, and therefore a combination of the treatments outlined below is often employed:

- Non-surgical: mechanical pressure therapy (day and night for up to 1 year), topical silicone gel sheets
- Surgical: revision of scar with closure by direct suturing, local Z-plasty or skin grafting to avoid excessive tension
- Intralesional steroid and local anaesthetic injections: using triamcinolone in combination with lignocaine.

Table 1.6

Features	Hypertrophic scars	Keloid scars
Appearance	Scar confined to wound margins	Scar extends beyond wound margins
Site	Across flexor surfaces and skin creases	Earlobes, chin, neck, shoulder, chest

Table 1.7

Features	Hypertrophic scars	Keloid scars
Age	Any age (commonly 8–20 years)	Puberty to 30 years
Gender	M = F	M = F
Race	All races	Black and Hispanic races

Table 1.8

Associations	Hypertrophic scars	Keloid scars
Biochemical	Normal rate of collagen synthesis but increased breakdown of collagen by collagenase activity	Increased rate of collagen synthesis (increased proline hydroxylase activity) and increased collagenase activity
Genetic	Not proven	Significant predisposition in Black and Hispanic races
Oxygen levels	Relative hypoxia – due to wound tension?	No link
Immunology	May be important, but no specific associations known	Increased IgG, IgM and C3 levels, and antinuclear antibodies to keloid fibroblasts

? ADVANCED QUESTIONS

(a) What other associations have been described with keloid and hypertrophic scars?

See Table 1.8.

Jean Louis Albert coined the name 'keloid' in 1806 in order to describe this 'overhealing' phenomenon, although they had been originally described in the *Smith Surgical Papyrus* (2500 BC).

FURTHER READING

Wolfram D, Tzankov A, Pülzl P, et al: Hypertrophic scars and keloids – a review of their pathophysiology, risk factors, and therapeutic management. *Dermatol Surg* 35(2):171–181, 2009.

CASE 14 | SQUAMOUS CELL CARCINOMA **

INSTRUCTION

'Examine this gentleman's leg.' (Fig. 1.23)

APPROACH

Sit or kneel in front of the patient to obtain the best view, and examine as for any lump.

VITAL POINTS

Inspect

- Usually occurs on areas of sun-exposed skin (where skin looks 'weathered')
- Appears vascular (red–brown)
- Raised and everted edge
- May be of considerable size (>1 cm)
- There may be erosion of the facial architecture if the tumour is advanced
- May have central ulceration.

Palpate

- Regional lymphadenopathy (may be due to metastases or secondary infection – only 5%

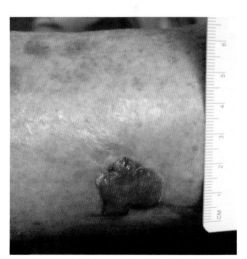

Figure 1.23 Squamous cell carcinoma (from Young C, Gladman M. *Examination Surgery*. Chatswood, NSW, Australia: Churchill Livingstone, 2013, with permission).

have metastasised by the time of presentation) (see Case 7).

Finish your examination here

Completion

Say that you would like to ask the patient about:

- Predisposing factors (see below)
- How the lesion affects his life, e.g. cosmetic symptoms.

? QUESTIONS

(a) What is your differential diagnosis?

Benign skin lesions:

- Keratoacanthoma
- Infected seborrhoeic wart
- Solar keratosis
- Pyogenic granuloma

Malignant skin lesions:

- Basal cell carcinoma
- Malignant melanoma (amelanotic).

(b) What are the predisposing factors for squamous cell carcinoma (SCC)?

Congenital:

- Xeroderma pigmentosum (see Case 16)

Acquired:

- Environmental agents, e.g. sunlight, ionising radiation, industrial carcinogens such as arsenic
- Pre-existing skin lesions, e.g. solar keratosis (see Case 27), Bowen's disease (see below)
- Infections, e.g. viral warts (human papilloma virus 5 and 8)
- Immunosuppression, e.g. in antirejection treatment post-transplant and in HIV infection – may develop multiple SCCs
- Chronic cutaneous ulceration, e.g. chronic burns, chronic venous ulcers (Marjolin's ulcer).

(c) What treatment options are available for SCC?

Primary lesion:

- Complete excision with 5-mm margins to achieve histologically negative wide and deep margins

- Mohs' staged chemosurgery with histological assessment of margins and electrodesiccation – for lesions of the eyelids, ears and nasolabial folds
- Radiotherapy – in unfit patients; where surgery would be disfiguring; in palliative, non-operable cases; for unresectable lesions

Nodal spread:

- Risk of lymph node metastases is small (<1%) but they occur more frequently in lesions:
  - >2 cm in diameter
  - >4 mm thick
  - that are poorly differentiated
  - that are recurrent
- Surgical block dissection – if palpable nodes or in cases of Marjolin's ulcers, although the benefit of prophylactic block lymph node dissection with Marjolin's ulcers is not proven
- Radiotherapy.

? ADVANCED QUESTION

(a) What do you know about the pathology of SCC?

The tumour arises from epidermal cells that normally migrate to the skin surface to form the superficial keratinising squamous layer. Full-thickness epidermal atypia is seen (vs. basal atypia only in solar keratosis) and tumour cells are seen to extend in all directions into the deep dermis and subcutaneous fat. The tumour itself may be well differentiated (with production of keratin), moderately differentiated or poorly differentiated.

Professor J. T. Bowen (1857–1941). American dermatologist. Bowen's disease is an intraepidermal carcinoma presenting as a single brown–red irregular plaque usually on the trunk that increases in size and may progress to invasive SCC. The condition is also associated with subsequent development of visceral malignancies, usually 5–7 years later, particularly if the affected area of skin has never been exposed to the sun. Excision with at least a 0.5-cm margin is recommended. Newer treatment options include topical diclofenac, topical imiquimod and photodynamic therapy. When seen on the penis, vulva or oral cavity, it is known as *erythroplasia of Queyrat* (French dermatologist *c.* 1900).

R. Marjolin (1812–1895). French surgeon.

FURTHER READING

Garcia-Zuazaga J, Olbricht SM: Cutaneous squamous cell carcinoma. *Adv Dermatol* 24:33–57, 2008.

www.britishskinfoundation.org.uk/standard .aspx?id=90 – general information about SCCs.

CASE 15 | MALIGNANT MELANOMA **

INSTRUCTION

'Examine the lesion on this lady's right leg.' (Fig. 1.24)

APPROACH

The patient should already be adequately exposed. Examine as for any lump (see Case 1).

VITAL POINTS

Inspect

- Found most commonly on the legs of young women and the trunk of middle-aged men, but location and characteristics depend on type
- Presence of naevi is the most common predictor of risk of malignant melanoma
- Commonest cancer of young adults aged between 20 and 39 years
- Commoner in women than men.

The four commonest types are:

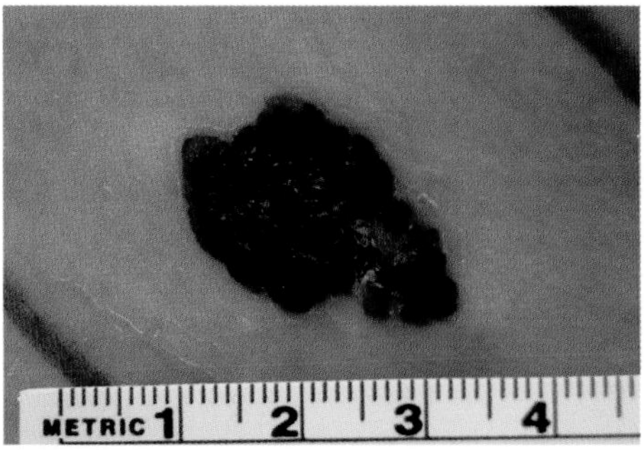

Figure 1.24 Malignant melanoma (from Young C, Gladman M. *Examination Surgery*. Chatswood, NSW, Australia: Churchill Livingstone, 2013, with permission).

SUPERFICIAL SPREADING MELANOMA

- Most common type (50–70%)
- Occurs most often on the legs of women and the backs of men
- Red, white and blue in colour
- Irregular edge
- Usually palpable but thin.

NODULAR MELANOMA

- Second most common type (15–50%)
- Occurs most often on the trunk
- Polypoid in shape and is raised
- Smooth surface
- Irregular edge
- Frequently ulcerated.

LENTIGO MALIGNA MELANOMA

- Arises in a lentigo maligna (Hutchinson's melanotic freckle – see below)
- Occurs most often on the face or dorsum of the hands and forearms
- Underlying lesion is flat and brown-to-black in colour with an irregular outline
- Malignant area in the lesion is usually thicker, and darker in colour.

ACRAL LENTIGINOUS MELANOMA

- Least common
- Occurs on hairless skin (such as subungual area, and palms of hands and soles of feet) and is more common in Oriental and Black races
- Irregular area of brown or black pigmentation.

There are other rarer types of melanoma (e.g. amelanotic melanoma, with no pigmentation and a poorer prognosis), but these are less likely to be encountered in the clinical cases. It is also possible to have intracranial melanoma as there is melanin in the substantia nigra, and also in the retina.

Features of a pigmented skin lesion suspicious of malignant melanoma change

- **A** – Asymmetry
- **B** – Border irregularity
- **C** – Colour variation within the lesion
- **D** – Diameter (large)
- **E** – Evolution (changing with time)
- Other concerning (late) features include: loss of normal surface markings around the lesion (e.g. skin creases); presence of ulceration; evidence of bleeding from the lesion; presence of a halo of brown pigment in the skin around the lesion; presence of satellite nodules of tumour around the lesion
- The appearances of nodular melanomas can be remembered by the acronym **EFG** (**E**levated; **F**irm; **G**rowing)

Finish your examination here

Completion

Say that you would like to:
- Examine the draining lymph nodes
- Ask the patient about symptoms from the lesion that may indicate malignancy, e.g. rapid increase in the size of a mole, itching, bleeding, change in colour, shape or thickness
- Ask the patient about predisposing factors (see below).

? QUESTIONS

(a) What is your differential diagnosis?

Benign skin lesions:
- Moles: increased numbers of melanocytes producing too much melanin (also called pigmented naevus)
- Freckles: normal numbers of melanocytes but each producing too much melanin
- Lentigo: increased numbers of melanocytes producing normal amounts of melanin
- Pigmented seborrhoeic keratoses

- Dermatofibromas (see Case 33)
- Thrombosed haemangiomas

Malignant skin lesions:
- Pigmented basal cell carcinomas (see Case 16).

(b) What are the predisposing factors for malignant melanomas?

Congenital:
- Xeroderma pigmentosum (see Case 16)
- Dysplastic naevus syndrome (also known as B-K mole or familial atypical multiple mole melanoma [FAMM] syndrome) – risk of developing malignant melanoma is 100% if two family members are affected
- Large congenital naevi
- Family history in first-degree relatives (increased risk by one and a half times)

Acquired:
- Sunlight (particularly ultraviolet light): especially in fair-skinned people with red hair
- Pre-existing skin lesions, e.g. lentigo maligna, more than 20 benign pigmented naevi (the latter increases the risk three times)
- Previous melanoma (increases the risk three and a half times).

(c) How do you stage malignant melanomas?

Historically, Clark's levels and Breslow's thickness were used, which are two pathological staging systems based on the depth of invasion of the tumour from the epidermis.

Clark's levels of invasion (Fig. 1.25) were described in 1969 (Table 1.9).

The second is Breslow's thickness (Fig. 1.26), described in 1970 (Table 1.10).

More recently, the AJCC/UICC tumour, nodes, metastases (TNM) system has replaced these (Table 1.11).

(d) What treatment options are available for malignant melanoma?

Surgical excision

Main lesion:

Wide excision of the primary lesion:

Stage	Lesion thickness	Margin
Tis		5 mm
T1	<1 mm	1 cm
T2	1–2 cm	1–2 cm
T3–4	>2 cm	2 cm

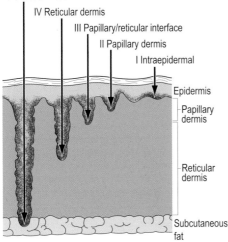

Figure 1.25   Clark's levels of melanoma invasion.

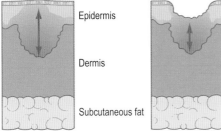

Figure 1.26   Breslow's thickness of malignant melanoma, which relates to thickness of the tumour itself.

Table 1.9

Clark's level	Extent of tumour	5-year survival (%)
I	Epidermis only	98
II	Invades papillary dermis	96
III	Fills papillary dermis	94
IV	Invades reticular dermis	78
V	Subcutaneous tissue invasion	44

Table 1.10

Breslow's thickness	10-year survival (%)
<0.76 mm	92
<3 mm	50
<4 mm	30
Lymph node involvement	<40 (8-year survival)

Table 1.11

T classification	Thickness
Tis	Melanoma in situ
T1	<1.0 mm
T2	1–2 mm
T3	2–4 mm
T4	>4 mm
N classification	**Number of metastatic nodes**
N0	No regional lymph nodes
N1	1 node
N2	2–3 nodes
N3	4 or more nodes
M classification	**Site**
M0	No distant metastases
M1a	Distant skin / lymph nodes
M1b	Lung
M1c	All other viscera

- Excision should be down to deep fascia

Nodal spread:

- Risk of metastasis increases from 8% for 1-mm tumours to 40% for tumours > 4 mm
- If clinically palpable nodes, lymph node biopsy or fine-needle aspiration cytology (FNAC)
- If lymph node metastases are proven the patient requires therapeutic block dissection
- Sentinel lymph node biopsy (SLNB) can be considered in:
  - Breslow thickness >1 mm (or >0.75 mm with ulceration present)
  - Clark level IV or V thickness >1 mm (or >0.75 mm with ulceration present)
  - Patients with a positive SLNB should have a therapeutic lymph node dissection

Palliation/adjuvant therapies

- The only drug with demonstrable efficacy for high-risk melanoma is interferon-alfa 2b therapy.

Prevention: *most important to mention this in your answer*

- Avoidance of causative factors, e.g. public education campaigns to reduce sun exposure.

? ADVANCED QUESTIONS

(a) What do you know about the pathology of malignant melanoma?

On microscopy, malignant melanomas consist of loose nests of melanocytes in the basal cell layer which invade the epidermis (leading to destruction and ulceration) and penetrate deeper into the dermis and subcutaneous fat.

(b) Do you know of any prognostic indicators for malignant melanoma?

Analysis of staging and survival data from 17 600 melanoma patients demonstrated that, for primary tumours (T), the most powerful predictors of survival were thickness and ulceration. Level of invasion had a significant impact only within the subgroup of thin (<1 mm) melanomas. In terms of lymph nodes (N), the number of metastatic nodes, whether nodal metastases were clinically occult or clinically apparent and the presence or absence of primary tumour ulceration also influenced survival. Finally, in the category of distant metastasis (M), non-visceral metastases are associated with a better survival compared with visceral metastases.

Sir John Hunter (1728–1793). First described malignant melanoma in 1787. (See Case 119.)

Sir Jonathan Hutchinson (1828–1913). English surgeon, London Hospital and Professor of Surgery, Royal College of Surgeons. He described a flat pigmented, brown-to-black melanocytic naevus with malignant potential that occurs on sun-damaged skin on the face, and on the dorsum of the hands and forearm. The freckle itself represents an increased number of melanocytes at the dermoepidermal junction. It occurs in the fifth to seventh decades, and after a period of time (10–30 years), it transforms into a malignant melanoma, heralded clinically by the development of a black or tan nodule. Also described Hutchinson triad (eighth-nerve deafness, notched teeth and interstitial keratitis in congenital syphilis).

FURTHER READING

Bataille V, de Vries E: Melanoma – part 1: epidemiology, risk factors, and prevention. *BMJ* 337:a2249, 2008.

Beahrs OH, Myers MH: *Manual for Staging of Cancer.* American Joint Committee Cancer. Philadelphia, 1983, Lippincott, p 117.

Thirlwell C, Nathan P: Melanoma – part 2: management. *BMJ* 337:a2488, 2008.

www.skincancerfacts.org.uk – information on all types of skin cancers for patients.

CASE 16 | BASAL CELL CARCINOMA **

INSTRUCTION

'Examine this gentleman's face.' (Fig. 1.27)

APPROACH

Sit or kneel in front of the patient in order to be at the same level as his face, and examine as for any lump.

VITAL POINTS

TOP TIP

✓ If you need to see the side of the patient's face, e.g. ear, stay still while sitting or kneeling and ask the patient to turn his head to the appropriate side – it looks unprofessional to move back and forth around the patient!

Inspect

- Occurs on hair-bearing sun-exposed skin of elderly people, especially around the eye
- Single or multiple
- Features of basal cell carcinomata (BCCs) depend on the clinical type and can be divided into:

RAISED ABOVE THE SKIN (Fig. 1.27)

- Nodular/nodulo-ulcerative
  - Most common type
  - Well-defined rolled, pearly edge
  - Central ulceration
- Cystic
  - Large cystic nodule

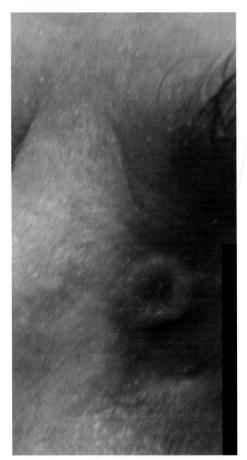

Figure 1.27 Basal cell carcinoma (from Young C, Gladman M. *Examination Surgery*. Chatswood, NSW, Australia: Churchill Livingstone, 2013, with permission).

NOT RAISED ABOVE THE SKIN

- Pigmented
  - Contains melanin
  - Can be confused with malignant melanoma (see Case 15)
- Sclerosing (also known as morphoeic)
  - Flat or depressed tumour
  - Ill-defined edge
  - May be ulcerated (occurs late)
- Cicatricial (also known as field-fire or bush-fire)
  - Multiple superficial erythematous lesions interspersed with pale atrophic areas
- Superficial
  - Erythematous scaly patches
  - Can be confused with Bowen's disease (see Case 14).

Palpate

- Fixation of the BCC deep to the skin is a sign of deep local invasion.

Finish your examination here

Completion

Say that you would like to:

- Examine for regional lymphadenopathy (but note that metastases are extremely rare, BCCs are locally aggressive)
- Ask the patient about predisposing factors (see below).

? QUESTIONS

(a) What is your differential diagnosis?

The two main differential diagnoses to consider are:

- Benign – keratoacanthoma – especially if it is sloughing at its centre (see Case 22)
- Malignant – squamous cell carcinoma – particularly the nodulo-ulcerative type with a rolled edge (see Case 14).

(b) What are the predisposing factors for basal cell carcinomas ?

- Congenital (rare):
  - Xeroderma pigmentosum (familial condition associated with failure of DNA transcription, leading to defective DNA repair) – also known as Kaposi's disease (see Cases 16 and 35)
  - Gorlin's syndrome (see below)
- Acquired (very common):
  - Sunlight (particularly ultraviolet light in the UVB range)
  - Carcinogens, e.g. cigarette smoke, arsenic
  - Previous radiotherapy
  - Malignant transformation in pre-existing skin lesions, e.g. naevus sebaceous.

(c) What treatment options are available for BCC?

Treatment options available are:

- Ideally, an excision margin of 3–5 mm with an adequate 0.5-mm microscopic clear margin.
- For tumours <6 mm a 4-mm margin and for tumours >6 mm a 6-mm margin will give a

95% local control rate at 5 years. Certain areas, e.g. inner canthus of eye, nasolabial fold, nasal floor and ear, require special attention.

- Frozen section may be necessary to ensure adequate excision
- Other approaches: radiotherapy and Mohs' surgery (see Case 14).

? ADVANCED QUESTIONS

(a) What do you know about the histology of BCC?

On microscopy, BCCs have many patterns, but the most common features are islands and nests of basaloid cells in the dermis (like those seen in the basal cell layer of the epidermis). The cells exhibit high mitotic rates and peripheral palisading (cell islands arranged radially with long axes in approximately parallel alignment). Often, there is ulceration of the epidermis.

(b) What do you know of the pathology of BCC?

The hedgehog signalling pathway is important in embryological development and is highly conserved through evolution. Recently patched, a member of the pathway was found to be important in Gorlin's syndrome. Inherited patched gene mutations underlie the syndrome, in which a key feature is multiple BCCs. The gene is also mutated in sporadic BCCs.

> *R. J. Gorlin (1923–2006).* American Professor of Oral Pathology, University of Minnesota. Gorlin's syndrome (naevoid basal cell epithelioma syndrome) is an autosomal-dominant condition presenting in early adult life with multiple basal cell carcinomas, keratocysts of the jaw, palmar and plantar pits, mesenteric cysts and scoliosis.

FURTHER READING

Epstein EH: Basal cell carcinomas: attack of the hedgehog. *Nat Rev Cancer* 8(10):743–754, 2008.

Gorlin RJ: Nevoid basal cell carcinoma syndrome. *Dermatol Clin* 13(1):113–125, 1995.

Roewert-Huber J, Lange-Asschenfeldt B, Stockfleth E, et al: Epidemiology and aetiology of basal cell carcinoma. *Br J Dermatol* 157(Suppl 2):47–51, 2007.

www.skincancerfacts.org.uk – information for patients on all skin cancers, including BCCs.

CASE 17 | PRESSURE SORES **

INSTRUCTION

'Have a look at this lady's back'. (Fig. 1.28)

APPROACH

Examine as for ulcers (see Case 112). It is important to bear in mind when examining the peripheral vascular system of patients in the circulatory bay that ulcers may be due to pressure necrosis as well as peripheral vascular disease.

VITAL POINTS

You should be able to pick up all of the points simply from inspection. The American National Pressure Ulcer Advisory Panel Classification should be kept in mind when describing your findings.

TOP TIP

☑ A classification of pressure sores

Stage 1: Abnormal area of skin with erythema that will not blanch – indicates extravasated blood from cutaneous capillary beds

Stage 2: Partial-thickness skin loss – a shallow abrasion wound

Stage 3: Full-thickness skin loss with fat at the base of the wound

Stage 4: Extensive soft-tissue loss through deep fascia, often with underlying muscle necrosis

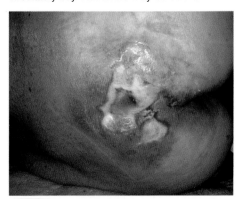

Figure 1.28 A pressure sore.

Completion

Say that you would like to take a history, looking for predisposing factors (see below).

? QUESTIONS

(a) Where are pressure sores most commonly found?

Pressure sores can occur over any bony prominence, the commonest areas being:

- Sacrum
- Greater trochanter
- Heel
- Lateral malleolus
- Ischial tuberosity
- Occiput.

(b) What conditions increase the risk of developing pressure sores?

Immobility and prolonged bed rest are the most important factors, particularly secondary to conditions such as:

- Cardiopulmonary disease
- Trauma
- Neurological disease, e.g. paraplegia
- Bone and joint disease
- Prolonged operative procedures, particularly if there are intraoperative episodes of hypotension.

Conditions that slow wound healing can increase the severity and risk of pressure necrosis:

- Metabolic disorders:
  - Diabetes mellitus
  - Deficiencies of vitamins and trace metals, e.g. vitamin C, zinc
- Drugs:
  - Steroids
  - Post-chemotherapy (also radiotherapy)
- Underlying disease:
  - Tissue hypoxia such as in peripheral vascular disease

- Renal failure
- Jaundice
- Carcinomatosis
- Infection.

? ADVANCED QUESTIONS

(a) How do you treat this condition?

- Prophylaxis: regular skin inspection, frequent turning of immobile patients (2–4-hourly), massage, toileting, the use of special mattresses and cushions which redistribute the pressure on at-risk areas
- Non-surgical: optimise tissue perfusion and oxygenation, treat infection as it arises, use various topical dressings as required and provide nutritional support. Specifically, vitamin C, zinc and multivitamins should be prescribed. Several other techniques, such as hyperbaric oxygen, hydrotherapy and ultrasound, are in use depending on local policy
- Surgical: debridement of dead tissue (which often does not require anaesthesia and can be performed by the tissue viability nurse) and reconstruction using a variety of fascial and muscle-containing composite flaps, e.g. buttock rotation flap for sacral sores.

(b) What do you know about the pathophysiology of pressure necrosis?

Prolonged weight bearing and mechanical shear forces act on areas of soft tissue overlying bony prominences, leading to both occlusion and tearing of small blood vessels, reduced tissue perfusion and ischaemic necrosis.

FURTHER READING

Reddy M, Gill SS, Rochon PA: Preventing pressure ulcers: a systematic review. *JAMA* 296(8):974–984, 2006.

Reddy M, Gill SS, Kalkar SR, et al: Treatment of pressure ulcers: a systematic review. *JAMA* 300(22):2647–2662, 2008.

CASE 18   GRAFTS AND FLAPS   **

INSTRUCTION

'Examine this patient's skin.' (Fig. 1.29)

It is important to be aware of the principles involved and the various types of grafts and flaps that may be encountered.

? QUESTIONS

(a) What is a skin graft?

A skin graft involves the transfer of skin from a donor site to a recipient site independent of a

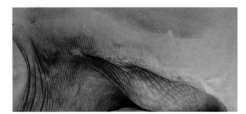

Figure 1.29 A skin graft.

blood supply. The graft 'takes' by acquiring a blood supply from a healthy donor bed. Skin grafts may either be full-thickness or partial-thickness, but contain the entire epidermis, with a portion of the underlying dermis. The dermis does not regenerate, but the epidermis regenerates from the adnexal elements of skin – hair follicles, sebaceous glands and sweat glands within the dermis.

(b) What tissues do skin grafts not take on?
- Unhealthy, necrotic and infected tissue
- Irradiated tissue
- Exposed cortical bone without periosteum
- Tendon without peritenon
- Cartilage without perichondrium.

(c) How do you harvest a skin graft?
- Use hand-held skin graft knives (e.g. Watson and Braithwaite modifications of the Humby knife) or electric- or gas-powered dermatomes, the latter producing a graft of even thickness from almost any site, with little expertise needed for operation
- Donor site is usually one that can be easily concealed, e.g. inner thigh, buttock or inner arm.

(d) What is a skin flap?
A skin flap consists of tissue, or tissues, transferred from one site of the body to another, while maintaining a continuous blood supply through a vascular pedicle.

(e) How do you classify skin flaps?
- Site: local or distant (also known as a 'free flap')
- Contents: can contain any tissue capable of transfer, including omentum and bowel
- Random or axial: the latter is based on a named artery or vein.

(f) What are the indications for flap reconstruction?
- Situations where skin grafts will not take (see above)
- When the aim is to reconstruct with tissue that is 'like for like' (bone, joint, tendon, nerve, epithelial lining, etc.) to promote optimal structure, function and cosmesis
- When blood supply has to be imported to areas of doubtful viability, e.g. pressure sores, complex trauma.

(g) What is the 'reconstruction ladder'?
This is the array of plastic surgical reconstruction techniques of increasing complexity that is available to the surgeon and which is used according to their suitability for individual patients:
- Healing by secondary intention (i.e. granulation) and then by primary intention (excision and closure) prior to reconstruction
- Skin graft
- Local flap
- Distant flap
- Composite flap
- Island flaps vs. pedicled flaps
- Free-tissue transfer
- Composite neurovascular free-tissue transfer.

FURTHER READING
Andreassi A, Bilenchi R, Biagioli M, et al: Classification and pathophysiology of skin grafts. *Clin Dermatol* 23(4):332–337, 2005.

CASE 19 | PTOSIS **

INSTRUCTION
'Examine this lady's face and tell me your diagnosis.' (Fig. 1.30)

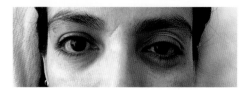

Figure 1.30 Unilateral ptosis.

APPROACH

This case is likely to be a spot diagnosis. Remember that the definition of ptosis is drooping of the upper eyelid associated with the inability to elevate the eyelid completely.

VITAL POINTS

Ptosis is best observed with the patient sitting up and the head being held by the candidate.

TOP TIP

- The upper eyelid is raised by the action of levator palpebrae superioris. This muscle is of dual origin and innervation (a favourite topic for surgical examiners):
  - Mainly skeletal muscle innervated by the third cranial nerve (oculomotor)
  - A thin sheet of smooth muscle (Müller's muscle) that is supplied by post-ganglionic sympathetic nerve fibres arising from cell bodies in the superior cervical ganglion
- Complete ptosis follows third-nerve palsy – the eyelid droops in all positions
- Partial ptosis follows an ipsilateral sympathetic nerve lesion – this is Horner's syndrome (ptosis, meiosis, anhydrosis and enophthalmos), which can be overcome on asking the patient to look up

Inspect

- Is it unilateral or bilateral?
- Note whether ptosis is partial or complete by asking the patient to look upwards
- Look at the size of the pupil
  - Small pupil in Horner's syndrome (look for other signs of Horner's; see above)
  - Large pupil in third cranial nerve palsy (look at the position of the eye [Fig. 1.31] – down and out in third-nerve palsy) and test the reaction of the pupil to light and accommodation – pupil does not react in third-nerve palsy.

Finish your examination here

Completion

Say that you would like to:
- Take a history from the patient to try to find the cause of the ptosis.

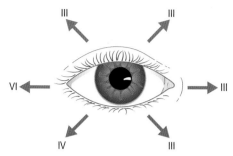

Figure 1.31 The actions of the third, fourth and sixth nerves on the eye movements of the right eye. III, oculomotor; IV, trochlear; VI, abducent.

? QUESTIONS

In surgical exams, ptosis is most likely to be due to Horner's syndrome, possibly secondary to:

- Lower brachial plexus injury (Déjerine-Klumpke paralysis; see Case 102)
- Pancoast's tumour of the lung (an apical lung carcinoma that invades the cervical sympathetic plexus, associated with shoulder and arm pain due to brachial plexus invasion of C8–T2, and a hoarse voice or bovine cough due to unilateral recurrent laryngeal nerve palsy and vocal cord paralysis).

(a) What causes of ptosis are you aware of?

Unilateral:
- Third cranial nerve palsy – complete ptosis
- Horner's syndrome – partial ptosis
- Syphilis

Bilateral:
- Congenital ptosis
- Myopathies – myasthenia gravis, dystrophia myotonica
- Syphilis.

(b) What surgical treatments are available?

A blepharoplasty can be performed: excess eyelid skin and fat are removed.

Henry Pancoast (1875–1939). Professor of Radiology, Pennsylvania, USA.

CASE 20 | FACIAL NERVE PALSY **

INSTRUCTION

'Have a look at this lady's face.'

APPROACH

In a surgical case, think of surgical causes, e.g. parotid gland tumours, old skull fracture – these result in lower motor neurone palsy of the seventh cranial nerve (facial nerve).

VITAL POINTS

Inspect systematically

- General: loss of facial expression
- Eyelids: on blinking, the affected side closes after the normal eyelid (Bell's sign – the eyeball moves vertically upwards on the abnormal side when the eye is closed)
- Eyes: widened palpebral fissure
- Nasolabial fold: flatter on affected side
- Mouth: the affected side droops and moves less when talking.

Test the muscles involved systematically

- Occipitofrontalis: 'raise your eyebrows' – spared in upper motor neurone facial nerve palsy as the forehead has bilateral cortical representation
- Orbicularis oculi: 'close your eyes as tightly as you can'
- Orbicularis oris: 'show me your teeth'
- Buccinator: 'puff out your cheeks'.

Look for an obvious cause

- Look for a scar over the parotid gland – indicating iatrogenic facial nerve damage
- Look for parotid gland enlargement
- Look in the external auditory meatus for herpes zoster (Ramsay Hunt syndrome; see below).

Completion

Say that you would like to:

- Take a history to determine the duration and effects of the condition on the patient

- Examine for taste with salt/sweet solutions (involvement of the chorda tympani, an afferent branch of the facial nerve)
- Test the patient's hearing (hyperacusis can result from involvement of the nerve to stapedius muscle, an efferent branch of the facial nerve).

? QUESTION

(a) What are the causes of facial nerve palsy?

- Intracranial:
  - Vascular – cerebrovascular accident
  - Tumour – acoustic neuroma
  - Infection – meningitis (rarely)
- Intratemporal:
  - Infection – acute and chronic otitis media, herpes zoster (Ramsay Hunt syndrome)
  - Idiopathic – Bell's palsy (see below)
  - Trauma – surgical, accidental, e.g. basal skull fracture
  - Tumour – paraganglioma, squamous cell carcinoma of external or middle ear, metastases, e.g. breast
- Extratemporal:
  - Tumour – parotid gland malignancy
  - Trauma – surgical, accidental, e.g. facial lacerations.

? ADVANCED QUESTION

(a) What are the branches of the facial nerve?
See Fig. 1.32.

- Motor:
  - Nerve to stapedius
  - Nerve to posterior belly of digastric
  - Five divisions within the parotid gland – temporal, zygomatic, buccal, mandibular and cervical – to supply the muscles of facial expression (such as orbicularis oculi, buccinator and orbicularis oris)
- Secretomotor – via greater superficial petrosal nerve to lacrimal, nasal and palatine glands
- Taste – via chorda tympani to anterior two-thirds of the tongue
- Sensory – uncommon sensory component of facial nerve carrying cutaneous impulses from the anterior wall of the external auditory meatus known as nervus intermedius or pars intermedia of Wrisberg.

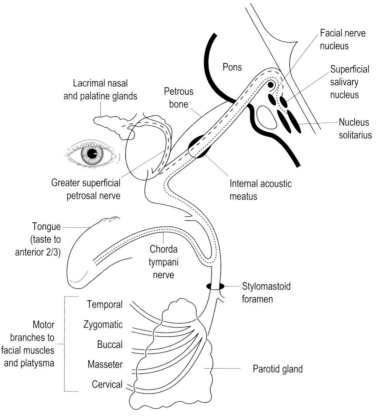

Figure 1.32   Branches of the facial nerve.

Sir Charles Bell (1774–1842). Scottish physiologist and Professor of Surgery, Edinburgh, who founded the Middlesex Hospital and Medical School, London. He described rapid, unilateral facial weakness associated with or preceded by an ache below the ear which worsens for 1–2 days and then resolves spontaneously within a few days in the majority (85%) of cases. Treatment involves the following:

- Physiotherapy (massage, electrical stimulation, splint to prevent drooping of the lower part of the face)

- Protection of the eye during sleep, wearing dark glasses during the day and use of artificial tears

- High-dose prednisolone to reduce nerve oedema which prevents weakness becoming paralysis – used if presentation is within a few days of onset.

J. Ramsay Hunt (1874–1937). Professor of Neurology, Columbia University, New York. He described involvement of the facial geniculate ganglion with herpes zoster resulting in lower motor neurone facial nerve palsy, severe ear pain and visible vesicles in the external auditory meatus, on the eardrum, on the soft palate or in the tonsillar fossa.

FURTHER READING

Sweeney CJ, Gilden DH: Ramsay Hunt syndrome. *J Neurol Neurosurg Psychiatry* 71(2):149–154, 2001.

Tiemstra JD, Khatkhate N: Bell's palsy: diagnosis and management. *Am Fam Physician* 76(7):997–1002, 2007.

CASE 21 | SALIVARY GLAND SWELLINGS **

INSTRUCTION

'This lady is complaining of a swelling on her left cheek. Examine it and tell me what you think.' (Fig. 1.33)

APPROACH

Sit or kneel in front of the patient in order to be at the same level as her face, and examine as for any lump (see Case 1).

VITAL POINTS

Inspect

* Swelling in the region of the parotid gland (which lies wedged between the

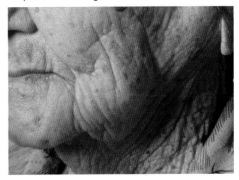

Figure 1.33 Parotid gland swelling (from Young C, Gladman M. *Examination Surgery*. Chatswood, NSW, Australia: Churchill Livingstone, 2013, with permission).

sternocleidomastoid muscle and the mandible) (Fig. 1.34) and the submandibular gland (at the angle of the jaw, wedged between the mandible and mylohyoid)
* Look for scars and the opening of a fistula (the latter can occur following parotidectomy or long-standing parotid traumatic injury)
* Stand back and look for facial asymmetry, which occurs if the seventh nerve is involved with a parotid lesion (see Case 20).

Palpate from behind

* Walk behind the patient and enquire about tenderness before palpating the swelling
* Is the swelling unilateral or bilateral?
* Is it fixed to the skin or underlying muscle? Ask the patient to clench her teeth, which tenses the masseter and makes the anterior border of the parotid gland more prominent
* Examine for other features as for any lump (see Case 2) – see below for features of malignancy
* Continue on to look for cervical lymphadenopathy using the 'down-and-up' routine (see Case 6).

Other tests

These tests may be described – in an examination you are unlikely to be asked to perform all of them:

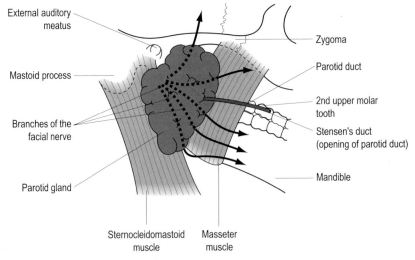

Figure 1.34 Anatomy of the right parotid gland.

External auditory meatus

Mastoid process

Branches of the facial nerve

Parotid gland

Zygoma

Parotid duct

2nd upper molar tooth

Stensen's duct (opening of parotid duct)

Mandible

Sternocleidomastoid muscle

Masseter muscle

- Look inside the mouth with a pen torch at the opening of the parotid duct (Stensen's duct), which can be found opposite the second upper molar and at the opening of the submandibular duct (Wharton's duct) on the floor of the mouth adjacent to the frenulum linguae – look for inflammation and pus, or the presence of a stone
- Palpate the parotid duct and submandibular duct openings wearing a pair of gloves, e.g. presence of stone
- Palpate the submandibular gland bimanually with a finger in the mouth and another finger below the angle of the jaw.

Finish your examination here

Completion

Say that you would like to:

- Test the facial nerve (see Case 20), which may be involved in malignant parotid tumours
- Perform a full ear, nose and throat examination.

? QUESTIONS

(a) What is the differential diagnosis of a unilateral swelling of the parotid gland?

See Table 1.12.

The acronym **SIN** will help you remember the causes of parotid gland enlargement affecting the gland.

(b) How would you diagnose a benign parotid tumour?

There are two important tumours – pleomorphic adenoma (commonest) and Warthin's tumour (second commonest) (Table 1.13)

Investigations:

- Fine-needle aspiration cytology for diagnosis
- Ultrasound/CT/MRI to exclude deep-lobe involvement.

Surgical treatment involves superficial parotidectomy (if superficial lobe of gland only involved) or total parotidectomy with preservation of the facial nerve (if deep lobe of gland or both lobes involved).

Table 1.13

Pleomorphic adenoma	Warthin's tumour
<50 years old	50 years old
	Smoking important risk factor
Tail of parotid, superficial to upper part of sternomastoid	Tail of parotid, superficial to upper part of sternomastoid
Facial nerve rarely involved	Facial nerve rarely involved

Table 1.12

Parotid gland pathology	Arising outside the parotid gland
Stones	Soft tissues
• Sialolithiasis	• Lipoma, sebaceous cyst
Infections/Inflammation/Infiltration	Dental origin
• Bacterial (*Staphylococcus*, *Streptococcus*, *Escherichia coli*, TB)	• Infection
	Muscular origin
• Viral (mumps, HIV)	• Hypertrophy of the masseter muscle
• Autoimmune (Sjögren's syndrome)*	Bony origin
• Sarcoidosis*	• Winged mandible
Neoplasia	• Transverse process of atlas/axis
Benign:	Neural origin
• Pleomorphic adenoma	• Facial nerve neuroma
• Warthin's tumour	Vascular origin
• Monomorphic adenoma	• Temporal artery aneurysm
• Oncocytoma	Systemic diseases
Malignant (primary/secondary):	• Alcoholic liver cirrhosis
• Adenocarcinoma	• Diabetes mellitus
• Lymphoma and leukaemia*	• Pancreatitis
• Squamous cell carcinoma	• Acromegaly
	• Malnutrition

*Can present as bilateral swellings.

(c) What clinical features would make you suspect that a parotid swelling is malignant in nature?

- Rapid growth and pain (on history)
- Hyperaemic, hot skin
- Hard consistency
- Fixed to skin and underlying muscle
- Irregular surface or ill-defined edge
- Facial nerve involvement.

(d) What is Sjögren's syndrome?

- Autoimmune condition – 90% occur in women at an average age of 50 years
- Intermittent or constant swelling of one or all of the salivary glands
- Clinical diagnosis based on the presence of at least two of the following triad:
  - Keratoconjuctivitis sicca (dry eyes)
  - Xerostomia (dry mouth)
  - Associated connective tissue disorders such as rheumatoid arthritis (50% of cases), scleroderma, systemic lupus erythematosus, polymyositis or polyarteritis nodosa
- If no associated connective tissue disorders are present, this is known as primary Sjögren's disease (note that Mikulicz syndrome is enlargement of the salivary and lacrimal glands secondary to sarcoidosis, lymphoma or tuberculosis, associated with dry mouth and dry eyes, but no arthritis)
- Pathology involves lymphocyte-mediated destruction of the exocrine glands secondary to B-cell hyper-reactivity and associated loss of suppressor T-cell activity
- Patients are at 40× increased risk of developing lymphoma, usually B-cell non-Hodgkin's type
- Several antibodies present, e.g. anti-salivary antibodies, rheumatoid factor, but two specific antibodies present – anti-SSA-Ro and anti-SSB-La
- Other investigations include Schirmer's test for xerophthalmia (strip of filter paper inserted into each fornix and hyposecretion confirmed by wetting of less than 5 mm in 5 min – normal is 15 mm), slit-lamp examination of the cornea and lip biopsy for histological examination of the minor salivary glands
- Treatment involves the use of artificial tears and saliva, systemic steroids and careful follow-up due to increased risk of lymphoma development.

? ADVANCED QUESTION

(a) What are the complications of parotidectomy?

Specific complications include:

- Immediate
  - Facial nerve transection (intraoperative)
  - Reactionary haemorrhage
- Early
  - Wound infection
  - Temporary facial weakness (neurapraxia)
  - Salivary fistula
  - Division of the greater auricular nerve – loss of sensation to the pinna
- Late
  - Wound dimple
  - Frey's syndrome (auriculotemporal syndrome) – increased sweating of the facial skin when eating, due to reinnervation of divided sympathetic nerves to the facial skin by fibres of the secretomotor branch of the auriculotemporal nerve.

L. Frey (1889–1944). Polish physician, Warsaw. She was killed by the Nazis.

J. von Mickulicz-Radecki (1850–1905). Professor of Surgery, Breslau, Germany.

O. W. A. Schirmer (1864–1917). German ophthalmologist.

H. S. C. Sjögren (1899–1986). Professor of Ophthalmology, Gothenburg, Sweden.

N. Stensen (1638–1686). Professor of Anatomy, Copenhagen, Denmark.

A. S. Warthin (1866–1931). Professor of Pathology, Ann Arbor, Michigan, USA.

T. Wharton (1614–1673). English physician, St Thomas's Hospital, London, UK.

FURTHER READING

Chandana SR, Conley BA: Salivary gland cancers: current treatments, molecular characteristics and new therapies. *Expert Rev Anticancer Ther* 8(4):645–652, 2008.

Notes on salivary gland tumours

- 80% of salivary gland tumours occur in the parotid gland: 80% of these parotid tumours are benign, with 80% of these benign tumours being pleomorphic adenomas

- In contrast, only 10% of salivary gland tumours occur in the submandibular gland, with only 60% of these submandibular tumours being benign (i.e. submandibular gland tumours are *twice* as likely to be malignant)
- The only known risk factor for salivary gland tumours is *exposure to radiation*
- The most common malignant salivary gland tumour is the mucoepidermoid tumour, which is most common in the parotid gland
- The most common malignant salivary gland tumour occurring in the submandibular gland, sublingual gland and the minor salivary glands is adenoid-cystic carcinoma
- The treatment of malignant salivary gland tumours involves total excision of the involved gland with preservation if possible of associated nerves (facial nerve in the case of the parotid gland and the lingual or hypoglossal nerves in the case of the submandibular gland) unless there is direct infiltration of the nerve by tumour. Adjuvant radiotherapy may also be used.

CASE 22 | KERATOACANTHOMA **

INSTRUCTION

'Examine this gentleman's hand.' (Fig. 1.35)

APPROACH

Examine as for any lump (see Case 1).

VITAL POINTS

- Found on sun-exposed parts of the body
- Commoner in males.

Inspect

- Dome-shaped with central crater (containing keratin)
- Normal skin colour (except for the central core, which is brown or black due to keratin).

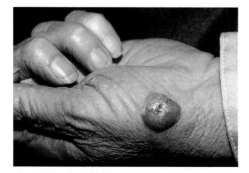

Figure 1.35 Keratoacanthoma (from James WD, Berger TG, Elston DM, et al. *Andrews' Diseases of the Skin*, 12th edn. Philadelphia, PA: Elsevier, 2016, with permission).

Palpate

- Firm consistency (except for the central core, which is hard)
- Fully mobile over deep tissues (as they occur in the skin).

Completion

Say that you would like to ask the patient:

- How the lump affects his life, e.g. cosmetic symptoms.

? QUESTIONS

(a) What is a keratoacanthoma?

A keratoacanthoma is a benign overgrowth of hair follicle cells that produces a central plug of keratin. It is rapidly growing, forming within 6 weeks and regressing after 6 weeks, leaving a depressed scar. Clinically and cytologically, keratoacanthomas may look similar to well-differentiated squamous cell carcinomas. Occasionally, rapidly growing malignant melanomas may appear similar.

(b) How would you treat this condition?

- Non-surgical: leave alone if asymptomatic (particularly in young patients)
- Surgical: complete excision of lesion with histology (particularly in elderly patients, where there should be a high index of suspicion for squamous cell carcinoma).

FURTHER READING

Schwartz RA: Keratoacanthoma: a clinico-pathologic enigma. *Dermatol Surg* 30(2 Pt 2): 326–333, 2004.

CASE 23 | NEUROFIBROMA **

INSTRUCTION

No specific instructions – neurofibromata can occur on any part of the body.

APPROACH

Examine as for any lump (Case 2).

VITAL POINTS

Inspect

- May be solitary or multiple (the latter being known as neurofibromatosis – see below)
- Pedunculated nodules
- If arising from deeper nerves, can result in severe deformity due to diffuse enlargement of the peripheral nerve with involvement of the skin (plexiform neurofibroma)
- Look for associated café-au-lait spots in neurofibromatosis (light brown macules which are greater than 1.5 cm in diameter – six or more suggest a diagnosis of neurofibromatosis) – if you see one or two, ask the patient to point out any others he may have anywhere else.

Palpate

- Soft ('fleshy') in consistency.

Completion

Say that you would like to ask the patient:
- How the lump(s) affects his life, e.g. cosmetic symptoms
- If multiple neurofibromata, say that you would like to test the cranial nerves (particularly the eighth) and measure the blood pressure (associated with phaeochromocytoma).

? QUESTIONS

(a) What is a neurofibroma?

A neurofibroma is a benign tumour derived from peripheral nerve elements.

(b) What is neurofibromatosis?

It is an autosomal-dominant condition characterised by the presence of multiple neurofibromas in combination with other dermatological manifestations (six café-au-lait spots). There are two types of neurofibromatosis:

- Type 1 (von Recklinghausen's disease) – defective gene on chromosome 17
- Type 2 (known as MISME syndrome – multiple inherited schwannomas, meningiomas and ependymomas – no relation to neurofibromatosis type 1) – defective gene on chromosome 22 with variable penetrance. Cutaneous signs are less often seen in this type.

(c) What complications can neurofibromata give rise to?

- Pressure effects, e.g. spinal cord and nerve root compression
- Deafness with involvement of the eighth cranial nerve
- Sarcomatous transformation: occurs only in von Recklinghausen's disease in 5–13% of cases
- Intra-abdominal effects: obstruction, chronic gastrointestinal bleeds
- Skeletal changes: can cause kyphoscoliosis, cystic changes and pseudoarthrosis.

(d) How would you treat a patient with a single neurofibroma?

- Non-surgical: leave alone if asymptomatic and if patient does not want intervention
- Surgical: indicated only if malignant growth suspected; post-excision, local regrowth is common as neurofibromata cannot be surgically detached from the underlying nerve.

? ADVANCED QUESTION

(a) What is the histological appearance of a neurofibroma?

- Consists of Schwann cells which appear as bundles of elongated wavy spindle cells
- Associated with collagen fibrils and myxoid material
- Often not encapsulated (unlike neurilemmomas – the other common benign tumour of peripheral nerves – which are always encapsulated).

Friedrich Daniel von Recklinghausen (1833–1910). Professor of Pathology, Strasbourg, Germany. Also described von Recklinghausen's disease of bone (osteitis fibrosa cystica, seen in hyperparathyroidism) and haemochromatosis.

FURTHER READING

Williams VC, Lucas J, Babcock MA, et al: Neurofibromatosis type 1 revisited. *Pediatrics* 123(1):124–133, 2009.

CASE 24   PAPILLOMA **

INSTRUCTION

'Examine this lesion on this gentleman's torso.' (Fig. 1.36)

APPROACH

Examine as for any lump (see Case 1).

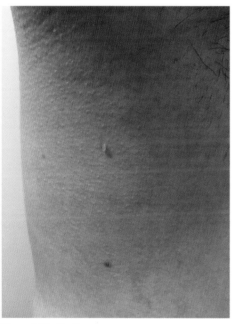

Figure 1.36 Papilloma.

VITAL POINTS

- Also known as skin tags or fibroepithelial polyps
- Can occur anywhere on the skin, particularly on the neck, trunk, face or anus
- Pedunculated swelling (may be sessile)
- Flesh-coloured
- Soft to palpation.

Completion

Say that you would like to ask the patient about:

- Similar lumps elsewhere
- How the lump affects his life, e.g. cosmetic symptoms
- Associated conditions – there is a link with pregnancy, diabetes and intestinal polyposis.

? QUESTIONS

(a) What is a papilloma?

A papilloma is an overgrowth of all layers of the skin with a central vascular core. They are increasingly common with age.

(b) How would you treat a papilloma?

The simplest surgical technique is to excise the papilloma with a sharp pair of scissors, controlling bleeding from the central vascular component with a single suture. Alternatively, diathermy can be used to control the bleeding at the same time as the excision.

CASE 25   PYOGENIC GRANULOMA **

INSTRUCTION

'Examine this patient's finger.' (Fig. 1.37)

(Pyogenic granulomata are found most commonly on the hands and face in children and young adults, and on the gums and lips in pregnant women.)

APPROACH

Examine as for any lump (see Case 1).

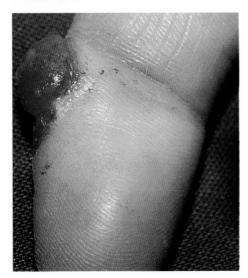

Figure 1.37 Pyogenic granuloma (from James WD, Berger TG, Elston DM, et al. *Andrews' Diseases of the Skin*, 12th edn. Philadelphia, PA: Elsevier, 2016, with permission).

VITAL POINTS

Inspect

- Bright-red or blood-encrusted hemispherical nodule
- May be sessile or pedunculated
- May be associated with a serous or purulent discharge
- Can be skin-coloured if long-standing (epithelialisation).

Palpate

- Soft in consistency ('fleshy')
- Slightly compressible (due to vascular origin)

- May bleed easily (so palpate only if the examiner asks you to).

Completion

Say that you would like to ask the patient:

- Whether he can remember a previous injury in this area (the association with trauma is now thought to be less strong, but show the examiner that you are aware that there is thought to be a link between the two)
- How long the lump took to appear (rapid growth in a few days)
- How the lump affects his life, e.g. pain, cosmetic symptoms, bleeding.

❓ QUESTIONS

(a) What is a pyogenic granuloma?

A pyogenic granuloma is a rapidly growing capillary haemangioma which usually measures less than 1 cm in diameter. It is neither pyogenic nor a granuloma.

(b) How would you treat this condition?

- Non-surgical: regression is uncommon, except those arising in pregnancy, and so they are best treated surgically, though occasionally cautery with silver nitrite can be attempted
- Surgical: curettage with diathermy of the base or complete excision biopsy (if recurrent, consider malignancy, e.g. amelanotic melanoma).

FURTHER READING

Giblin AV, Clover AJ, Athanassopoulos A, et al: Pyogenic granuloma – the quest for optimum treatment: audit of treatment of 408 cases. *J Plast Reconstr Aesthet Surg* 60(9):1030–1035, 2007.

CASE 26 | SEBORRHOEIC KERATOSIS ★★

INSTRUCTION

'Have a look at this lady's back.' (Fig. 1.38)

APPROACH

Examine as for any lump (see Case 1).

VITAL POINTS

- Commonly found on the trunk and face but can occur anywhere
- Single or multiple
- Round or oval in shape
- 'Stuck-on' appearance
- Varying degree of pigmentation – light brown to black (in Black people, seborrhoeic

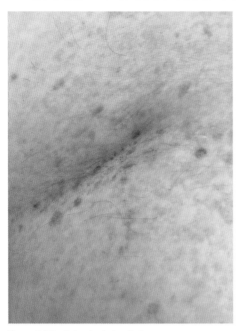

Figure 1.38   Seborrhoeic keratosis.

keratoses on the face are known as dermatosis papulosa nigra)
- Surface appears velvety or warty
- Can be picked off the skin, leaving behind pink skin and one or two surface capillaries that bleed slightly (*do not attempt to do this in the exam!*).

Completion

Say that you would like to ask the patient:
- About similar lesions elsewhere (note that sudden onset of multiple seborrhoeic

keratoses is associated with visceral malignancy – this is known as the Leser–Trélat sign)
- How the lesion affects her life, e.g. cosmetic symptoms, catches on clothes.

? QUESTIONS

(a) What is a seborrhoeic keratosis?

A seborrhoeic keratosis is a benign overgrowth of the basal cell layer of the epidermis. Histologically, it is characterised by:
- Hyperkeratosis (thickening of the keratin layer)
- Acanthosis (thickening of the prickle cell layer)
- Hyperplasia of variably pigmented basaloid cells.

This condition can be confused clinically with acanthosis nigricans.

(b) How would you treat this condition?

- Non-surgical: since it is a benign lesion, it can be managed conservatively
- Surgical: as the keratosis lies above the level of the surrounding normal epidermis, it can be treated by superficial shaving or cautery.

> *E. Leser (1828–1916).* German surgeon.
> *W. Trélat (1828–1890).* French surgeon.

CASE 27   SOLAR (ACTINIC) KERATOSIS   ★★

INSTRUCTION

'Have a look at this patient's arm.' (Fig. 1.39)

(Solar keratoses are commonly found on sun-exposed parts of the face and dorsum of the hands of elderly people.)

APPROACH

Examine as for any lump (see Case 1).

VITAL POINTS

- Usually multiple
- Yellow-grey or brown in colour
- Begin with thickening of skin which can become unsightly and catch on clothing
- Scaly surface
- Can occur as a 'solar horn' on the pinna of the ear – these are also benign.

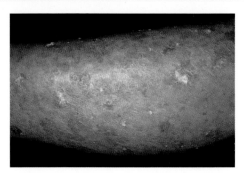

Figure 1.39 Solar keratosis (from Bolognia JL, Schaffer JV, Duncan KO et al. *Dermatology Essentials*. Philadelphia, PA: Saunders, 2014, with permission).

Completion

Say that you would like to ask the patient about:

- Similar lesions elsewhere
- How the lesion affects his life, e.g. cosmetic symptoms.

? QUESTIONS

(a) What are solar keratoses?

Solar keratoses are extremely common, and the populations most at risk are older individuals with chronic sun exposure and light skin. The condition is related to squamous cell carcinoma of the skin and they are considered precursors of an early form in cancer in situ (Bowen's disease). They are characterised by the following histological appearances:

- Basal layer atypia only (vs. atypia in all layers of the epidermis in squamous cell carcinoma – see Case 14).
- Hyperkeratosis (thickening of the keratin layer)
- Focal parakeratosis (thinning of the granular layer)
- Irregular acanthosis (thickening of the prickle cell layer)

(b) What is the risk of progression to invasive squamous cell carcinoma?

If untreated, 25% progress to invasive squamous cell carcinoma.

(c) How would you treat this condition?

- Non-surgical: cryotherapy, topical application of 5-fluorouracil (cytotoxic agent), retinoic acid (to reverse the damaging effects of sunlight)
- Surgical: shaving of affected skin.

FURTHER READING

Dinehart SM: The treatment of actinic keratoses. *J Am Acad Dermatol* 42(1/2):25–28, 2000.

CASE 28 | DIGITAL CLUBBING *

INSTRUCTION

'Examine this patient's hands.' (Fig. 1.40)

APPROACH

This case is a spot diagnosis. As for any case involving the hands, expose to above the elbows and ask the patient to place his hands palm upwards on a pillow (if available). If the instruction is to inspect the nails, then just look at them without going through this routine.

VITAL POINTS

Inspect

- Exaggerated anteroposterior and longitudinal curvature to fingernails (Fig. 1.41)

- Loss of angle between nail and nail bed (this can be more clearly seen by approximating the dorsal aspects of the terminal phalanges of the fingers of both hands after flexing at the interphalangeal joints, and is known as Lovibond's sign or the 'diamond sign')
- 'Drumstick' or 'parrot-beak' appearance of the nail (also known as '*doigts Hippocratique*').

Palpate

- Increased bogginess/fluctuation of nail bed – elicit this by supporting the patient's finger with your two thumbs and use your index fingers to demonstrate fluctuance.

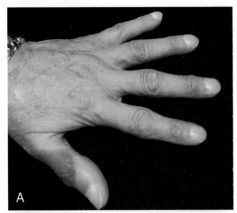

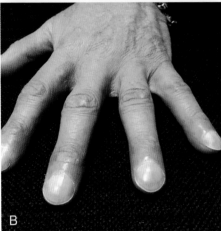

Figure 1.40   (A, B) Bilateral digital clubbing.

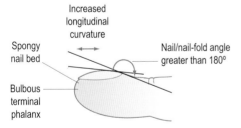

Figure 1.41   Digital clubbing.

Completion

Say that you would like to:

- Palpate the wrist joints for tenderness in hypertrophic pulmonary osteoarthropathy – rapid painful digital clubbing is nearly always due to bronchial carcinoma
- Examine the toes to look for digital clubbing

- Take a history and examine the patient to elicit the duration of digital clubbing, e.g. is it from birth, and to look for underlying causes (see below).

TOP TIP

☑ Note that the correct term is 'digital clubbing' – the word clubbing on its own may have several connotations, e.g. something done on a Friday night (or, more worryingly, to a seal)!

? QUESTION

(a) What are the causes of digital clubbing?

The most common cause of clubbing is *idiopathic*. The other causes can be divided into:

- Gastrointestinal:
  - Liver cirrhosis (especially primary biliary cirrhosis)
  - Inflammatory bowel disease (especially Crohn's disease)
  - Malabsorption (coeliac disease, tropical sprue)
  - Gastrointestinal lymphoma
- Respiratory:
  - Bronchial carcinoma (most commonly squamous cell)
  - Chronic suppurative lung disease (abscess, bronchiectasis, cystic fibrosis, empyema)
  - Fibrosing alveolitis
  - Mesothelioma
- Cardiac:
  - Cyanotic congenital heart diseases (e.g. Fallot's tetralogy, transposition of the great arteries)
  - Infective endocarditis
  - Atrial myxoma (rare)
- Rare causes:
  - Familial, e.g. 'hazel nails' (usually seen before puberty), pachydermoperiostitis (idiopathic familial hypertrophic pulmonary osteoarthropathy with post-pubertal digital clubbing, bone changes, increased sweating of palms and soles and marked thickening of the skin, forehead and scalp)
  - Graves' disease (pseudoclubbing – also known as thyroid acropathy)
  - When unilateral, as a consequence of an axillary artery aneurysm and brachial arteriovenous malformation.

? ADVANCED QUESTIONS

(a) What do you know about the pathophysiology of digital clubbing?

Several theories have been put forward to try to explain the mechanisms behind digital clubbing:

- The current favoured explanation is failure of platelet precursors to become fragmented into platelets within the pulmonary circulation – they are easily trapped in the peripheral vasculature and release platelet-derived growth factor and vascular endothelial growth factor, leading to promotion of vascularity and ultimately clubbing
- Vasodilatation of nail-bed vessels secondary to an unidentified mediator (candidates include ferritin, bradykinin, prostaglandin and 5-hydroxytryptamine), which is normally inactivated in the lung but may persist in those with digital clubbing where inactivation is defective
- Increased growth hormone
- Organs supplied by the vagus are affected by digital clubbing – vagotomy can reverse digital clubbing in bronchial carcinoma
- Tumour necrosis factor.

(b) How do you grade digital clubbing?

- Grade I: increased glossiness and cyanosis of the skin at the root of the nail associated with increased fluctuation at the base of the nail bed
- Grade II: loss of angle between nail and nail bed (see above)
- Grade III: drumstick appearance of nail (see above)
- Grade IV: bony changes involving the wrists and ankles, sometimes the elbow and knees (hypertrophic pulmonary osteoarthropathy).

Hippocrates (460–379 BC). Greek physician, born in Kos, commonly thought of as the founder of medicine.

E. L. A. Fallot (1850–1911). Professor of Hygiene and Legal Medicine, Marseilles, France. He described congenital cyanotic heart disease due to a combination of: (1) ventricular septal defect; (2) right ventricular outflow tract obstruction; (3) right ventricular hypertrophy; and (4) overriding aorta.

FURTHER READING

Myers KA, Farquhar DR: Does this patient have clubbing? *JAMA* 286(3):341–347, 2001.

Spicknall KE, Zirwas MJ, English JC 3rd: Clubbing: an update on diagnosis, differential diagnosis, pathophysiology, and clinical relevance. *J Am Acad Dermatol* 52(6):1020–1028, 2005.

Note

Hippocrates first described digital clubbing over 2400 years ago!

CASE 29 | BRANCHIAL CYST *

INSTRUCTION

'Examine this patient's neck.'

APPROACH

Approach as for neck examination (see Case 6).

VITAL POINTS

- Usually presents in a young adult in the third decade
- Equally common in males and females
- Found in anterior triangle of neck in front of the upper or middle third of the sternocleidomastoid

- Smooth, firm swelling that is ovoid in shape with its long axis running forwards and downwards
- Fluctuant on palpation
- Usually opaque on transillumination (due to desquamated epithelial cell contents)
- May be hard and fixed to surrounding structures in the presence of established or recurrent infection
- Look carefully for the opening of a fistula in this area (a branchial fistula runs between the tonsillar fossa and the anterior border of the sternocleidomastoid).

TOP TIP

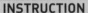

☑ There are three surgical definitions that you should be able to roll off your tongue:

- Cyst: an abnormal sac with an epithelial lining, containing gas, fluid or semisolid material

- Sinus: a blind-ending track, typically lined by epithelial or granulation tissue, which opens on to an epithelial surface

- Fistula: an abnormal communication between two epithelial surfaces (or endothelial surfaces, e.g. arteriovenous fistula).

Completion

Say that you would like to ask the patient about:

- Associated symptoms, e.g. pain, symptoms of infection

- The effect of the lump on his life.

? QUESTIONS

(a) What is a branchial cyst?

A branchial cyst is thought to develop because of a failure of fusion of the embryonic second and third branchial arches. An alternative, and currently popular, hypothesis is that it is an acquired condition due to cystic degeneration in cervical lymphatic tissue. The cysts are lined by squamous epithelium.

(b) How would you diagnose a branchial cyst?

- Clinical examination
- Imaging – especially ultrasound
- Fine-needle aspiration – opalescent fluid containing cholesterol crystals or pus

(c) How would you treat a branchial cyst?

- The cyst may be surgically excised – whole if possible, although this may be difficult if there has been previous infection

- Bonney's blue dye can be injected into the fistula/sinus, allowing accurate surgical excision and therefore reducing recurrence rates

- Complicating infections may be treated with antibiotics

- Complications include recurrence of the cyst and development of a chronic, discharging sinus.

FURTHER READING

Tracy TF Jr, Muratore CS: Management of common head and neck masses. *Semin Pediatr Surg* 16(1):3–13, 2007.

www.pedisurg.com/PtEduc/Branchial_Cleft_Cyst.htm – information for parents on their children's neck lumps.

CASE 30 | DERMOID CYST *

INSTRUCTION

No specific instruction – can occur in various sites. (Fig. 1.42)

APPROACH

Examine as for any lump (see Case 1).

VITAL POINTS

Inspect

- Smooth spherical swelling
- Soft and may fluctuate
- Non-tender
- Look for associated scar from previous injury (especially in adults).

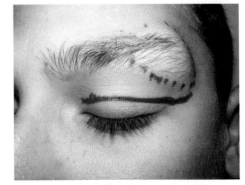

Figure 1.42 Dermoid cyst. With permission from Excision of Orbital Dermoid Cysts via Upper Eyelid Incision: A Review of 24 Cases. Journal of Current Surgery Volume 4, Number 4, December 2014, pages 110–112

TOP TIP

Dermoid cysts lie deep to the skin in the subcutaneous tissues. They differ from lipomas as they are not within the fat layers, and from sebaceous cysts as they are not attached to skin.

Completion

Say that you would like to ask the patient:

- How the cyst affects his life, e.g. cosmetic symptoms
- Whether he has suffered an injury previously (if you suspect that it is an acquired cyst).

? QUESTIONS

(a) What is a dermoid cyst?

- A dermoid cyst is a skin-lined cyst deep to the skin. They may be congenital or acquired
- Congenital – due to developmental inclusion of epidermis along lines of fusion of skin dermatomes and are therefore found commonly at:
  - The medial and lateral ends of the eyebrows (internal and external angular dermoid cysts)
  - The midline of the nose (nasal dermoid cysts)
  - The midline of the neck and trunk

Suspect if you see a *child* or *young adult* in the exam.

- Acquired – due to forced implantation of skin into subcutaneous tissues following an injury. Normally found in areas of the body prone to injury such as fingers. Suspect if you see an *adult* in exam.

(b) How would you treat this condition?

- Congenital – surgical treatment involves complete excision, but the full extent of the cyst should be established with suitable radiographic views (X-ray or CT scan)
- Acquired – surgical treatment involves complete excision of the cyst.

FURTHER READING

Turkyilmaz Z, Karabulut R, Bayazit YA, et al: Congenital neck masses in children and their embryologic and clinical features. *B-ENT* 4(1):7–18, 2008.

CASE 31 THYROGLOSSAL CYST *

INSTRUCTION

'Examine this lady's neck.' (Fig. 1.43)

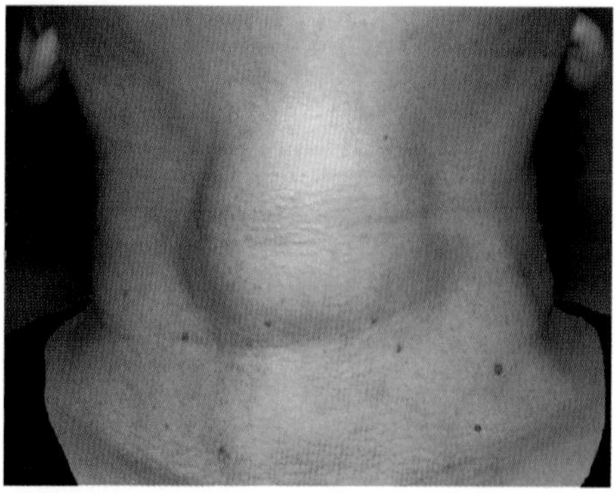

Figure 1.43 Thyroglossal cyst (from Young C, Gladman M. *Examination Surgery*. Chatswood, NSW, Australia: Churchill Livingstone, 2013, with permission).

APPROACH

Approach as you would a neck examination (see Case 6).

Inspect (from the front)

- Site of the lump – note that 75% are in the midline, 25% are either a little to the right or the left
- Smooth and rounded
- Other features on inspection of the lump, e.g. size, skin changes (you may see the opening of a thyroglossal sinus with seropurulent discharge, which follows rupture or incision of a thyroglossal cyst), scars (see Case 8).

Protrusion of the tongue

- Ask the patient to open her mouth and stick her tongue out as far as possible

- If the lump moves on protrusion of the tongue, it is likely to be a thyroglossal cyst (this is because the cyst is usually related to the base of the tongue by a patent or fibrous track which runs through the central portion of the hyoid bone) – a lump from the thyroid gland does not move on protrusion of the tongue.

Swallowing

- Place a glass of water in the patient's hands; ask her to take a sip of water, hold it in her mouth and swallow when you ask her to
- As she swallows, inspect the lump – if it moves on swallowing, it is likely to originate from the thyroid gland
- Note that thyroglossal cysts also move on swallowing, so ask the patient to stick her tongue out before proceeding with the thyroid gland examination (see Case 8).

Palpate (from the back)

Repeat the two above tests, this time palpating the cyst gently from behind the patient to ensure that the diagnosis is correct.

Finish your examination here

Completion

Say that you would like to:

- Take a history from the patient, particularly concentrating on how the lump affects her life, e.g. cosmetic symptoms.

? QUESTIONS

(a) What is your differential diagnosis?

The differential diagnosis includes other midline neck lumps:

- Thyroid nodules and masses (including pyramidal lobe)
- Enlarged lymph nodes
- Other cysts – dermoid and epidermoid
- Subhyoid bursae.

(b) What do you know about the epidemiology of thyroglossal cysts?

- Rare
- Worldwide distribution
- Equally common in males and females
- Rarely present at birth; 40% present in the first decade and can even present late in the ninth decade.

(c) How do you treat a thyroglossal cyst?

- Treatment is essentially surgical
- Inject patent track with dye at the start of the operation
- Operation of choice is Sistrunk's operation, which involves *en bloc* excision of the cyst and the duct remnants from the foramen caecum to the pyramidal lobe, including the central portion of the hyoid bone.

? ADVANCED QUESTIONS

(a) What is the embryological origin of a thyroglossal cyst?

- Results from persistence of part of the thyroglossal tract, which marks the developmental descent of the thyroid gland
- At the 4th week of development, the thyroid appears as a midline diverticulum and descends ventrally to the pharynx between the developing second arch as a duct (which normally involutes)
- The origin of the tract can persist as a midline dimple – the foramen caecum – at the junction of the vallate and filiform papillae of the tongue.

(b) What are the pathological features of thyroglossal cysts?

- Lined by stratified squamous or ciliated pseudostratified columnar epithelium
- May also contain thyroid or lymphoid tissue, which can undergo malignant change
- If malignancy occurs, usually of thyroid papillary type.

FURTHER READING

Foley DS, Fallat ME: Thyroglossal duct and other congenital midline cervical anomalies. *Semin Pediatr Surg* 15(2):70–75, 2006.

CASE 32 RADIOTHERAPY MARKS *

INSTRUCTION

'Have a look at this lady's lower back.' (Fig. 1.44)

You may also encounter such marks on patients who have undergone treatment for breast cancer. If this is the case, proceed as for breast examination (see Case 63).

APPROACH

As this is a spot diagnosis, the patient should be adequately exposed to the waist – if the patient is covered up, explain what you are going to do and obtain sufficient exposure.

VITAL POINTS

Inspect

• For evidence of abdominal scars, including port sites if a midline laparotomy is not evident and stoma closure.

Current radiotherapy

• India-ink marks
• Erythema
• Desquamation
• Skin markings to delineate area of treatment.

Previous radiotherapy

• Telangiectasia.

Completion

Say that you would like to:
• Take a history to determine the duration and side-effects of radiotherapy on this lady.

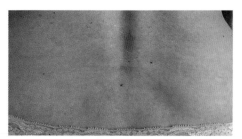

Figure 1.44   Radiotherapy marks.

? ADVANCED QUESTIONS

(a) How does radiotherapy work?

High-energy X-rays interact with tissues to release electrons of high kinetic energy, which cause secondary damage to adjacent DNA via an oxygen-dependent mechanism. The damage is either reparable or irreparable, the latter manifesting itself as chromosomal abnormalities preventing mitosis. Normal tissues have a greater ability to repopulate in response to radiation-induced cell depletion than tumours.

(b) Which normal tissues are particularly affected by radiotherapy?

Tissues with rapid turnover:
• Epidermal layers of the skin
• Small intestine
• Bone marrow stem cells

Tissues with a limited ability to repopulate:
• Spinal cord
• Gonads – oocytes and spermatocytes.

(c) What are the side-effects of radiotherapy?

Early:
• General: malaise, fatigue, loss of appetite, nausea and vomiting
• Skin: as above
• Bone marrow suppression: particularly if irradiation to the pelvis and long bones
• Gastrointestinal: diarrhoea

Late:
• Skin: as above
• Lungs: pneumonitis, pulmonary fibrosis
• Heart: ischaemic heart disease
• Arteries: radiation arteritis, especially the carotids post head and neck radiotherapy; this leads to subsequent stenosis and distal ischaemia
• Spinal cord: myelopathy
• Visceral damage: constricted fibrotic bladder, bowel obstruction secondary to strictures and adhesions, renal impairment due to depletion of renal tubular cells
• Gonadal damage: infertility
• Thyroid: hypothyroidism due to depletion of thyroid follicular cells
• Eyes: cataracts
• Secondary malignancies: increased risk of solid tumours and also of leukaemias (the

risk of the latter being 1–2% at 15 years, with an even higher risk if chemotherapy with alkylating agents is used in conjunction).

(d) How are the side-effects of radiotherapy minimised?

- Lead shields to protect the eyes and gonads
- Dose fractionation – to allow recovery of normal host tissues

- Prior chemotherapy – to increase sensitivity of tumour to radiotherapy
- Regional hypothermia – useful in superficial tumours and bulky non-vascular tumours
- Radiolabelled antibodies – delivering high levels of radiation locally to the tumour.

CASE 33   DERMATOFIBROMA   *

INSTRUCTION

'Examine this lady's legs.' (Fig. 1.45)

APPROACH

Examine as for any lump (see Case 1).

VITAL POINTS

Inspect

- Can occur anywhere, but are more common on the lower limbs of young to middle-aged women

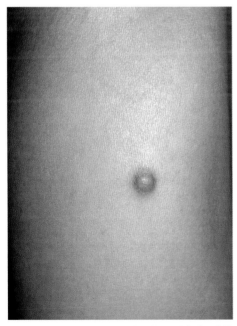

Figure 1.45 Dermatofibroma (from Huang P-Y, Chu C-Y, Hsiao C-H Multiple eruptive dermatofibromas in a patient with dermatomyositis taking prednisolone and methotrexate. *J Am Acad Dermatol* 57:S81–S84, 2007, with permission).

- Small pink or brown pigmented hemispherical nodules
- Smooth in appearance.

Palpate

- Firm woody feel (characteristic)
- They are part of the skin and are therefore fully mobile over deep tissues.

Completion

Say that you would like to ask the patient:

- What symptoms she is experiencing from the lump, e.g. cosmetic.

? QUESTIONS

(a) What is a dermatofibroma?

A dermatofibroma (also known as a fibrous histiocytoma) is a benign neoplasm of dermal fibroblasts. Previous theories that dermatofibromas are a reaction to a previous injury or insect bite have now fallen out of favour. Recent thinking favours the concept that it is a result of an abortive immunoreactive process, featuring dermal dendritic cells as initiators of the disease.

(b) What is the differential diagnosis?

It is important to exclude malignant tumours such as:

- Malignant melanoma (see Case 15)
- Basal cell carcinoma (see Case 16).

(c) How would you treat this condition?

- Non-surgical: leave alone if asymptomatic and if patient does not want intervention
- Surgical: simple excision followed by histology.

FURTHER READING

Nestle FO, Nickoloff BJ, Burg G:
Dermatofibroma: an abortive immunoreactive process mediated by dermal dendritic cells? *Dermatology* 190(4):265–268, 1995.

www.skinsite.com/info_dermatofibromas.htm – information for patients.

CASE 34 | HIDRADENITIS SUPPURATIVA *

INSTRUCTION

'Examine this patient's groin.' (Fig. 1.46)

APPROACH

Examine as for any lump/ulcer (see Case 1).

VITAL POINTS

- The skin is thickened and may be ulcerated; 'watering-can' sinuses may be seen
- Look for signs of any active current infection (tenderness/increased temperature/ erythema).

COMPLETION

Say that you would like to ask the patient about:

- Symptoms arising from this condition and how they affect the patient

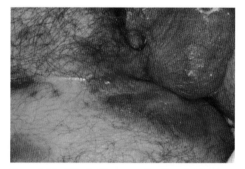

Figure 1.46 Hidradenitis suppurativa (from Gawkrodger D, Ardern Jones M *Dermatology*, 5th edn. Edinburgh: Churchill Livingstone, 2012, with permission).

- Any other affected areas, e.g. axilla
- Predisposing factors, e.g. diabetes mellitus.

? QUESTIONS

(a) What is hidradenitis suppurativa?

Hidradenitis suppurativa, also known as acne inversa, is now considered a disease of follicular occlusion rather than an inflammatory or infectious process of the apocrine glands. Abscesses form recurrently and this causes the characteristic permanent disfiguring of the skin. It usually affects young women, with a prevalence of 0.3–0.4% in industrialised countries.

(b) How would you treat hidradenitis suppurativa?

Hidradenitis can be extremely uncomfortable, cosmetically unpleasant and distressing for the patient; they are also problematic to treat satisfactorily.

- Medical treatments include long-term antibiotics, oral/lesion-injected corticosteroids, and tumour necrosis factor-alpha inhibitors such as infliximab (Remicade) and adalimumab (Humira)
- Surgical procedures include incision and drainage under antibiotic cover of localised abscesses, de-roofing of tunnels and radical excision with full-thickness skin grafting usually harvested from the groins or abdomen of larger lesions.

FURTHER READING

Alikhan A, Lynch PJ, Eisen DB: Hidradenitis suppurativa: a comprehensive review. *J Am Acad Dermatol* 60(4):539–561, 2009.

CASE 35 | KAPOSI'S SARCOMA *

INSTRUCTION

'Have a look at this skin lesion.'

APPROACH

Examine as for any lump (see Case 1).

VITAL POINTS

Inspect

- Purple papules or plaques
- Solitary or multiple
- Can be found anywhere on skin or on mucosa of any organ, but usually found on the limbs, mouth, tip of the nose or palate.

Completion

Say that you would like to:

- Take a history, e.g. ethnic origin, previous transplant
- Ask the patient about underlying immunocompromise.

? QUESTIONS

(a) What do you know about Kaposi's sarcoma?

- Derived from capillary endothelial cells or from fibrous tissue
- Linked to human herpesvirus 8 – also known as Kaposi's sarcoma herpesvirus.

(b) How would you treat this condition?

- Leave alone if asymptomatic and if patient does not want intervention
- Intervene only when extensive or for cosmetic reasons:
  - Local radiotherapy
  - Chemotherapy – interferon-α, doxorubicin, intralesional vinblastine

Mention that Kaposi's is usually present in advanced HIV infection and so formal diagnosis should be sought and adequate antiretroviral therapy as indicated.

? ADVANCED QUESTION

(a) What varieties do you know of Kaposi's sarcoma?

- Classic Kaposi's sarcoma:
  - Initially described in Ashkenazi Jews
  - Found on the legs of elderly men
  - Confined to skin
  - Not fatal
- AIDS-associated Kaposi's sarcoma
  - Found in one-third of patients with AIDS (diagnostic of AIDS)
  - More common in homosexual patients
  - One-third develop a second malignancy, e.g. leukaemia, lymphoma
- Endemic (central African) variety
  - Aggressive invasive tumour
  - Ultimately fatal
  - Good response to chemotherapy
- Transplantation-associated Kaposi's sarcoma
  - Following high-dose immunosuppressive therapy
  - Often regress when treatment stopped.

Moricz Kaposi (1837–1902). Hungarian dermatologist. Also described the rash in systemic lupus erythematosus as a 'butterfly rash' and xeroderma pigmentosum (Kaposi's disease).

FURTHER READING

Schwartz RA, Micali G, Nasca MR, et al: Kaposi sarcoma: a continuing conundrum. *J Am Acad Dermatol* 59(2):179–206, 2008.

CASE 36 | PHARYNGEAL POUCH *

INSTRUCTION

'Examine this gentleman's neck.'

APPROACH

Approach as for neck examination (see Case 6).

VITAL POINTS

- Most commonly seen in the elderly
- May be very little to find except for a cystic swelling low down in the anterior triangle of the neck (Fig. 1.47)
- Deep palpation produces a squelching sound due to free fluid in the pouch
- Halitosis is a frequent feature, as food is regurgitated into the neck.

Completion

Say that you would like to ask the patient about:

- Associated symptoms, e.g. regurgitation leading to coughing, dysphagia
- Complications (see below)
- The effect of the lump on his life.

Ask to listen to the patient's chest.

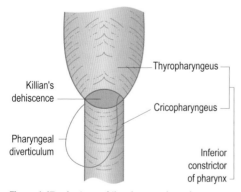

Figure 1.47 Anatomy of the pharyngeal pouch.

Killian's dehiscence

Thyropharyngeus

Cricopharyngeus

Pharyngeal diverticulum

Inferior constrictor of pharynx

? QUESTIONS

(a) What is a pharyngeal pouch?

A pharyngeal pouch is formed by the herniation of pharyngeal mucosa (known as a pulsion diverticulum) through its muscular coat at its weakest point (Killian's dehiscence) between the thyropharyngeal and cricopharyngeal muscles that make up the inferior constrictor. Patients are usually symptom-free for a long period of time followed by dysphagia and hoarseness, associated with regurgitation of undigested foods and associated weight loss.

(b) What are the complications of a pharyngeal pouch?

- Chest infection – due to pulmonary aspiration
- Diverticular neoplasia – in less than 1% of cases.

(c) What investigations would you perform to help you in your diagnosis?

- Barium swallow – usually diagnostic
- Rigid endoscopy – if neoplasia suspected.

(d) How would you treat a pharyngeal pouch?

- Non-surgical: leave alone if small and asymptomatic
- Surgical:
  - Minimally invasive surgery: Dohlman's procedure – endoscopic diathermy resection of the posterior pharyngeal wall or endoscopic stapling – less risk of fistula formation and consequent mediastinitis
  - Surgical excision: simple inversion and oversewing (diverticulopexy) – as pouch is left in situ, risk of missing a possible diverticular carcinoma or diverticulectomy.

FURTHER READING

Aly A, Devitt PG, Jamieson GG: Evolution of surgical treatment for pharyngeal pouch. *Br J Surg* 91(6):657–664, 2004.

CASE 37 | CYSTIC HYGROMA *

INSTRUCTION

'Examine this patient's neck.'

APPROACH

Approach as for neck examination (see Case 6) – note these patients are more frequently found in paediatric cases.

VITAL POINTS

- 50–65% are present at birth, but occasionally may present in late childhood or adulthood
- Located in the posterior triangle of the neck
- Lobulated cystic swelling
- Soft and fluctuant
- Compressible (usually into another part of the cyst)
- 'Brilliantly transilluminable'.

Completion

Say that you would like to:

- Look in the oropharynx (a large cyst may extend deeply beneath the sternocleidomastoid muscle into the retropharyngeal space)
- Ask the patient how the lump affects his life.

? QUESTIONS

(a) What is a cystic hygroma?

A cystic hygroma is a congenital cystic lymphatic malformation found in the posterior triangle of the neck. It is probably a developmental anomaly formed during the coalescence of primitive lymph elements. It consists of thin-walled, single or multiple interconnecting or separate cysts which insinuate themselves widely into the tissues at the root of the neck.

(b) What are the complications of a cystic hygroma?

Complications include cosmetic symptoms but important problems are encountered in the perinatal period:

- Before delivery:
  - May obstruct delivery
- After delivery:
  - Respiratory obstruction
  - Obstruction of swallowing.

(c) What investigations would you perform to help you in your diagnosis?

Investigations are mainly radiological:

- Chest X-ray – to map the caudal extent of the cystic hygroma
- CT/MRI scanning – especially if complex.

(d) How would you treat a cystic hygroma?

- Non-surgical:
  - Aspiration ± injection of sclerosant
- Surgical:
  - Excision – may be partial (to relieve symptoms) or complete (as a one-stage procedure).

FURTHER READING

Bloom DC, Perkins JA, Manning SC: Management of lymphatic malformations. *Curr Opin Otolaryngol Head Neck Surg* 12(6):500–504, 2004.

CASE 38 | CHEMODECTOMA *

INSTRUCTION

'Examine this patient's neck.'

APPROACH

Approach as for neck examination (see Case 6).

VITAL POINTS

- Located in the anterior triangle of the neck, at the angle of the jaw
- Be gentle when examining in this area, as pressure on the carotid bifurcation can induce a vasovagal attack
- Usually the lump is solid and firm

- Pulsatile but not expansile in nature – be extra gentle as soon as you realise it is pulsatile! May be due to:
  - Transmitted pulsation from the adjacent carotid arteries
  - An overlying palpable external carotid artery
  - True expansile pulsation from a soft or very vascular tumour
- Due to intimate relationship with the carotid arteries, the lump can be moved from side to side but not up and down
- May be bilateral.

? QUESTIONS

(a) What is a chemodectoma?

A chemodectoma is a tumour of the paraganglion cells of the carotid body located at the bifurcation of the common carotid artery. They are usually benign (but locally invasive), but occasionally, they are malignant with potential to metastasise to local lymph nodes.

(b) What investigations would you perform to help you in your diagnosis?

- Duplex ultrasound
- Angiography – shows a hypervascular mass displacing the bifurcation of the carotid arteries
- CT/MRI – to delineate the extent of the tumour.

(c) How would you treat a chemodectoma?

- Surgical:
  - Surgical excision (with preoperative embolisation if the tumour is large)
  - Ultrasonic surgical dissection may also be used
- Radiotherapy:
  - For patients unfit for surgery
  - For large tumours.

FURTHER READING

Sajid MS, Hamilton G, Baker DM; Joint Vascular Research Group: A multicenter review of carotid body tumour management. *Eur J Vasc Endovasc Surg* 34(2):127–130, 2007.

CASE 39   FURUNCLES   *

INSTRUCTION

'Examine this patient's neck.' (Fig. 1.48)

APPROACH

Examine as for any lump (see Case 1). These are common in A&E but are rare in examinations.

VITAL POINTS

- Can affect any hair-bearing area of the skin, particularly the face, neck, buttocks, groins and axillae
- Small pus-containing swelling (when the contents become solid, it is known as a boil)
- Tender on palpation
- May be multiple.

Completion

Say that you would like to ask the patient about:

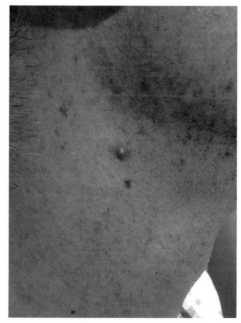

Figure 1.48 Furuncle.

- Other affected areas
- Predisposing factors such as diabetes mellitus, steroid treatment and other immunodeficiencies.

Ask to test the urine or blood for sugar.

? QUESTIONS

(a) What is a furuncle?

A furuncle results from infection of hair follicles with *Staphylococcus aureus*.

(b) How would you treat this condition?

- Non-surgical: risk-factor modification, e.g. establishment of good diabetic control and, for recurrent infections, eradication of nasal carriage of *Staphylococcus aureus* with

antiseptics and/or antibiotics, e.g. chlorhexidine and mupirocin
- Surgical: incision and drainage for large and painful boils.

(c) What is a carbuncle?

A carbuncle is an extensive infection of hair follicles by the same organism, with involvement of adjacent follicles and development of draining sinuses. It is associated with diabetes and is treated with a combination of systemic antibiotics and surgical incision.

FURTHER READING

Bernard P: Management of common bacterial infections of the skin. *Curr Opin Infect Dis* 21(2):122–128, 2008.

CASE 40 | PYODERMA GANGRENOSUM *

INSTRUCTION

No specific instruction – lesion can be on any part of the body but usually found on the trunk, lower limbs or face. It can commonly be associated with abdominal stomas (Fig. 1.49).

APPROACH

Examine as for ulcers (see Case 2).

VITAL POINTS

Inspect

- Ulcer with necrotic base
- Irregular bluish-red overhanging edges

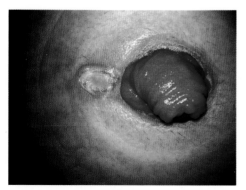

Figure 1.49 Pyoderma gangrenosum.

- Associated with surrounding erythematous plaques with pustules.

Completion

Say that you would like to:

- Take a history and examine the patient for evidence of:
  - Ulcerative colitis (the presence of pyoderma gangrenosum is related to disease activity)
  - Crohn's disease
  - Rheumatoid arthritis.

? QUESTIONS

This is likely to continue on to questions concerning inflammatory bowel disease, particularly ulcerative colitis (Case 50).

? ADVANCED QUESTIONS

(a) What other associations of pyoderma gangrenosum do you know of?

- Idiopathic (50%)
- Myeloproliferative disorders, e.g. polycythaemia rubra vera, myeloma
- Autoimmune hepatitis
- More common in males than females.

(b) What is your differential diagnosis?

- Autoimmune:
  - Rheumatoid vasculitis
- Infectious:
  - Tertiary syphilis
  - Amoebiasis
- Iatrogenic:
  - Warfarin necrosis
- Unknown:
  - Behçet's disease.

(c) How would you treat this condition?

- Medical: treat underlying condition, saline cleansing, high-dose oral or intralesional steroids ± cyclosporin
- Surgical: serial allograft followed by autologous skin graft or muscle flap coverage when necessary.

Hulusi Behçet (1889–1948). Professor to the Clinic of Dermatology and Syphilis, Turkey. Behçet's disease is a multi-organ disease of unknown (? viral) aetiology causing arthritis, pyoderma, ulcers in the mouth, scrotum and labia, eye problems such as hypopyon (pus in the anterior chamber of the eye) and iritis, and with central nervous system involvement, e.g. meningoencephalitis. Most common geographically along the Silk Road and is linked with HLA-B51.

FURTHER READING

Callen JP, Jackson JM: Pyoderma gangrenosum: an update. *Rheum Dis Clin North Am* 33(4):787–802, vi, 2007.

CASE 41 | VASCULAR MALFORMATIONS *

INSTRUCTION

'Examine this patient's chest.' (Fig. 1.50)

Note: lesions can be on any part of the body but are usually found on the trunk, lower limbs or face.

GENERAL

These are unlikely cases, but a few points are described below in case they appear in your examinations. Some of these conditions may occur in paediatric short cases or OSCEs.

TYPES

- Capillary – account for two-thirds of all cases and include naevi, port-wine stains, telangiectasia and spider naevi
- Predominantly venous – venous angioma
- Predominantly lymphatic – lymphangioma circumscriptum (see Case 132).

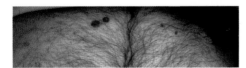

Figure 1.50 Vascular malformations – Campbell de Morgan spot.

COMMON FEATURES

- Develop as an abnormal proliferation of the embryonic vascular network
- Hamartomas
- May ulcerate
- May induce hyperkeratosis in the overlying stratum corneum layer of the skin.

SPECIFIC LESIONS

Campbell de Morgan spots

- Small red capillary naevus
- Develop on the trunk in middle age
- No clinical significance.

Spider naevus (also known as naevus araneus)

- Form of telangiectasis
- Central arteriole with leg-like branches which blanch on central pressure
- Found over upper torso, head and neck in adults (thought to be within the drainage area of the superior vena cava)
- Associated with chronic liver disease and pregnancy
- More than five is considered as pathological in chronic liver disease.

Telangiectasis

- Dilatation of normal capillaries
- Can be secondary to skin irradiation (see Case 32)
- Can be part of hereditary haemorrhagic telangiectasia (Osler–Rendu–Weber syndrome) – rare autosomal-dominant disease (with incomplete penetrance) in which overt and occult haemorrhage can occur presenting as haematuria, haematemesis, melaena, epistaxis or iron-deficiency anaemia.

Port-wine stain (also known as naevus vinosus)

- Purple-blue naevus found on face, lips and mucous membranes of the mouth
- Present from birth and does not change in size thereafter
- Found on limbs in association with Klippel–Trenaunay syndrome (see Case 111)
- Sturge–Weber syndrome is the association of a facial port-wine stain with a corresponding haemangioma in the brain, leading to contralateral focal fits.

Strawberry patch (cavernous haemangioma)

- Bright-red raised strawberry-like lesion
- Present from birth, but 60% undergo spontaneous resolution by the age of 3 years
- Only treated if obscuring a visual field or spontaneous resolution not occurring.

Campbell de Morgan (1811–1876). Full surgeon to the Middlesex Hospital in London, who believed the spots were a sign of cancer.

Sir William Osler (1849–1919). Canadian-born Professor of Medicine at McGill, Pennsylvania, Johns Hopkins and Oxford. Also described Osler's nodes (cutaneous nodules in infective endocarditis) and Osler–Vaquez disease (polycythaemia rubra vera).

Henry Jules Louis Marie Rendu (1844–1902). Parisian physician at the Necker Hospital.

William Allen Sturge (1850–1919). English physician and pathologist at the Royal Free Hospital.

Frederick Parkes Weber (1863–1962). English physician.

CASE 42 | INGUINAL HERNIA ***

INSTRUCTION

'Examine this gentleman's right groin.' (Fig. 2.1)

APPROACH

Expose the patient from umbilicus to knees.

VITAL POINTS

Differential diagnosis of a lump in the groin

Use the acronym **L-SHAPE:**

- **L**ymph node/**L**ipoma of the cord
- **S**aphenovarix/**S**kin lesions (sebaceous cyst/lipoma, etc.)
- **H**ernia – inguinal/femoral
- **A**neurysmal dilatation of the femoral artery
- **P**soas abscess/bursa
- **E**ctopic/undescended testis.

TOP TIP

✓ Should the hernia be examined with the patient lying down or standing up? The answer is that it doesn't matter. It is generally considered to be easier to define the anatomy with the patient supine, and if the hernia can be detected with the patient on the couch, then examine the patient there. If no lump can be felt, or if no couch is available, then stand the patient up first.   ✓

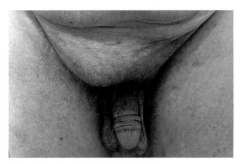

Figure 2.1   Inguinal hernia.

TOP TIP

✓ Don't forget that the same opening instruction may apply to the examination of the scrotum, and it may be a scrotal lump rather than a hernia. If you cannot see a visible swelling, proceed by asking the patient where the lump is.   ✓

TOP TIP

✓ An inguinal hernia arises above and medial to the pubic tubercle. By contrast, a femoral hernia arises below and lateral to it (Fig. 2.2).   ✓

TOP TIP

✓ Be completely conversant with the anatomy of the inguinal region and the location of surface anatomy (Figs 2.2 and 2.3).

- Midinguinal point – point halfway along a line joining the anterior superior iliac spine and the midline – location of femoral artery

- Midpoint of the inguinal ligament – halfway along the inguinal ligament (i.e. between the pubic tubercle and anterior superior iliac spine) – deep inguinal ring.

✓ Accordingly, the femoral pulse is located medial to the deep inguinal ring.   ✓

THE OBJECTIVES OF THE EXAMINATION ARE TO:

1. Confirm that the lump is a hernia
2. Differentiate an inguinal from a femoral hernia
3. If it is an inguinal hernia, establish whether it is direct or indirect.

Inspect

- Look at the groin for old surgical scars (is the hernia recurrent?) – this requires *very careful* inspection to identify old, small scars that are frequently hidden in groin creases and/or by hair
- If the hernia is obvious, then begin to examine it

- If it cannot be seen then ask the patient to cough and observe for the appearance of a lump
- If it is *still* not obvious, ask: 'Have you noticed a lump in your groin?' and get the patient to demonstrate it
- Fulfil objective (1) above and confirm that the lump is a hernia by:
  - Asking the patient to cough, while observing for an expansile cough impulse
  - Getting the patient to reduce the hernia if possible. If the patient cannot achieve this, attempt to reduce the lump yourself by applying *gentle pressure* in the direction of the inguinal canal. If you cannot reduce the lump it is either (1) *not* a hernia or (2) incarcerated (irreducible).

Palpate

- Begin by defining the anatomy (Figs 2.2 and 2.3)
- Palpate the pubic tubercle and the anterior superior iliac spine. The former can reliably be located by palpating in the midline downwards from the umbilicus until the symphysis pubis is reached (Fig. 2.4). Then move laterally to identify the tubercle
- Place one finger on each to demonstrate that the inguinal ligament runs between the two (Fig. 2.5)
- Ask the patient to cough for the second time and demonstrate that the hernia arises above this line, medial to the pubic tubercle (Fig. 2.2). This fulfils objective (2) (see above) and confirms that the hernia is inguinal and not femoral

- If it wasn't obvious on inspection alone, demonstrate that the lump has an expansile cough impulse: place one hand over the lump and ask the patient to cough
- It is only possible to fulfil objective (3) above if the hernia is reducible. With the hernia fully reduced, try to control the hernia at the deep inguinal ring:
  - Redefine the inguinal ligament again and place one finger 1 cm craniad to the midpoint of the inguinal ligament (halfway along the inguinal ligament) (Fig. 2.6).
  - Ask the patient to cough for the third and final time. If the hernia is controlled by your finger at the deep inguinal ring it is an *indirect* inguinal hernia. If the hernia is not controlled and reappears, then it is a *direct* inguinal hernia.

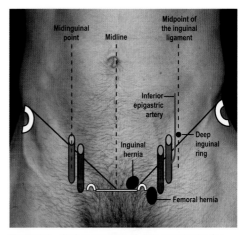

Figure 2.2 Surface anatomy of groin examination for herniae.

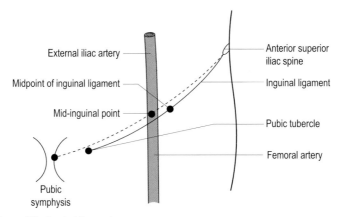

Figure 2.3 Anatomy of the inguinal ligament.

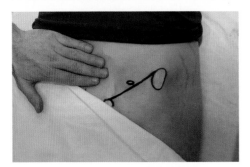

Figure 2.4 Palpation of the symphysis pubis.

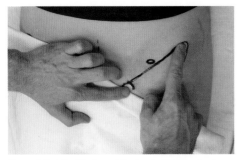

Figure 2.5 Identification of the inguinal ligament using bony landmarks.

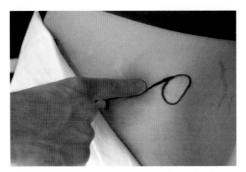

Figure 2.6 Attempting to control the reduced hernia at the deep ring.

- Remember that the accuracy of clinical examination in distinguishing a direct from an indirect hernia may be low (56% of direct herniae were wrongly classified by consultant surgeons as indirect on clinical examination in one such study; see Further Reading)
- Other aspects of the lump (as for any lump) may be defined at this stage, e.g. skin changes

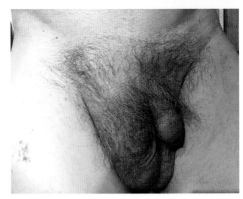

Figure 2.7 Inguinoscrotal hernia.

- Decide whether the lump is confined to the inguinal region or descends into the scrotum as an inguinoscrotal hernia (Fig. 2.7).

Completion

Complete your examination by asking to examine the scrotum for incidental scrotal lumps and to examine the contralateral groin for herniae.

? QUESTIONS

(a) What is the difference between a direct and an indirect inguinal hernia?

Indirect inguinal herniae:

- Are the remnants of a patent processus vaginalis
- Arise from the abdominal cavity *lateral* to the inferior epigastric vessels at operation, passing obliquely through the deep inguinal ring and travelling through the inguinal canal with the spermatic cord
- May continue through the superficial inguinal ring into the scrotum.

Direct inguinal herniae:

- Are the result of a weak posterior wall to the inguinal canal
- Arise medial to the inferior epigastric vessels at operation.

This weakness causes the abdominal contents to bulge through the wall into the inguinal canal, but the hernia is not within the spermatic cord.

(b) What are the contents of the spermatic cord?

Three arteries:

- Artery to vas deferens (from inferior vesicular artery)
- Testicular artery (from aorta)
- Cremasteric artery (from inferior epigastric artery)

Three nerves:

- Ilioinguinal nerve (L1) on the front of the cord
- Nerve to cremaster (from genitofemoral nerve)
- Autonomic nerves (sympathetic fibres from T10)

Three other structures:

- Vas deferens
- Pampiniform plexus of veins (drains right testis into inferior vena cava and left testis into renal vein)
- Lymphatics (drain the testis to the para-aortic lymph nodes).

(c) What would you tell patients about their recovery from inguinal hernia repair?

- Early mobilisation is important
- They should keep the area clean and wash carefully, especially after the clips/sutures have been removed
- They may need to be off work for 6 weeks if their job involves heavy lifting
- They should avoid prolonged coughing (control chronic obstructive pulmonary disease preoperatively)
- They should take laxatives if they get constipated postoperatively.

? ADVANCED QUESTIONS

(a) How would you perform a hernia repair?

Be prepared to discuss a method of hernia repair you have learned. The main points to remember are:

- Testicular damage should be mentioned as a specific risk factor
- The operation can be performed under local or general anaesthetic and often as a day case

- The Royal College of Surgeons of England has recommended the Lichtenstein mesh repair and the Shouldice repair
- Laparoscopic repair is increasingly recognised as having a role in the repair of bilateral and/or recurrent herniae.

(b) What are the complications of inguinal hernia repair?

Complications should be divided into *immediate* (first 24 h), *early* (within the first month) and *late* (later than the first month) and further into *general* for any procedure and *specific* for this procedure.

Specific complications to mention:

- Urinary retention
- Bruising – occurs in 30%
- Pain – often very severe and patients should be discharged with adequate analgesia; chronic groin pain persists in 5% of patients
- Haematoma – 10%
- Infection – 1%
- Ischaemic orchitis – 0.5% (caused by thrombosis of the pampiniform plexus draining the testis)
  - Previous vasectomy is a predisposing cause
  - Dissection beyond (more medial than) the pubic tubercle is one operative risk and so this practice should be avoided
- Recurrence – should be <0.5%
  - Normally due to inadequate ring and posterior wall closure
  - Occasionally due to over-tight sutures.

FURTHER READING

Cameron AE: Accuracy of clinical diagnosis of direct and indirect inguinal hernia. *Br J Surg* 81(2):250, 1994.

Liem MS, van Vroonhoven TJ: Laparoscopic inguinal hernia repair. *Br J Surg* 83(9):1197–1204, 1996.

McGreevy JM: Groin hernia and surgical truth (editorial). *Am J Surg* 176(4):301–304, 1998.

CASE 43 | ABDOMINAL EXAMINATION – GENERAL APPROACH ***

INSTRUCTION

'Examine this patient's abdominal system/ abdomen.'

APPROACH

TOP TIP

☑ Should I begin with the hands?

☑ Listen carefully to the examiner's instructions. If you are told to examine the *abdominal system,* then begin with the hands and conduct a complete examination of the entire patient. By contrast, if you are told to examine the *abdomen,* begin with the abdominal examination itself (commence at 'Exposure the patient's abdomen' below); do *not* annoy your examiner by asking whether you should begin with the hands!

TOP TIP

EXPOSURE OF THE PATIENT

☑ The exposure of the abdomen is very important and opinions differ as to how much of the abdomen needs to be exposed (and at what point) during the clinical examination. Clearly, if there is an inguinal hernia or a scrotal lump, this will be missed if the external genitalia are not exposed. By contrast, a patient who has an epigastric hernia need not have his or her dignity compromised.

☑ You are not expected to say, 'I would expose the patient from nipple to knees'; this sounds colloquial and unprofessional in front of a patient and misses the point – that the degree of exposure depends on the case and how much the examiner expects of you.

☑ We would advocate beginning by positioning the patient flat on the bed, but keeping the groin covered until later on, starting your examination looking for peripheral stigmata of gastrointestinal disease.

TOP TIP

INSPECT AND THEN INSPECT AGAIN

☑ Assuming that you have been instructed to undertake an examination of the entire abdominal system, you should inspect the patient *twice:* first, before you begin noting the general condition of the patient, the presence of infusions/catheters/drains, etc. and then second, just prior to inspecting the abdomen itself, to inspect more closely for scars, caput medusae, etc.

VITAL POINTS

Inspect for peripheral stigmata of abdominal disease

HANDS

- Take the patient's right hand and look for signs of chronic liver disease (see Case 46) and inflammatory bowel disease (see Case 50)
- Look for digital clubbing (see Case 28) by inspecting the angle between the nail bed and fold (Fig. 2.8) and by performing Schamroth's test (Fig. 2.9); a small diamond-shaped 'window' is normally apparent between the nail beds when the distal phalanges are opposed. If this window is obliterated, the test is positive and clubbing is present. Clubbing is confirmed by the following:
- Fluctuation and softening of the nail bed (increased ballotability)

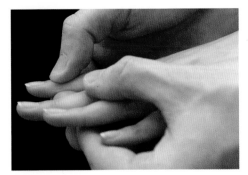

Figure 2.8 Examining for digital clubbing by inspecting the angle between the nail bed and fold.

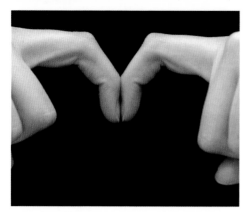

Figure 2.9 Schamroth's test to establish the presence of digital clubbing.

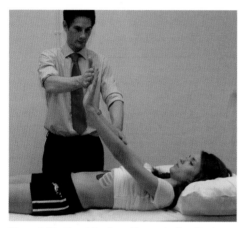

Figure 2.10 Examining for evidence of a liver flap by extending the outstretched wrists.

- Loss of the normal <165° angle between the nail bed and the fold
- Increased convexity of the nail fold
- Thickening of the finger distally (resembling a drumstick)
- Shiny aspect and striation of the nail and skin
- Gastrointestinal disease associated with digital clubbing includes inflammatory bowel disease, malabsorption and cirrhosis, especially primary biliary cirrhosis
- Look for koilonychia (spoon-shaped nails in iron-deficiency anaemia) and pallor of the palmar creases in anaemia
- Check for a liver flap with both of the patient's hands (you can ask the patient to put his hands out in front of him and cock his wrists back as if he is stopping traffic) (Fig. 2.10); in practice, this is a late sign of

hepatic encephalopathy and these patients will not be in examinations.

EYES

- Look at the conjunctivae for pallor (anaemia can only be confirmed following haemoglobin measurement) and at the sclerae for jaundice (see Case 44).

MOUTH

- Look in the mouth (and smell) for oral manifestations of chronic gastrointestinal disease, e.g. hepatic foetor, pallor of the mucous membranes (see Case 72 for full description of mouth signs in abdominal disease).

NECK

- Palpate the neck for supraclavicular lymphadenopathy – Virchow's node (also known as Troisier's sign) is found in the supraclavicular fossa between the sternal and clavicular heads of the sternocleidomastoid muscle.

TRUNK

- Inspect the rest of the arms and upper chest wall for spider naevi, which are in the distribution of drainage of the superior vena cava (see Case 41)
- Briefly inspect the back, by asking the patient to roll towards and away from you.

Expose the patient's abdomen

- If it is a man, ask him to remove his shirt
- If it is a woman, keep the bra on but expose the rest of the chest
- Expose down to the symphysis pubis, keeping the genitalia covered.

Stand back from the couch

Stand at the end or to the side of the couch, and inspect the abdomen thoroughly, looking for:

- Distension
- Scars (see Case 62)
- Visible pulsation
- Ask the patient to take a deep breath in and hold it, seeing the transmitted pulsation of an abdominal aortic aneurysm

- Ask the patient to cough or lift the head off the bed, demonstrating any herniae – especially important if scars are present.

Palpate

Kneel down next to the patient's right side and ask if there is any pain anywhere, before beginning to palpate the abdomen. Look at the patient's face the whole time when attempting to elicit any tenderness. Palapation of the entire abdomen is performed *twice*. The first time is superficial palpation trying to elicit tenderness. The second time is deeper palpation to determine if there are any masses.

- Commence furthest away from you and palpate the nine regions of the abdomen with the four fingers of your right hand held together
- Begin with light, superficial palpation looking for tenderness. When you arrive in the epigastric region, *pause for pulsation*, testing for an abdominal aortic aneurysm (see Case 117)
- Continue with deep palpation in the same nine regions, feeling for any masses – often this is done using two hands interlocked above each other
- Palpate the liver (see Case 46) and spleen (see Case 49) in turn
- Attempt to ballot the kidneys (see Case 61).

Percuss

- If there is hepatosplenomegaly the spleen and liver should be percussed
- If there is any abdominal distension you should percuss for ascites (see Case 57).

Auscultate (Fig. 2.11)

- Over the liver for a bruit
- In the left iliac fossa for bowel sounds

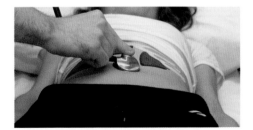

Figure 2.11 Auscultation of the abdomen.

- Over the abdominal aorta and iliac vessels for bruits.

Continue

If you have not found any abnormality, expose the external genitalia and proceed to examining the scrotum (see Case 51) and groin for herniae (see Case 42). Do not forget to palpate the femoral pulses.

Finish your examination here

Make sure to cover the patient back up and ensure the patient is comfortable.

Completion

Say that you would like to:
- Review the observation chart (temperature, blood pressure, pulse and respiratory rate)
- Examine the lower limbs for peripheral oedema
- Examine the external genitalia and groin (if not already done)
- Perform a digital rectal examination (see Case 75)
- Dipstick the urine.

TOP TIP

☑ The term 'per rectal' is incorrect; 'digital rectal examination' is more appropriate.

C. E. Troisier (1844–1919). Professor of Pathology, Paris. Also described haemochromatosis (Troisier syndrome).

R. L. K. Virchow (1821–1902). Professor of Pathology, Würzberg and Berlin. Also described Virchow space (perivascular space of Virchow–Robin), Virchow cell (lepra cell) and the Virchow triad of thrombogenesis.

L. Schamroth (1924–1988). Professor of Cardiology, Baragwanath Hospital, South Africa. A leading authority on electrocardiography and cardiac arrhythmias and originally demonstrated finger clubbing on himself!

CASE 44   SURGICAL JAUNDICE   ★★★

INSTRUCTION 1

'Ask this patient some questions about his jaundice.' (Fig. 2.12)

APPROACH

Direct your questions to finding out whether the cause of his jaundice is likely to be pre-hepatic, hepatic or post-hepatic. Remember that, in the surgical short case, post-hepatic is the most likely cause and this is the easiest to diagnose from the history:

- Have you noticed any change in the colour of your urine?
- Have you noticed any change in the colour of your stools?
- Have you noticed yourself feeling itchy?

If the patient has noticed pale stools and dark urine, then explore possible causes:

- Weight loss, change in bowel habit, loss of appetite and back pain are associated with primary and secondary intra-abdominal malignancies
- Younger age, previous biliary colic or episodic right upper quadrant pains may indicate gallstones.

Continue by asking some questions differentiating the other types of jaundice, and possibly to identify any risk factors for hepatic jaundice, such as foreign travel (hepatitis A), blood transfusion (hepatitis B and C), sore throat (Epstein–Barr virus), alcohol intake and use of certain drugs such as the oral contraceptive pill and phenothiazines.

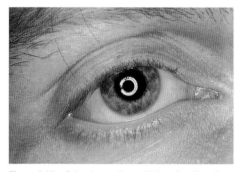

Figure 2.12 Sclera in a patient with jaundice (from Gaw A, Murphy MJ, Srivastava R et al. *Clinical Biochemistry*, 5th edn. Edinburgh: Churchill Livingstone, 2013, with permission).

INSTRUCTION 2

'Examine this gentleman's abdominal system.'

APPROACH

Expose the patient as previously (Case 43) and begin by examining the hands.

VITAL POINTS

- Look for signs of chronic liver disease (see Case 46).
- Confirm the presence of jaundice by looking at the sclera (see Top Tip)
- Examine the neck for Virchow's node (see Case 43).

Inspect

- The abdomen may be distended with ascites
- There may be distended veins around the umbilicus if there is portal hypertension (caput medusae; see Case 130).

TOP TIP

☑ When examining the eyes for jaundice or pallor, only look into one eye (the sign will be bilateral if present). It is easier to use your left thumb to lower the patient's lower eyelid and ask the patient to look towards the ceiling in order to get the best opportunity to inspect the sclera and conjunctiva.

☑ If you suspect a jaundiced sclera but you are unsure, continue to examine the patient's soft palate with a pen torch. Bilirubin is avidly taken up by tissues that are rich in elastin. Consequently, discoloration of the soft palate is a sensitive indicator of the presence of jaundice.

Palpate

- Palpate the abdomen as previously (see Case 43)
- Palpate carefully in the right upper quadrant identifying any tenderness or masses, remembering Courvoisier's law: 'in the presence of painless jaundice, if the gallbladder is palpable in the right upper quadrant, the cause is unlikely to be due to gallstones'. Interpretation: stones in the

gallbladder tend to cause contraction, not distension, so duct stones are unlikely to be the causes of the (obstructive) jaundice. Rather, the cause is more likely to be a head of pancreas lesion (cancer) resulting in increased pressure within the biliary tree with secondary distension of the gallbladder.

Finish your examination here

Completion

Say that you would like to:

- Complete the abdominal examination (see Case 43) by checking the hernial orifices, examining the external genitalia, performing a digital rectal examination (see Case 75) and examining the lower limbs for peripheral oedema
- Check the temperature to see whether the potential obstruction has been complicated by infection
- Dipstick the urine for raised levels of bilirubin.

? QUESTIONS

(a) How can jaundice be classified?

Jaundice is yellow discoloration of the skin and mucous membranes caused by the accumulation of bile pigments. The causes can be classified (Table 2.1) into:

- Pre-hepatic
- Hepatic
- Post-hepatic.

(b) What level does the serum bilirubin need to rise to before jaundice can be detected on clinical examination?

Normal bilirubin is <17 mmol/L and it usually has to reach at least three times this before the sclera is discoloured (i.e. >50 mmol/L). Very high levels of bilirubin are usually associated with hepatic jaundice.

(c) Assuming this patient has obstructive jaundice, how should he be investigated?

Urine should be tested for raised bilirubin (Fig. 2.13).

Blood tests:

- Full blood count: evidence of anaemia in gastrointestinal malignancies; associated infection
- Renal function: any evidence of hepatorenal syndrome
- Liver function tests: see below
- Clotting: functional assessment of hepatic impairment.

Radiological investigations:

- Ultrasound will show:
  - Presence of underlying liver disease
  - Degree of dilatation of the common bile duct (>8 mm is abnormal)
  - Presence of gallstones
  - Presence of lymphadenopathy or a pancreatic mass
- CT / MRI scan
- Endoscopic retrograde cholangiopancreatography
- Magnetic resonance cholangiopancreatography.

Table 2.1   Causes of jaundice and effects on liver function tests

	Pre-hepatic	Hepatic	Post-hepatic
Major causes	Haemolysis Hereditary, e.g. Gilbert's syndrome	Hepatitis Decompensated chronic liver disease Drugs	Gallstones Carcinoma head of pancreas Lymph nodes
Bilirubin type	Unconjugated	Conjugated	Conjugated
Bilirubin increase	++	+++/++++	++
ALT	+/++	++/+++	+/++
ALP	−/+	+/++	++/+++

ALT, alanine aminotransferase (similar rises with aspartate aminotransferase); ALP, alkaline phosphatase.

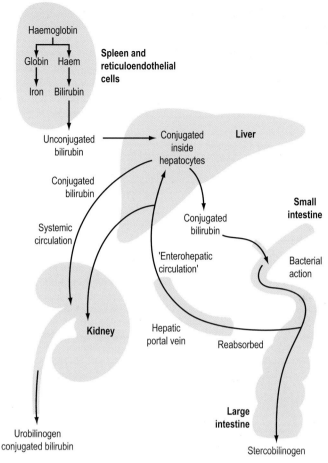

Figure 2.13   Pathway for bilirubin excretion.

(d) How might the liver function tests help in distinguishing the types of jaundice?

This is particularly important in OSCEs, where you may be asked to interpret liver function test results (Table 2.1).

? ADVANCED QUESTIONS

(a) What are the causes of postoperative jaundice?

- Pre-hepatic jaundice can occur due to haemolysis, especially following a transfusion
- Hepatic jaundice can result from the use of halogenated anaesthetics, sepsis or intra- or postoperative hypotension

- Post-hepatic jaundice can occur due to biliary injury (such as in laparoscopic cholecystectomy).

Nicolas Augustin Gilbert (1858–1927). French physician who worked on the classification of liver disease.

FURTHER READING

www.nlm.nih.gov/medlineplus/ency/article/000210.htm – online medical encyclopaedia explaining the various causes of jaundice.

CASE 45 | STOMA ★★★

INSTRUCTION

'Inspect this abdomen and comment on what you see.' (Fig. 2.14)

APPROACH

Expose the patient as in Case 43. Do not start at the hands, as you have been given a specific direction to inspect the abdomen.

VITAL POINTS

Inspect

- Site (right iliac fossa, left iliac fossa, etc.) (Fig. 2.15)

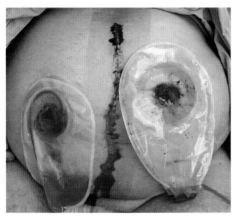

Figure 2.14 Abdominal stoma.

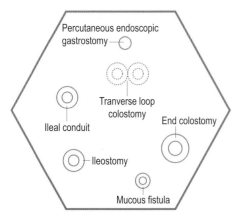

Figure 2.15 Relevant sites for stomas on abdominal wall.

- Whether it is covered by a bag or whether the bag has been removed
- Appearance – if the bag has been removed, then comment on:
  - Mucosal lining – does it look healthy?
  - Presence of a spout or flush with the skin
  - End (one opening) or loop (an afferent and efferent portion of bowel with one common opening or two separate openings)
- Contents – if there is a bag covering the stoma, then describe the bag and comment on:
  - Urine
  - Formed stool
  - Semi-formed or liquid stool
- Move on to describe the rest of the abdominal wall and remember there is likely to be a scar, which you should also describe (see Case 62)
- Are there any other drains/healed stoma sites?

Palpate

If you are only asked to inspect, then do not touch the patient at any time, even to move the stoma bag out of the way – there may be a good reason why you should not touch it.

Finish your examination here

Completion

Say that you would like to:

- Continue to examine the rest of the abdomen to look for reasons why the stoma may have been formed in the first place.

❓ QUESTIONS

(a) What are the indications for forming a stoma?

- Feeding, e.g. feeding gastrostomy/ jejunostomy
- Lavage, e.g. appendicostomy
- Decompression – bypass of an obstructing bowel lesion distal to the stoma

- Diversion
  1. Protection of a distal bowel anastomosis
     - Anastomosis with high chance of dehiscence, e.g. low rectal anastomoses
  2. Urinary diversion following cystectomy
- Exteriorisation
  - When performing an anastomosis is unsafe, e.g. peritoneal contaminated/unstable patient
  - Permanent stoma, e.g. abdominoperineal resection of rectum.

(b) How would you prepare a patient who is going for surgery which will involve forming a stoma?

- Psychosocial and physical preparation
- Explanation of indications and complications
- This includes seeing a specialist stoma therapist preoperatively, who would normally mark the site
- Marking of the stoma site – *with the patient standing up* as he or she must be able to see the stoma
  - The stoma must be within the rectus abdominis muscle
  - Away from scars, skin creases or abdominal folds (especially in obese patients)
  - Away from bony points or waistline of clothes
  - At a site that is easily accessible to the patient, e.g. not under a large fold of fat.

(c) What are the complications of forming a stoma?

Complications can always be divided into 'specific to the procedure' vs. 'general to any surgical procedure', and also into immediate (<24 h), early (<1 month) and late (>1 month).

Specific complications:

- Ischaemia/gangrene
- Haemorrhage
- Retraction
- Prolapse/intussusception
- Parastomal hernia
- Stenosis
- Skin excoriation

General complications – related to underlying disease:

- Stoma diarrhoea – related to water and electrolyte imbalances, hypokalaemia being the commonest and most important consequence
- Nutritional disorders
- Stones – both gallstones and renal stones increase in frequency following an ileostomy
- Psychosexual
- Residual disease, e.g. Crohn's and parastomal fistula.

(d) How can you tell the difference between an ileostomy and a colostomy?

See Table 2.2 and Figures 2.16 and 2.17.

(e) How would you rehabilitate a patient following the placement of a stoma?

- Diet should be normal
- Bag should be changed once or twice a day

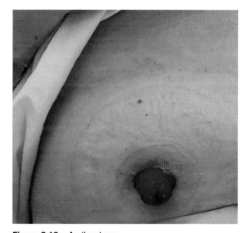

Figure 2.16   An ileostomy.

Table 2.2

	Ileostomy	Colostomy
Site	Right iliac fossa	Left iliac fossa
Surface	Spout (contents are erosive and can damage local skin)	Flush with skin
Contents	Watery – small-bowel content	Formed faeces
Examples of permanent stomas	Post-panproctocolectomy	Abdominoperineal resection of rectum
Examples of temporary stomas	Loop ileostomy over low anastomosis of anterior resection	Hartmann's procedure (end colostomy)

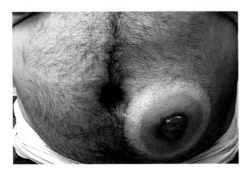

Figure 2.17   A colostomy.

(needs to be emptied more frequently than this if it is urine or small-bowel content/ liquid faeces)

• Psychological and psychosexual support.

FURTHER READING

Cheung MT: Complications of an abdominal stoma: an analysis of 322 stomas. *Aust N Z J Surg* 65(11):808–811, 1995.

Shellito PC: Complications of abdominal stoma surgery. *Dis Colon Rectum* 41(12):1562–1572, 1998.

www.colostomyassociation.org.uk – British Colostomy Association website – help and information for patients who are just about to have a colostomy.

CASE 46 | HEPATOMEGALY ***

INSTRUCTION

'Examine this patient's abdominal system.' (Fig. 2.18)

APPROACH

Expose the patient as per Case 43 and begin by examining the hands.

VITAL POINTS

Inspect

Look for the peripheral stigmata of chronic liver disease. In the hands:

• Digital clubbing – feature associated with cirrhosis of the liver, especially of primary biliary cirrhosis (see Cases 28 and 43)
• Leukonychia – 'white nails' associated with liver disease and fungal infection and can be congenital
• Terry's lines – whitening of the proximal nail bed with loss of the lunula with preservation of normal pink nail bed colour distally. Indeed, it is often noticed as prominent 'pink lines' distally just below the free (white) edge of the nail (Fig. 2.19), rather than whitening more proximally – seen in cirrhosis
• Palmar erythema – vasodilatation due to non-metabolised oestrogens
• Dupuytren's contracture – (see Case 79)
• Liver flap – ask the patient to hyperextend the hands, holding the arms straight out in

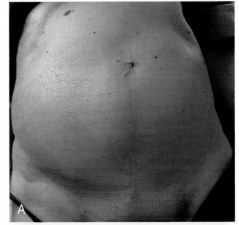

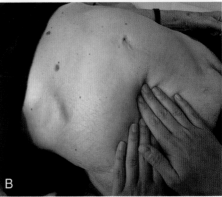

Figure 2.18   (A, B) Hepatomegaly.

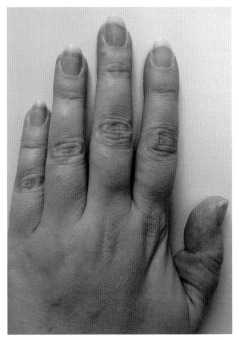

Figure 2.19   Terry's lines.

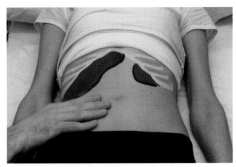

Figure 2.20   Palpation of the liver, beginning immediately above the right anterior superior iliac spine, in the right iliac fossa.

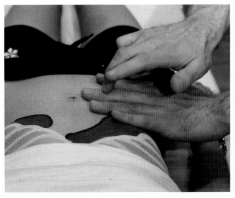

Figure 2.21   Percussion of the upper edge of the liver.

front and cocking the wrists back 'as if you are trying to stop traffic' – look for flapping of the hands (see Case 43).

In the rest of the arms, and upper trunk:

- Spider naevi
- Tattoos (risk factor for transmission of hepatitis B and C virus)
- Scratch marks – icterus, or itch, is a sign of post-hepatic jaundice
- Gynaecomastia (see Case 67)

In the face and neck:

- Pale conjunctiva
- Yellow sclera (see Case 44)
- Inside the mouth – smell for hepatic foetor
- Palpate the supraclavicular fossa for lymphadenopathy.

Inspection of the abdomen

- The abdomen may be swollen due to ascites, and there may be a fullness in the right upper quadrant
- Note the presence of distended abdominal veins, which may occur in portal hypertension (caput medusae; see Case 130).

Examination of the liver

- Palpate the liver, beginning immediately above the right anterior superior iliac spine, in the right iliac fossa (Fig. 2.20). Ask the patient to breathe in and move your hand proximally between each breath in order to detect the liver edge, coming down onto the hand in inspiration
- Define the distance in fingerbreadths from the costal margin at which the liver edge first appears
- Palpate the edge of the liver again, noting the presence of nodules and whether the edge is firm or smooth
- Percuss the upper edge of the liver, beginning at the top of the right hemithorax; the percussion note usually becomes dull at the level of the fifth rib (Fig. 2.21)
- At this point, auscultate the liver for a bruit (heard in hepatocellular carcinoma and alcoholic hepatitis)

- Check next for splenomegaly (see Case 49)
- Check for ascites if the abdomen is distended (see Case 57).

TOP TIP

☑ Demonstrate to the examiner that the mass in the right upper quadrant is an enlarged liver using the acronym **SPRUE** (SPRUE = gastrointestinal disease – causes of gastrointestinal visceral enlargement). The same acronym can also be used to confirm the presence of splenomegaly (see Case 49).

- **S**ite of enlargement: from the right costal margin towards the right iliac fossa
- **P**ercussion note: dull
- **R**espiration movement: it descends
- **U**nable to get above it
- **E**dge: may be smooth or irregular

Finish your examination here

Completion

Say that you would like to:
- Complete the abdominal examination (see Case 43)
- Check for peripheral and sacral oedema (which occur in hypoalbuminaemia).

? QUESTIONS

(a) How would you investigate this patient?

Blood tests:
- Full blood count – e.g. raised white cell count in infection
- Liver function – hypoalbuminaemia, evidence of hepatic dysfunction
- Clotting – functional hepatic impairment
- C-reactive protein/erythrocyte sedimentation rate – increased in infection/inflammation and in malignancy

Radiological investigations:
- Ultrasound is the first-line radiological investigation – used to define the liver architecture, give an idea of the size and may identify the pathology
- Contrast-enhanced CT and/or MRI may also be useful, especially to investigate solid lesions further.

(b) What are the causes of hepatomegaly?

Physiological:
- Reidel's lobe
- Hyperexpanded chest

Infections:
- Viral: viral hepatitis, Epstein–Barr virus, cytomegalovirus
- Bacterial: tuberculosis, liver abscess
- Protozoal: malaria, histoplasmosis, amoebiasis, hydatid, schistosomiasis

Alcoholic liver disease:
- Fatty liver (although more commonly seen these days in the context of obesity/diabetes mellitus)
- Cirrhosis (other causes of cirrhosis also lead to hepatomegaly, but these are less common)

Metabolic diseases:
- Wilson's disease
- Haemochromatosis
- Cellular infiltration, e.g. amyloid

Malignant disease:
- Primary/secondary solid tumours (secondary are more common)
- Lymphoma
- Leukaemia

Congestive:
- Right heart failure
- Tricuspid regurgitation (causes a pulsatile liver)
- Budd–Chiari syndrome.

TOP TIP (SEE CASE 49)

- **C**ongestive: right-heart failure, Budd–Chiari syndrome
- **H**aematological: reticuloses
- **I**nfection: viral, bacterial, protozoal
- **A**myloid
- **S**torage disorders: Wilson's disease, haemochromatosis
- **M**asses: primary/secondary neoplasia
- **A**utoimmune/**A**lcohol (fatty liver/cirrhosis).

? ADVANCED QUESTIONS

(a) What is the significance of an arterial bruit or venous hum over the liver?

An arterial bruit may indicate alcoholic hepatitis, and carcinoma. A venous hum is associated with portal hypertension and if this is secondary to cirrhosis with a patent umbilical vein (or varices in the falciform ligament), this is known as the Cruveilhier–Baumgarten syndrome.

(b) What is portal hypertension?

Defined as portal vein pressure of more than 10 mmHg (normal 5–10 mmHg). Portal blood flow through the liver is greatly reduced or even reversed in the most severe cases. The causes can broadly be divided into:

- Extrahepatic: caused by increased resistance to flow, e.g. portal or splenic vein thrombosis
- Intrahepatic: due to cirrhosis, right heart failure, sarcoidosis and schistosomiasis (the latter is the most important cause worldwide – ova of the parasite colonise and obstruct the portal venules).

W. Baumgarten (1873–1945). Born in St Louis, Missouri, was one of the founding members of the American Association of Physicians.

Jean Cruveilhier (1791–1874). French pathologist, who also described gastric ulcers.

M. Epstein (born 1921). Professor of Pathology in Bristol, investigated Burkitt's lymphoma and identified this virus as important in its pathogenesis.

B. Riedel (1846–1916). German surgeon and pathologist.

R. Terry. British physician.

FURTHER READING

Garcia N Jr, Sanyal AJ: Portal hypertension. *Clin Liver Dis* 5(2):509–540, 2001.

www.british-liver-trust.org.uk – patient-centred website with information about viral hepatitis and regional liver support groups.

CASE 47 | INCISIONAL HERNIA ★★★

INSTRUCTION

'Examine this lady's abdomen.' (Fig. 2.22)

APPROACH

Begin by exposing and examining the abdomen itself.

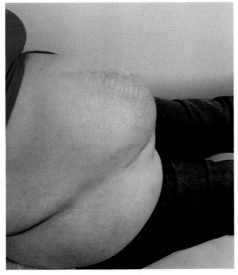

Figure 2.22 Incisional hernia.

VITAL POINTS

Inspect

- The patient may be overweight
- There will be a scar over the abdominal wall – describe the scar (see Case 62) and be sure to note the presence of any other scars, drain sites or old stomas
- Ask the patient to lift her head off the bed and note any bulging out of the scar
- Ask the patient to cough and, again, tell the examiner that you have demonstrated an element of weakness associated with the scar.

Palpate

- Begin by palpating the patient's scar, asking whether there is any tenderness
- Note the presence of any nodularity and feel for the presence of a defect under all, or part of, the length of the incision
- Ask the patient to cough and feel the weakness in the scar allowing the intra-abdominal contents to come out into your hand
- Determine whether the defect is the whole length of the scar or not

- If the hernia was already present before the patient coughed (typically a very large defect), ask the patient whether she can push the lump back inside the abdomen.

Auscultate

- Listen for bowel sounds if there is a large incarcerated hernia.

Finish your examination here

Completion

Say that you would like to:

- Complete the rest of the abdominal examination, and wait to see whether the examiner wants you to do so (implying there may be a second problem for you to identify).

? QUESTIONS

(a) What is an incisional hernia?

- Extrusion of peritoneum and abdominal contents through a weak scar or accidental wound on the abdominal wall
- Represents a partial wound dehiscence where the skin remains intact.

(b) What are the complications of incisional hernia?

- Intestinal obstruction (often intermittent)
- Incarceration
- Strangulation
- Skin excoriation
- Persistent pain.

(c) What factors predispose to incisional hernia?

Preoperative:

- Age
- Immunocompromised state (including renal failure, diabetes, steroid use)
- Obesity
- Malignancy
- Abdominal distension from obstruction or ascites

Operative:

- Poor technical closure of the wound
- Placing drains through wounds

Postoperative:

- Wound infection
- Wound haematoma
- Postoperative atelectasis and chest infection.

? ADVANCED QUESTIONS

(a) What are the treatment options for this patient?

Most patients don't need formal repair of their incisional hernia. Surgical repair carries a risk of wound haematoma and infection, dehiscence and recurrent hernia. In addition, many patients have concurrent medical problems (like obesity and chronic obstructive pulmonary disease), increasing their anaesthetic risk.

Non-surgical:

- Use of a truss or corset
- Weight loss and management of other risk factors

Surgical:

- Prior to surgery
  - Cardiac and respiratory disease should be controlled first
  - Other risk factors should be optimised
  - Preoperative weight loss should be encouraged
- Surgical treatment principles are:
  - Dissection of the hernial sac from surrounding tissues and definition of tissue bordering the defect on all sides for at least 3 cm
  - Reduction of hernial sac contents
  - Attention to the fascial defect
    - If small (<1 cm), direct closure using a Keel or Mayo repair
    - If large, a tension-free mesh repair should be performed. A sublay (space is created to place the mesh deep to the fascia layers of the anterior abdominal wall) technique is associated with lower recurrence than the inlay (mesh literally bridges the gap in the fascia) and onlay (mesh is placed on top of/superficial to the fascia) techniques
    - Adequate overlapping (>5–>8 cm) of mesh over normal tissues to allow for mesh shrinkage/contraction during healing
  - Layered closure technique with sutures (especially if there is no tissue loss)
  - Large hernia may require the placing of postoperative drains.

FURTHER READING

Khaira HS, Lall P, Hunter B, et al: Repair of incisional hernias. *J R Coll Surg Edin* 46(1):39–43, 2001.

Luijendijk RW, Hop WC, van den Tol MP, et al: A comparison of suture repair with mesh repair for incisional hernia. *N Engl J Med* 343(6):392–398, 2000.

CASE 48   UMBILICAL/PARAUMBILICAL HERNIA   ***

INSTRUCTION

'Examine this patient's abdomen.' (Fig. 2.23)

APPROACH

Expose the patient and begin examination of the abdomen itself.

VITAL POINTS

Inspect

- The patient may be overweight
- From the side or end of the couch ask the patient to lift the head off the bed and then to cough noticing the bulge appearing around or above the umbilicus
- Note any associated ulceration or skin damage
- Note the presence of an overlying scar indicating a recurrent hernia
- Point out the presence of a lump underlying the umbilicus, pushing the umbilicus out from the abdominal wall.

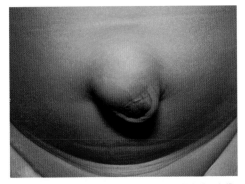

Figure 2.23 Umbilical hernia (from Quick CRG, Reed JB, Harper SJF et al. *Essential Surgery*, 5th edn. Edinburgh: Elsevier, 2013, with permission).

Palpate

- Try to determine the size of the defect
- If there is a lump, ask the patient to 'push it back in' (do not attempt to do this yourself – the lump may be irreducible because loops of adherent omentum divide the sac into multilocular cavities)
- Ask the patient to cough, demonstrating an expansile cough impulse.

Finish your examination here

Completion

Say that you would like to:

- Continue with the rest of the abdominal system examination.

? QUESTIONS

(a) What is the pathogenesis of umbilical herniae?

These are due to a defect through the linea alba (the union of the rectus sheath in the midline) adjacent to the umbilicus and usually due to obesity stretching the fibres.

True umbilical herniae occur through the umbilical scar (cicatrix) (Fig. 2.24) and are usually congenital in origin and particularly common in patients of Afro-Caribbean origin.

Paraumbilical herniae occur around the umbilical scar (Fig. 2.24). They are uncommon before the age of 40 years and can become large. Peristalsis can be observed through the skin when the defect is large.

The neck of the sac is often tight and held with a fibrous band – this increases the rate of incarceration and strangulation. Rarely, spontaneous discharge of the contents can

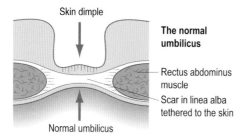

Skin dimple

The normal umbilicus

Rectus abdominus muscle

Scar in linea alba tethered to the skin

Normal umbilicus

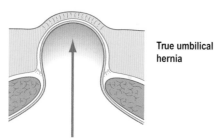

True umbilical hernia

Scar stretched and umbilicus everts

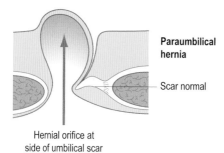

Paraumbilical hernia

Scar normal

Hernial orifice at side of umbilical scar

Figure 2.24 Umbilical and paraumbilical herniae.

occur through the skin, resulting in an enterocutaneous fistula (see Case 71).

(b) Tell me about umbilical herniae in children

Minor defects in neonates are common but usually repair spontaneously. In older children, umbilical herniae are more common; they tend to have a narrow neck and folds of peritoneum stuck within this neck, which can occasionally strangulate. Most cases resolve before puberty and should only be repaired in symptomatic children.

(c) What differences are there in adults?

Acquired umbilical herniae may be caused by:

- Pregnancy
- Ascites

- Ovarian cysts
- Fibroids
- Bowel distension

More commonly, they require surgical repair.

? ADVANCED QUESTIONS

(a) How would this hernia be repaired?

It is important to mention the importance of treating concurrent medical problems prior to surgery; many of these patients have significant comorbidity, which increases their anaesthetic risk. Where possible, the hernia should be repaired, as the risk of strangulation is high.

Surgical technique:

- Mayo's 'vest-over-pants' operation is the most widely accepted repair for these herniae if small and primary:
- A horizontal ellipse of stretched supra- or infraumbilical skin is excised, deepening the incision to the rectus sheath and identifying the fibrous band which is the neck of the sac
- The sac is dissected free from surrounding tissues, which may include release from the cicatrix
- The contents are reduced with or, more commonly without, excision of the hernial sac
- The hernial defect is repaired:
  - The lower edge of the rectus is sutured behind the upper edge, so that the two flaps overlap using interrupted mattress non-absorbable sutures
  - As with incisional hernia, the use of a sublay (extraperitoneally beneath the rectus sheath) mesh is preferable for large defects and is associated with reduced recurrence rates compared to onlay/inlay meshes.

Charles Horace Mayo (1865–1939) and *William James Mayo (1861–1939)*. Brothers who founded the Mayo Clinic in Rochester, Minnesota.

FURTHER READING

Skinner MA, Grosfeld JL: Inguinal and umbilical hernia repair in infants and children. *Surg Clin North Am* 73(3):439–449, 1993.

CASE 49 | SPLENOMEGALY ***

INSTRUCTION

'Examine this gentleman's abdominal system.'
(Fig. 2.25)

APPROACH

Expose the patient as for the abdominal
examination (see Case 43).

VITAL POINTS

Peripheral stigmata

- Pallor (pale nail beds/conjunctivae, skin
  folds, mucous membranes)
- Lymphadenopathy
- There may also be stigmata of rheumatoid
  disease (see Case 81).

Inspect

- A fullness underneath the left costal margin
  may be seen.

Palpate and percuss

Begin palpating for the spleen at the right iliac
fossa (i.e. to the right of and below the
umbilicus), moving your fingers towards the
costal margin on the left-hand side as the
patient breathes in each time (Figs 2.26 and
2.27). The spleen is palpable below the costal
margin on the left. Characteristically, the
defining features confirming that a left upper
quadrant mass is due to splenomegaly are
(using the acronym **SPRUE**; see Case 46):

- **S**ite of enlargement – from the left costal
  margin towards the umbilicus
- **P**ercussion note – dull (remember that the
  spleen underlies ribs 9–11 and while you are
  remembering that fact, note also that it is 1 ×
  3 × 5 inches in size and that it weighs 7 oz.,
  i.e. 1 × 3 × 5 and 7 and 9–11)

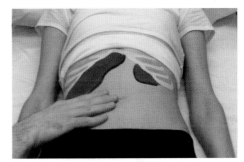

Figure 2.26   Palpating for the spleen beginning to the
right of and below the umbilicus.

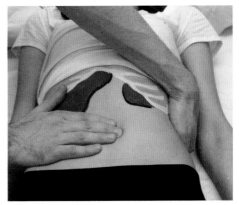

Figure 2.27   Attempting to make a spleen more easily
palpable by insertion of the examining left hand around
the lower left ribcage.

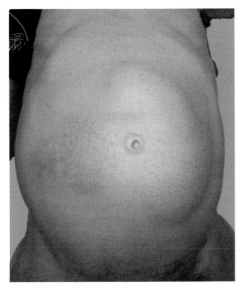

Figure 2.25   Splenomegaly (from Young C, Gladman M.
Examination Surgery. Chatswood, NSW, Australia:
Churchill Livingstone, 2013).

- **R**espiration movement – it descends
- **U**nable to get above it or ballot it (differentiating it from the kidney)
- **E**dge – a notch may be palpable on the superomedial surface.

TOP TIP

☑ If the spleen is difficult to palpate, reach your left hand around the lower left ribcage and lift forwards as the patient breathes in – this manoeuvre may make a slightly enlarged spleen more easily palpable.

TOP TIP

☑ Use the following acronym **CHIASMA** for the causes of splenomegaly (the same acronym and causes are relevant for hepatomegaly: see Case 46).

- **C**ongestive: portal hypertension, hepatic vein obstruction
- **H**aematological: reticuloses
- **I**nfection: viral, bacterial, protozoal
- **A**myloid
- **S**torage disorders: Gaucher's disease
- **M**asses: primary/secondary neoplasia
- **A**utoimmune: Felty's syndrome

Finish your examination here

Completion

Say that you would like to:

- Examine the rest of the abdomen, particularly for hepatomegaly
- Listen to the heart for murmurs, and examine for other stigmata of infective endocarditis
- Enquire about foreign travel and symptoms of possible haematological malignancy.

? QUESTIONS

(a) What are the causes of splenomegaly?

Infective:

- Acute: Epstein–Barr virus, cytomegalovirus, HIV, infective endocarditis
- Chronic: toxoplasmosis, malaria, brucella, leishmaniasis, schistosomiasis

Haematological disease:

- Haemolytic anaemia
- Myeloproliferative disorders (especially myelofibrosis)
- Sickle cell disease/thalassaemia
- Leukaemia (especially chronic myeloid leukaemia)
- Lymphoma

Portal hypertension:

- Cirrhosis
- Hepatic, portal or splenic vein thrombosis

Systemic diseases:

- Amyloidosis
- Sarcoidosis
- Rheumatoid arthritis (also remember Felty's syndrome; see below).

(b) What are the causes of massive splenomegaly?

- Myelofibrosis
- Chronic myeloid leukaemia
- Malaria
- Tropical splenomegaly
- Kala-azar (visceral leishmaniasis)

(c) What are the indications for splenectomy?

- Trauma
- Hypersplenism:
  - Autoimmune thrombocytopenia/ haemolytic anaemia (Evan's syndrome)
  - Hereditary spherocytosis
  - Thrombotic thrombocytopenia
  - Sickle cell/thalassaemia
  - Myelofibrosis, rarely in chronic myeloid leukaemia, Hodgkin's if symptomatic splenomegaly / hypersplenism is present.

? ADVANCED QUESTIONS

(a) What are the functions of the spleen?

- Produces IgM, to capture and process foreign antigen
- Filters especially capsulated microorganisms, e.g. *Pneumococcus*
- Sequesters and removes old red blood cells and platelets
- Recycles iron
- Pools platelets (30% of total platelets within spleen).

(b) What immunisations would you need to organise in the event of performing a splenectomy?

Protocol depends on local guidelines but essentially:

- Pneumococcal vaccine
- *Haemophilis influenzae* type B vaccine
- Meningococcal vaccine
- Repeat pneumococcus vaccine once at 5 years
- Timing:
  - Ideal: >2 weeks preoperative
    - If postoperative: delay 2 weeks if possible, although better to give sooner than 2 weeks if follow-up is unlikely
- Consideration for annual flu vaccine / lifelong penicillin or penicillin
- Warn about risk of malaria, especially *Plasmodium falciparum*

(c) What are the appearances of the blood film after a splenectomy?

- Increased platelet count and large platelets
- Increased neutrophils
- Nucleated red cells with Howell–Jolly bodies and target cells
- Tend to mount more of a leukocytosis in response to infection.

Augustus Roi Felty (1895–1963). American physician who described the combination of splenomegaly, lymphadenopathy and leucopenia.

Philippe Charles Ernest Gaucher (1854–1918). French dermatologist. He originally described Gaucher's disease, the most common of the lysosomal storage diseases, in 1882. It is caused by a hereditary deficiency of the enzyme glucocerebrosidase (also known as acid β-glucosidase), leading to an accumulation of its substrate, the fatty substance glucocerebroside (also known as glucosylceramide).

FURTHER READING

Baccarani U, Donini A, Terrosu G, et al: Laparoscopic splenectomy for haematological diseases: review of current concepts and opinions. *Eur J Surg* 165(10):917–923, 1999.

Farid H, O'Connell TX: Surgical management of massive splenomegaly. *Am Surg* 62(10):803–805, 1996.

Glasgow RE, Mulvihill SJ: Laparoscopic splenectomy. *World J Surg* 23(4):384–388, 1999.

CASE 50   INFLAMMATORY BOWEL DISEASE   ***

INSTRUCTION

'Examine this lady's abdominal system.'

APPROACH

Expose the patient as in Case 43 and begin by examining the hands.

VITAL POINTS

Inspect for peripheral stigmata of gastrointestinal disease

- General signs of malnutrition or weight loss
- In the hands, look for:
  - Digital clubbing
  - Pale skin creases if anaemic
- In the eyes look for:
  - Pale conjunctivae if anaemic, uveitis, iritis, episcleritis

- Around the mouth look for:
  - Aphthous ulceration, often severe, deep ulcers
- If the patient is an inpatient, comment on the:
  - Intravenous lines, blood transfusions and fluids
  - Central venous pressure line
  - Urinary catheter.

Inspect abdominal signs

Comment on all the signs on the abdominal wall, including:

- Scars (see Case 62) – in cases of complicated Crohn's disease these may be multiple, and not typical – just describe the anatomical location of each scar
- Stomas (see Case 45) or healed stoma sites

- Enterocutaneous fistulae (more common in Crohn's disease)
- Abdominal drains or healed drain sites.

Palpate

- In acute exacerbations, the abdomen may be distended and tense
- There may be a mass, most commonly in the right iliac fossa (see Case 55)
- Note the site of any tenderness
- The patient may have hepatomegaly.

Percuss

If the abdomen is distended the percussion note may be hyper-resonant, reflecting dilatation of subacutely obstructed (small) bowel.

Auscultate

Bowel sounds may be increased in acute exacerbations – likely to be normal in the exam itself.

Finish your examination here

Completion

Say that you would like to:

- Complete the abdominal system examination (as in Case 43, inspection of the perineum and the digital rectal examination are particularly important)
- Examine for systemic manifestations of inflammatory bowel disease:
  - Large joint monoarthritis and sacroiliitis
  - Pyoderma gangrenosum
  - Erythema nodosum (usually over the extensor surfaces of the limbs).

? QUESTIONS

(a) What investigations would you perform?

Stool tests:

- A stool culture should be performed in new cases/exacerbations of inflammatory bowel disease to exclude infection
- Faecal calprotectin – elevated levels indicate the migration of neutrophils to the intestinal mucosa, which occurs during inflammation, such as seen in inflammatory bowel disease.

Blood tests:

- Full blood count may show anaemia and leukocytosis
- Electrolytes may show evidence of dehydration or hypokalaemia
- Liver function tests
- C-reactive protein and erythrocyte sedimentation rate may be raised, which can also be used to monitor progress of the disease

Endoscopy:

- An ileocolonoscopy with regional biopsies throughout the entire bowel is the investigation of choice

Radiology:

- Depending on the exact symptoms, a small-bowel follow-through study is useful in assessing jejunal/ileal Crohn's disease. Occasionally, a barium enema is useful for assessing the large bowel
- Abdominal MRI (MR Enterography) is increasingly used for the assessment of Crohn's disease, especially in younger patients, in an attempt to reduce ionising radiation exposure.

(b) What are the extraintestinal manifestations of inflammatory bowel disease?

Use the acronym **ULCERATIVE**:

- **U**rinary calculi – especially oxalate (Crohn's)
- **L**iver – fatty change, chronic active hepatitis, cirrhosis, sclerosing cholangitis, primary biliary cirrhosis, cholangiocarcinoma
- **C**holelithiasis – decreased bile acid reabsorption
- **E**pithelium – erythema nodosum / multiforme; pyoderma gangrenosum (see Case 40)
- **R**etardation of growth and sexual maturation (children)
- **A**rthralgias – arthritis, ankylosing spondylitis – independent of disease activity
- **T**hrombophlebitis – migratory
- **I**atrogenic – steroids, blood product transfusion, biological agents, surgery
- **V**itamin deficiencies
- **E**yes – uveitis, chorioretinitis, iridocylitis

To complete the acronym, the intestinal complications can be remembered using **COLITIS**:

- **C**ancer – risk increased by duration (>10 years), age of onset, pancolitis
- **O**bstruction – rare with ulcerative colitis; more common with Crohn's, especially post-surgery

- Leakage, i.e. perforation –uveitis, chorioretinitis, iridocylitis
- Iron deficiency – from (chronic) haemorrhage
- Toxic megacolon – more common in ulcerative colitis (3%)
- Inanition – severe wasting / weight loss due to malabsorption and decreased oral intake
- Stricture / fistula – occurs in 40% of Crohn's.

(c) What is the definition of severe exacerbation of inflammatory bowel disease?

Truelove classification:

- Gastrointestinal symptoms:
  - Passage of bloody stools >6 times per day
- Systemic signs:
  - Tachycardia (>90 bpm)
  - Pyrexia (>37°C)
- Laboratory findings:
  - Anaemia (Hb <10.5 g/dL)
  - C-reactive protein >30.

? ADVANCED QUESTIONS

(a) What are the indications for surgery in inflammatory bowel disease?

Acute severe ulcerative colitis

Use the following acronym **MPS** (as in **M**edical **P**rotection **S**ociety, whom you may be calling if you forget these indications!) as an aide-mémoire.

- (Toxic) **M**egacolon (transverse diameter of colon of at least 6 cm on a plain abdominal X-ray) – high risk of perforation and faecal peritonitis
- **P**erforation – rare in the absence of toxic dilatation and raises possibility of Crohn's disease. The mortality is 40%!
- **S**evere gastrointestinal bleeding.

Chronic ulcerative colitis

Use the 3 **Ms**:

- **M**edical management failure to control symptoms
- **M**alignant transformation, including severe dysplasia on biopsies
- **M**aturation failure in children.

Surgery for Crohn's disease

Essentially, to treat complications not amenable to medical therapy:

- Intra-abdominal abscesses that cannot be drained radiologically

- Enterocutaneous fistulae (but see notes in Case 71)
- Stenosis causing obstructive symptoms
- Control of acute/chronic bleeding.

(b) What are the surgical options for managing ulcerative colitis?

Subtotal colectomy with ileostomy (± mucous fistula) formation:

- Operation of choice for acute severe colitis
- All of the colon is resected except the distal sigmoid and rectum, which is retained. If the rectosigmoid stump is very diseased, the surgeon may choose to bring it up into the wound to form a mucous fistula, particularly if it is too fragile to be closed safely or if the general condition of the patient is poor. A compromise to the latter is to close the stump and locate it in the subcutaneous tissues but superficial to the fascia, so that if it 'blows' and leaks, there is no peritoneal contamination or its associated physiological complications.

Proctocolectomy and permanent ileostomy (= panproctocolectomy):

- Rectum and anus excised with all of the colon
- As it involves the construction of a *permanent* stoma, it is only performed for patient choice or when the patient (and specifically, the anus) is not suitable for a restorative procedure (e.g. advanced age, impaired anal sphincter function).

Restorative proctocolectomy:

- This is the procedure of choice for most patients as it avoids a permanent stoma
- The surgery may involve three stages, although increasingly these may be combined
- A neorectum is created by fashioning an ileal reservoir
- Stage 1: resection of colon and/or rectum (many patients have already undergone subtotal colectomy and ileostomy formation as an emergency procedure, in which case this stage involves completion proctectomy only)
- Stage 2: construction of an ileal reservoir, which is anastomosed to the anus (ileal pouch anal anastomosis) – this is usually covered with a diverting-loop ileostomy proximal to the pouch, although some surgeons, under the right circumstances, omit the diverting stoma and the need for another operation

- Stage 3: closure of a diverting-loop ileostomy if constructed following satisfactory water-soluble contrast study.

(c) What are the surgical options for Crohn's disease?

- Up to 80% of patients with distal ileal disease require surgical intervention within a 5-year period. The operation of choice is a limited ileocaecectomy, including only a few centimetres of macroscopically normal bowel at each end
- When operating for Crohn's of the small intestine, as much bowel should be preserved as possible, as 50% of patients will require repeat surgery within the next 10 years
- Intra-abdominal abscesses should be drained

- Occasionally a proctocolectomy and permanent end ileostomy may be needed for refractory colonic Crohn's or in the presence of dysplasia
- Pouch surgery is generally contraindicated in Crohn's disease.

> *Burrell Bernard Crohn (born 1884).* US physician working in New York who became the president of the American Gastroenterology Society, presenting a paper in 1932 which described Crohn's disease.

FURTHER READING

www.nacc.org.uk – website of the UK National Association for Colitis and Crohn's Disease, a charity for patients with inflammatory bowel disease.

CASE 51   EXAMINATION OF THE SCROTUM – GENERAL APPROACH **

INSTRUCTION

'Examine this gentleman's scrotum.'

APPROACH

It is important to listen to the stem of the question, as there will be a clue as to whether the problem is in the groin or in the scrotum itself. If asked to examine the groin then begin with the inguinal hernia examination (see Case 42), unless there is an obvious mass or swelling in the hemiscrotum.

If the patient is lying on a bed then examine him supine, remembering to ask him to stand up at the end to ensure that you do not miss a varicocele. If he is standing or sitting in a chair, then examine him standing.

VITAL POINTS

The objectives of the examination are to:

- Confirm that the swelling is confined to the scrotum (i.e. you can get above it)
- Establish whether the testis and epididymis are identifiable
- Determine whether the lump transilluminates.

Inspect

The key distinction in these cases is whether the problem arises from the groin (is it an indirect inguinoscrotal hernia? see Fig. 2.7) or is of scrotal origin:

- Inspect the groin and scrotum
- Scrotal incisions may be difficult to see as they are frequently made in the median raphe in between the two hemiscrotums
- Check in the groins, identifying any oblique groin incisions, which may have been used to approach the testes.

Palpate

Ask the patient if he has any pain and watch his face while palpating the scrotum:

- Ensure that the swelling is confined to the scrotum by demonstrating that you can get above it
- Attempt to palpate each testis one at a time, commencing on the side with the lump if evident on inspection. Establish whether the testis and epididymis are separate from the lump or indefinable
- When palpating the testis, place the fingers of one hand behind the testis, supporting it, while examining the surface of the testis with the finger and thumb

- Palpate the normal contour of the testis, identifying the epididymis and the ductus deferens as well
- The surface of the testis is normally firm and regular
- Lumps and irregularity, and especially any hard masses, are abnormal and should precipitate further investigation. If a lump is identified, attempt to transilluminate it.

Lumps in the groin can easily be distinguished by answering the objectives of the examination, as set out above (see Cases 52, 53, 54 and 70 for details).

Finish your examination here

Completion

Say that you would like to:

- Continue to examine the rest of the abdomen and groin (see specific cases)
  - The lymph drainage of the testes is to the para-aortic nodes, which are retroperitoneal and unless extremely large will not be palpable
  - Inguinal lymphadenopathy is not likely to result from testicular pathology. However, the skin of the scrotum and penis does drain to the inguinal nodes, and if there is pathology involving the scrotal skin or a squamous cell carcinoma of the penis there may be inguinal lymphadenopathy.

CASE 52 | HYDROCELE **

INSTRUCTION

'Examine this gentleman's scrotum.' (Fig. 2.28)

APPROACH

See Case 51.

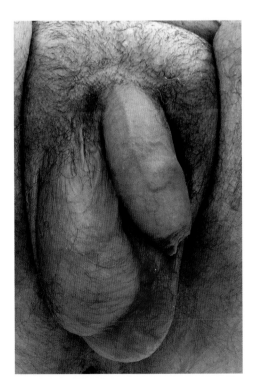

Figure 2.28 Hydrocele.

VITAL POINTS

Inspect

The scrotum may be very swollen if the hydrocele is large.

Palpate

The identifying characteristics of the mass are:

- Distinct from the superficial inguinal ring (you can 'get above' the mass)
- Usually inseparable from the testis (although a hydrocele of the cord will be separate) and uniformly enlarged
- Firm – often tense
- Usually it is possible to transilluminate.

Hydroceles vary enormously in size and some patients who come along to examinations have chronic hydroceles which may be very large – it may be that some other medical problem makes surgical intervention hazardous.

Finish your examination here

Completion

Say that you would like to:

- Examine the contralateral scrotum.

? QUESTIONS

(a) What is a hydrocele?

Excess accumulation of fluid in the processus vaginalis. During the descent of the testis from the posterior abdominal wall in utero, it carries a fold of peritoneum, the processus vaginalis. This normally forms the tunica vaginalis, one of the adult coverings of the testis, and the remainder of the connection from the abdomen is obliterated. If this obliteration does not occur, and fluid accumulates in any part of this peritoneum-derived covering, a hydrocele forms.

(b) What is the anatomical classification of hydroceles?

- Vaginal hydrocele: fluid accumulates in the tunica vaginalis, which surrounds the testis but does not extend up into the cord
- Hydrocele of the cord: fluid accumulates around the spermatic cord and therefore the mass appears around the ductus deferens. This may be very difficult to distinguish from an irreducible inguinal hernia, as it may extend up to and beyond the superficial inguinal ring into the groin. If in doubt, traction on the testis causes a hydrocele of the cord to be pulled downwards
- Congenital hydrocele: the proximal part of the processus vaginalis has not obliterated, the sac communicates directly with the peritoneum and the hydrocele is filled with peritoneal fluid
- Infantile hydrocele: a situation in between the congenital hydrocele and hydrocele of the cord; the processus vaginalis is obliterated at the deep ring and so the hydrocele does not communicate with the abdomen but it remains patent in both the cord and scrotum.

? ADVANCED QUESTIONS

(a) What are the treatment options?

Non-surgical:

- 'Watch and wait' – a small hydrocele may require no treatment other than reassurance, but an underlying malignancy should be excluded (clinically and with ultrasound)
- Aspiration – the hydrocele fluid can be aspirated to relieve symptoms, although it tends to reaccumulate

Surgical:

- Lord's plication – small incision through the scrotum to lift out the testis; the sac is plicated with a series of interrupted sutures to the junction of the testis and epididymis
- Jaboulay's operation – the sac is everted through a longitudinal incision, the excess sac is excised and the remainder replaced behind the cord.

(b) What is a secondary hydrocele?

Although most hydroceles are the result of a patent processus vaginalis, the vaginal type can be secondary to a number of local pathologies:

- Testicular tumours
- Torsion
- Orchitis
- Trauma
- Following inguinal hernia repair.

Peter Lord. Contemporary surgeon, formerly at Wycombe General Hospital, England, also named the 'Lord's stretch', for treatment of anal fissure (now obsolete due to unacceptable risk of anal sphincter injury), and 'Lord's directors', instruments used to assist knot tying within the abdominal cavity.

FURTHER READING

Davenport M: ABC of general paediatric surgery. Inguinal hernia, hydrocele, and the undescended testis. *BMJ* 312(7030):564–567, 1996.

CASE 53   EPIDIDYMAL CYST   **

INSTRUCTION

'Examine this gentleman's scrotum.' (Fig. 2.29)

APPROACH

As in Case 51.

VITAL POINTS

Inspect

- Unless the cyst is unusually large the scrotum will appear normal.

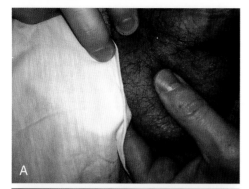

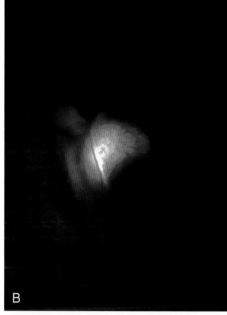

Figure 2.29 Epididymal cyst. (A) Palpation of the cyst as separate from the testis and within the epididymis (B) Transillumination.

Palpate

The identifying characteristics of the mass are:

- Distinct from the superficial inguinal ring (you can 'get above' the mass)

- Separate from the testis – within the epididymis
- Firm, and may be loculated
- May be brilliantly transilluminable, unless they contain sperm (spermatocele), in which case they do not transilluminate as well / at all.

Finish your examination here

Completion

Say that you would like to:

- Examine the contralateral hemiscrotum.

? QUESTIONS

(a) How are epididymal cysts caused?

They are often multiple and most commonly arise in the head of the epididymis. Occasionally they occur as a complication of vasectomy, in which case they are full of sperm and are termed spermatoceles.

(b) How should they be managed?

Non-surgical:

- If the cyst is not troublesome, it should not be removed, especially in younger men, because there is risk of operative damage and postoperative fibrosis causing subfertility.

Surgical:

- Very large or painful cysts can be removed and occasionally excision of the entire epididymis is indicated to prevent frequent recurrence of painful cysts.

CASE 54 | VARICOCELE **

INSTRUCTION

'Examine this gentleman's scrotum.'

APPROACH

As in Case 51.

VITAL POINTS

Inspect

The scrotum will usually appear normal but the testis on the side of the varicocele may hang lower than the other side.

Palpate

The varicocele does not usually appear until the patient is standing up; all scrotal examinations should include an examination of the patient standing to exclude a varicocele. Ask the patient to cough while palpating the varicocele.

The mass is characterised by:

- Distinct from the superficial inguinal ring (you can 'get above' the mass)
- Being separate from the testis
- 'Bag of worms' feel on palpation
- Does not transilluminate
- May have a palpable cough impulse.

Finish your examination here

Completion

Say that you would like to:

- Examine the contralateral hemiscrotum.

? QUESTIONS

(a) What is the aetiology of varicoceles?

- Varicoceles are dilated tortuous varicose veins in the pampiniform plexus, the network of veins that drains the testis (draining eventually into the testicular vein)
- They usually occur in up to 15% of younger men, often around puberty, and are thought to have an anatomical basis
- If they appear suddenly in older men, underlying retroperitoneal disease should be sought, including renal carcinoma extending into the left renal vein – clinically these may be suggested by varicoceles that do not disappear on lying supine.

? ADVANCED QUESTIONS

(a) Why are 98% of varicoceles left-sided?

- The left spermatic vein is more vertical where it connects to the left renal vein
- The left renal vein can be compressed by the colon
- The left testicular vein is longer than the right
- It frequently lacks a terminal valve which serves to try to prevent back-flow in the vein.

(b) What are the treatment options?

Non-surgical:

- Transfemoral radiological embolisation of the testicular vein, using either a spring coil or sclerosant

Surgical:

- Surgical treatment is often advised as the problem usually gets worse with age and there is a risk of infertility
- Palomo operation – exposure of the testicular vein by the high retroperitoneal approach, through an incision above and medial to the anterior superior iliac spine and ligation of all the surrounding veins
- Inguinal approach – similar principle with ligation of the veins in the inguinal canal
- Laparoscopic ligation is also possible.

FURTHER READING

Cornud F, Belin X, Amar E, et al: Varicocele: strategies in diagnosis and treatment. *Eur Radiol* 9(3):536–545, 1999.

Jarow JP: Effect of varicocele on male fertility. *Hum Reprod Update* 7(1):59–64, 2001.

www.netdoctor.co.uk/diseases/facts/hydrocele – review of both hydrocele and varicocele.

CASE 55 | RIGHT ILIAC FOSSA MASS **

INSTRUCTION

'Examine this lady's abdomen.'

APPROACH

Expose the patient and begin, as in Case 43, by examining the hands.

VITAL POINTS

Inspect peripheral signs

In the hands look for:

- Digital clubbing (inflammatory bowel disease)
- Pale skin creases (anaemia, e.g. chronic bleeding from colonic carcinoma)

- Arteriovenous fistula at the wrist (transplanted kidney)

In the eyes look for:

- Pale conjunctivae (anaemia)
- Sclera (jaundice)

In the neck, palpate:

- Lymphadenopathy, especially noting the presence of a Virchow's node in the left supraclavicular fossa (Case 43).

Inspect abdominal signs

Note the presence of any scars from previous surgery and asymmetry may suggest an abdominal mass – especially note the presence of scars indicating renal transplantation (see Case 56).

Palpate

Begin palpating the abdomen as in Case 43. When you locate the mass, differentiate the mass before continuing with the rest of the abdominal examination. Note the:

- Size
- Edge – well defined or poorly defined
- Surface – smooth/irregular/nodular
- Relations – does it arise from the pelvis or are you able to place a hand between the pelvis and the mass?
- Attachment to skin
- Attachment to the abdominal wall muscles – ask the patient to lift the head up off the bed while you palpate the mass.

Finish your examination here

Completion

Further examination would depend on your diagnosis but say that you would like to:

- Complete the rest of the abdominal system examination.

? QUESTIONS

(a) What are the causes of a mass in the right iliac fossa?

The best way to classify this answer is to think of the different anatomical compartments / layers and structures within the right iliac fossa – this avoids leaving out any important causes. There are four main compartments:

1. Arising from the skin and soft tissues:
    - Sebaceous cyst
    - Lipoma
    - Sarcoma
2. Peritoneal cavity
    Arising from the bowel:
    - Carcinoma of the caecum
    - Crohn's mass in the terminal ileum
    - Tuberculosis of the terminal ileum
    - Appendicular mass or abscess
    Arising from the gynaecological organs:
    - Ovarian tumours (benign and malignant)
    - Fibroid uterus
3. Retroperitoneal cavity
    Arising from the male reproductive system:
    - Incompletely descended testis (Fig. 2.30)
    - Ectopic testis (Fig. 2.31)

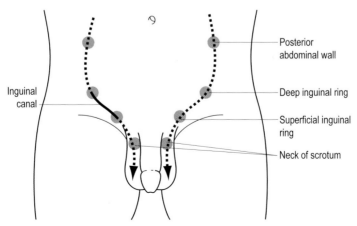

Posterior abdominal wall

Inguinal canal

Deep inguinal ring

Superficial inguinal ring

Neck of scrotum

Figure 2.30　Incompletely descended testis.

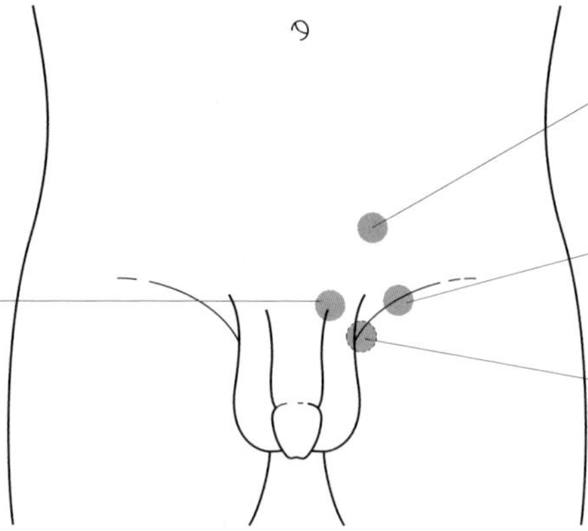

Figure 2.31 Ectopic testis.

Arising from the urological system:
- Transplanted kidney
- Ectopic kidney
- Bladder diverticulum

Arising from blood vessels:
- External iliac or common iliac artery aneurysm
- Lymphadenopathy

4. Posterior abdominal wall
- Psoas abscess (may track along the iliopsoas to 'point' in the groin).

(b) What radiological investigations would be helpful in distinguishing the possible causes?

- Ultrasound would be the first investigation – this would distinguish a bowel mass from an ovarian or uterine mass, and would identify any lymph nodes or abnormal blood vessels
- Abdominal wall masses are better seen with CT scan, and this would also be useful in looking at the extent of intra-abdominal malignant disease
- Intravenous contrast-enhanced CT scanning would clarify lower abdominal and pelvic vasculature.

Differential diagnosis of a mass in the left iliac fossa

This is a very similar list to the one above; the only change is in the 'arising from the bowel' section:

- Diverticular mass (often tender)
- Carcinoma of the colon
- Faecal mass.

CASE 56 | TRANSPLANTED KIDNEY **

INSTRUCTION

'Examine this gentleman's abdomen.'

APPROACH

Expose the patient as in Case 43 and begin by examining the hands.

VITAL POINTS

Inspect peripheral signs

- There may be signs of anaemia (pale palmar skin creases, pale conjunctivae)

- A scar may be visible over the wrist at the site of a Brescia–Cimino arteriovenous fistula (see Case 133)
- There may be signs of steroid use (e.g. bruising, thin skin).

Inspect the abdomen

- Note the swelling in the right or left iliac fossa
- There will be a specific scar over the iliac fossa; a curved incision is used to perform the transplant
- Note also the presence of previous nephrectomy scars and points of access of old (peritoneal) dialysis catheters.

Palpate

Note the mass in the right or left iliac fossa – the mass is superficial and well defined as the transplanted kidney is placed outside the peritoneum, covered only by the external and internal oblique and transversus abdominis muscles. It should only be palpated very gently.

Finish your examination here

? QUESTIONS

(a) What are the major indications for renal transplantation?

Renal transplantation is indicated in end-stage renal failure. The commonest reasons in the UK are:

- Diabetes mellitus
- Hypertensive renal disease
- Glomerulonephritis
- Polycystic kidney disease.

? ADVANCED QUESTIONS

(a) How is 'matching' of transplanted kidneys performed?

Matching is performed at two levels:

- ABO compatibility
- HLA compatibility – matching at the HLA-DR locus is most important, followed by matching at the HLA-B locus and then at the HLA-A locus

In patients who are HLA- and ABO-matched, the 1-year donor kidney survival rate is 90%. Blood transfusions prior to transplant should be avoided, as this carries the risk of HLA sensitisation.

(b) What occurs in 'transplant rejection'?

Rejection is genetically modified and also relates to HLA incompatibility. It can be divided into:

- Hyperacute: within hours of surgery – due to pre-formed antibodies in a sensitised recipient
- Accelerated acute: 1–4 days postoperatively – due to a secondary immune response as a consequence of activation of memory T cells
- Acute – 5 days to 2 weeks after surgery – cell-mediated immunity-related; renal epithelial cells are destroyed by a lymphocyte interstitial infiltrate
- Chronic – humoral mechanisms more important, tubular atrophy and interstitial fibrosis are the histological features.

(c) How might you be aware that transplant rejection is occurring?

The features that may be expected are:

- Tenderness over the graft
- Reduction in urine output
- Rising creatinine.

(d) Describe the vascular supply of the transplanted kidney

- The donor renal artery is anastomosed to either the internal or external iliac artery (Fig. 2.32)
- The donor renal vein is anastomosed to the external iliac vein
- The ureter is anastomosed separately to the patient's bladder
- The renal pelvis is the most anterior structure, then artery and the vein most posterior.

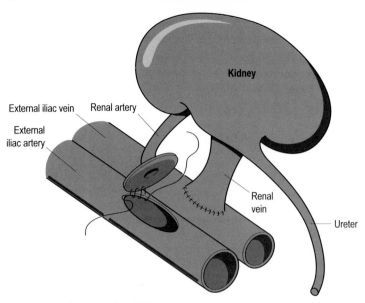

Figure 2.32 Vascular supply of the transplanted kidney.

FURTHER READING

Paduch DA, Barry JM, Arsanjani A, et al:
Indication, surgical technique and outcome of
orthotopic renal transplantation. *J Urol*
166(5):1647–1650, 2001.

Tejani A, Emmett L: Acute and chronic rejection.
Semin Nephrol 21(5):498–507, 2001.

CASE 57 | ASCITES **

INSTRUCTION

'Examine this gentleman's abdomen.' (Fig. 2.33)

APPROACH

Expose the patient and begin to examine the
abdomen as in Case 43.

VITAL POINTS

Inspect

- The abdomen may be distended if the
  ascites is gross – distension will be
  noticeable laterally in the flanks, as fluid
  accumulates in the paracolic gutters when
  the patient is supine
- Begin at the hands, noting any peripheral
  stigmata of chronic liver disease (see Case 46).

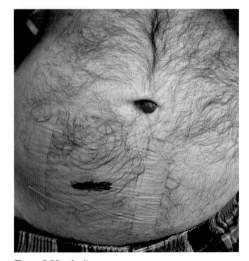

Figure 2.33 Ascites.

Specific tests for ascites

- Flank dullness – percussion over the flanks is dull because of accumulated fluid in the paracolic gutters
- Shifting dullness – while examining from the right, begin percussing in the midline and move laterally towards the right and define the position where the percussion note first becomes dull. Next, ask the patient to roll away from you on to the left side, whilst keeping your finger on the same point on the abdomen. Wait for the fluid to resettle and then demonstrate the percussion note has become resonant again (Fig. 2.34)
- Fluid thrill – with large volumes of ascites, a transmitted thrill can be felt. Ask the patient to place his hand parallel to the body over the umbilicus, resting firmly on the abdomen (Fig. 2.35). Tap gently (with a percussing action) with your right hand on to his left flank, feeling the transmitted pulsation with your left hand resting on the right flank (Fig. 2.36).

TOP TIP

☑ It can be extremely difficult to palpate the liver in patients with ascites. If possible, percuss the abdomen for fluid before continuing to examine for organomegaly – the examiner may stop you at this point.

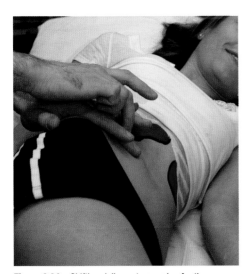

Figure 2.34 Shifting dullness to examine for the presence of ascites.

Finish your examination here

Completion

Say that you would like to:

- Examine the rest of the abdomen looking for other problems, and in particular evidence of intra-abdominal malignancy
- Continue to look for ankle and sacral oedema (signs of hypoalbuminaemia)
- Examine the chest for signs of right heart failure.

? QUESTIONS

(a) What are the causes of ascites?

Common:

- Chronic liver disease
- Right heart failure

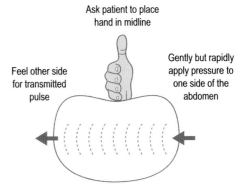

Ask patient to place hand in midline

Feel other side for transmitted pulse

Gently but rapidly apply pressure to one side of the abdomen

Figure 2.35 Fluid thrill.

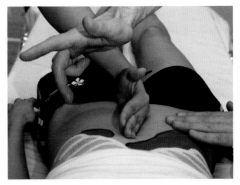

Figure 2.36 Testing for the presence of a fluid thrill in the presence of ascites.

- Intra-abdominal malignancy
- Hypoalbuminaemia

Uncommon:

- Nephrotic syndrome
- Tuberculosis
- Chylous ascites.

Table 2.3

Transudate (protein <30 g/L)	Exudate (protein >30 g/L)
Cardiac failure	Cirrhosis
Tricuspid regurgitation	Malignancy
Constrictive pericarditis	Lymphatic rupture or damage

? ADVANCED QUESTIONS

(a) How would you perform an ascitic tap?

The procedure should be performed under sterile conditions and if the ascites is not clinically apparent or easy to locate, it should be done by a radiologist under ultrasound guidance to prevent inadvertent injuries to intra-abdominal structures:

- Local anaesthetic is infiltrated and the site marked. A safe site is in the iliac fossa lateral to the linea semilunaris (this avoids the inferior epigastric vessels) and should be in an area dull to percussion (fluid rather than air underneath)
- A narrow-gauge needle should be introduced first to check the position before a larger-gauge cannula is inserted into the abdomen
- When in position, a plastic tube can be connected to a urine bag in order to collect the ascitic fluid from the abdominal cavity
- Samples of fluid are taken for:
  - Cytology (presence of any malignant cells)
  - Protein (difference between exudate and transudate – an exudate has protein content of >30 g/L)
  - Microbiology (to exclude bacterial peritonitis as a complication).

(b) With which conditions would an exudate be expected?

See Table 2.3.

(c) What are the indications for the use of a shunt in the management of ascites?

The mainstay of treatment of ascites is to treat the underlying condition and to place the patient on a weight reduction programme, with the help of diuretics, and a low-sodium diet. In diuretic-resistant ascites, shunting may be performed in a number of ways:

- Peritoneovenous shunting (LeVeen shunt), where a subcutaneous Silastic catheter is used to drain the fluid into the jugular vein
- The Denver shunt is a modification, adding a small subcutaneous pump that can be compressed externally
- Transjugular intrahepatic portosystemic stent shunt (TIPS), a side-to-side shunt stenting a channel between a branch of the portal vein and the hepatic vein.

Note that interventional radiology techniques have largely replaced the surgically difficult open techniques.

FURTHER READING

Suzuki H, Stanley AJ: Current management and novel therapeutic strategies for refractory ascites and hepatorenal syndrome. *QJM* 94(6):293–300, 2001.

Yu AS, Hu KQ: Management of ascites. *Clin Liver Dis* 5(2):541–568, viii, 2001.

CASE 58 | EPIGASTRIC MASS **

INSTRUCTION

'Examine this patient's abdominal system.'

APPROACH

Expose the patient and begin, as in Case 43, with the hands.

VITAL POINTS

Inspect peripheral signs

- Look for signs of anaemia in the hands and eyes
- Look for evidence of jaundice
- Palpate the supraclavicular fossa for lymphadenopathy (especially for a Virchow's node in the left supraclavicular fossa).

Inspect abdominal signs

- Comment on the presence of any scars
- There may be epigastric fullness.

Palpate

Begin palpating as in Case 43, but stop when you find the mass and describe the mass fully before moving on. Comment on the:

- Size
- Surface
- Edge
- Consistency
- Relations – to the skin, to the costal margin, to the abdominal muscles
- Could the mass be hepatomegaly or splenomegaly?

Finish your examination here

Completion

Say that you would like to:

- Carry on to complete the rest of the abdominal examination.

? QUESTIONS

(a) What is the differential diagnosis?

As with right iliac fossa masses (see Case 55), the best way to think about this answer is to consider the possible diagnoses anatomically in layers / compartments. You are less likely to forget any of the potential answers.

1. Arising from the skin and soft tissues:
   - Sebaceous cysts
   - Sarcoma
   - Lipoma
   - Hernia (epigastric)
2. Peritoneal cavity
   Arising from the gastrointestinal tract (begin with the stomach and move distally):
   - Carcinoma of the stomach
   - Hepatomegaly
   - Carcinoma of the pancreas (remember Courvoisier's law – a palpable gallbladder in the presence of jaundice is not likely to be due to gallstones)
   - Pancreatic pseudocyst
3. Retroperitoneal cavity
   Arising from the vascular system:
   - Abdominal aortic aneurysm (see Case 117)
   - Retroperitoneal lymphadenopathy.

Ludwig Georg Courvoisier (1843–1918). Professor of Surgery, Basle, Switzerland.

CASE 59   PLEURAL EFFUSION   **

INSTRUCTION

'Examine this patient's respiratory system.'

APPROACH

Expose the patient from the waist up and sit at 45° on the bed. Begin by examining the hands for peripheral stigmata of chronic pulmonary disease.

VITAL POINTS

Inspect

In the hands and wrists, look for:

- Digital clubbing
- Nicotine (tar) staining of the fingers
- Pale palmar skin creases secondary to anaemia
- Hypertrophic pulmonary osteoarthropathy

In the neck, note:

- Position of the jugular venous pulse
- Presence of supraclavicular lymphadenopathy
- Whether the trachea is central

Inspect the chest wall for:

- Scars
- Abdominal breathing

Note the respiratory rate while you are completing the peripheral examination.

Palpate

- Check expansion of the chest wall, noting whether it is equal bilaterally.

Percuss

- Percuss the chest wall from the upper zone down, comparing the percussion note on both sides
- Repeat the process on the posterior chest wall (where effusions will be easier to hear)
- The percussion note is 'stony dull' on the side of the effusion.

Auscultate

- Auscultate using the bell over the apices and the diaphragm elsewhere
- Diminished breath sounds will be heard over the effusion
- Vocal resonance will also be reduced

- Bronchial breathing may be heard if there is associated consolidation of the lung parenchyma.

Finish your examination here

Completion

Say that you would like to:

- Examine the sputum pot
- Check the temperature
- Examine for potential causes of a pleural effusion (see below).

? QUESTIONS

(a) How may pleural effusions be classified?

The protein content of a sample of effusion fluid is measured and the classification depends on this value:

- Transudate = protein <30 g/L
- Exudate = protein >30 g/L

(b) What are the causes of a pleural effusion?

See Table 2.4.

? ADVANCED QUESTIONS

(a) How would you diagnose and treat a pleural effusion?

When the diagnosis has been made and confirmed with a plain radiograph of the chest, a sample should be taken for:

Table 2.4

Transudate	Exudate
Cardiac failure	Malignancy
Medical disorders leading	Primary lung tumour:
to hypoalbuminaemia:	Secondary (especially breast, gastrointestinal, ovary)
Cirrhosis	Lymphoma
Nephrotic syndrome	Chylothorax secondary to malignant infiltration of lymph
	Cardiovascular:
	Pulmonary embolus/infarct
	Dressler's syndrome (post myocardial infarct)
	Infections:
	Pneumonia
	Tuberculosis
	Subphrenic abscess
	Systemic diseases:
	Rheumatoid arthritis
	Systemic lupus erythematosus

- Biochemistry (including protein)
- Microbiology
- Cytology

Pleural taps are most easily performed in the mid-scapular line with the patient leaning forward over a table *within the zone of clinical signs* (stony dull to percussion/reduced breath sounds etc.). Closed-needle biopsy of the pleura can also be performed – combined with cytology, this will diagnose 90% of malignancies and 75% cases of tuberculosis.

Treatment:

- If the patient remains symptomatic the fluid should be drained with a 14-gauge cannula
- Occasionally the pleural space may be obliterated (pleurodesis) using various chemicals
- Surgical pleurodesis may also be performed using video-assisted thorascopic surgery.

(b) Under what situations would a chest drain be required to manage a pleural effusion?

Exudates that recur after aspiration require drainage and they may be placed on low suction (2.5–5 kPa); unlike drainage of a pneumothorax, these drains may be interrupted periodically to allow mobilisation. The drain is left until the volume of fluid is <100 mL/day and there is radiological re-expansion of the lung.

> *William Dressler (1890–1969).* Cardiologist, Maimonides Hospital, New York. He described fever, chest pain, pericardial and pleural rub developing 2–10 weeks after a myocardial infarction. It is thought to be due to an antibody reaction to heart muscle.

FURTHER READING

Ferrer J, Roldan J: Investigation of pleural effusion. *Eur J Radiol* 34(2):76–86, 2000.

Peak GJ, Morcos S, Cooper G: The pleural cavity. *BMJ* 320:1318–1321, 2000.

CASE 60 | DYSPHAGIA **

INSTRUCTION

'Have a look at this lady's hands and ask her a few questions about her swallowing.' (Fig. 2.37)

APPROACH

It is useful to group your questions in terms of aetiologies and to let the examiner know you are conscious of the possible more serious pathologies.

VITAL POINTS

- Are you having difficulty swallowing liquids, or solids or both?

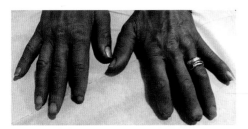

Figure 2.37 Hands in a patient with CREST syndrome.

- Did the problem start suddenly or was the onset gradual?
- Do you ever regurgitate food?
- Can you eat a full meal?
- How long have you had this problem for?
- Where does the food stick – in the back of the throat, bottom of the neck or bottom of the chest?
- Do you ever get any pain – when you swallow or at other times?
- Have you had any weight loss?
- Have you had a chest infection recently?
- Specific to this case (CREST syndrome), you should also ask whether she has noticed any of the following:

  Calcinosis – skin changes / thickening / nodules

  Raynaud's phenomenon (see Case 123) – colour changes of the hands / feet in different weather conditions

  (O)**E**sophageal dysmotility – already done above; typically patients drink fluids to help swallow food

  Sclerodactyly – thickening / tightening / ulceration of the skin of the fingers (Fig. 2.37)

  Telangiectasias – dilated, red blood vessels.

? QUESTIONS

(a) What are the causes of dysphagia?
See Table 2.5.

(b) Which of these conditions are predisposing factors for the development of oesophageal carcinoma?

- Barrett's oesophagus
- Strictures (especially chemical)
- Achalasia
- Plummer–Vinson syndrome.

(c) How do carcinomas of the oesophagus present?

- The characteristic presentation is insidious with progressive weight loss and dysphagia
- The patient initially has difficulty swallowing solids and often describes the food getting stuck in the lower part of the oesophagus
- The patient may also describe odynophagia – pain on swallowing
- Occasionally patients present with aspiration pneumonia.

(d) What other conditions cause odynophagia?

- Infections within the oesophagus (especially candidiasis, herpes simplex)
- Pharyngitis
- Occasionally ulceration over the lower third of the oesophagus.

? ADVANCED QUESTIONS

(a) How would you investigate a patient with a suspected dysmotility problem?

A barium swallow may be useful:

- In diffuse oesophageal spasm, a motor disorder of smooth muscle, below the aortic arch, normal coordinated peristalsis is replaced by multiple spontaneous contractions and this gives the characteristic 'corkscrew' oesophagus appearance
- Achalasia is a motility disorder due to loss of ganglia in the myenteric plexus, causing incomplete relaxation of the lower oesophageal sphincter; the oesophagus has a 'rat's tail' appearance on the barium swallow and there is no gas bubble in the stomach

Endoscopy:

- If the diagnosis is in doubt, endoscopy with biopsies and brushings should be performed to exclude a carcinoma

Test of physiological function:

- 24-h oesophageal pH studies (to exclude reflux) and manometry.

(b) What is the pathophysiology of dysphagia in patients with CREST syndrome?

Oesophageal dysmotility in patients with CREST syndrome is thought to result from atrophy of the gastrointestinal tract wall smooth muscle. This change may occur with or without pathological evidence of significant tissue fibrosis.

Table 2.5   Causes of dysphagia

Mechanical obstruction	Coordination abnormalities
Within the lumen:	**Motility disorders:**
Foreign body	CREST syndrome
Oesophageal web: Plummer–Vinson syndrome (Paterson–Brown–Kelly syndrome)	Diffuse oesophageal spasm
	Achalasia
In the wall:	**Neurological disease:**
Carcinoma of the oesophagus	Myasthenia gravis
Oesophagitis (due to burns or chronic reflux)	Bulbar palsy, including motor neurone disease
Barrett's oesophagus	Cerebrovascular accident (with involvement of
Benign oesophageal stricture	the ninth, 10th or 12th cranial nerves or a
Post-radiation/chemical strictures	coordination difficulty)
Outside the wall:	
Retrosternal goitre	
Lung carcinoma	
Pharyngeal pouch	

A. Brown-Kelly (1865–1941). British ENT surgeon; also described congenital stenosis as well as problems with motility.

D. R. Paterson (1863–1939). ENT surgeon at the Cardiff Royal Infirmary, described the association of glossitis, anaemia and dysphagia.

H. S. Plummer (1874–1936). US physician working at the Mayo Clinic, who investigated the therapeutic use of oxygen in respiratory disease and was interested in the diagnostic and therapeutic use of bronchoscopy and endoscopy.

P. P. Vinson (1890–1959). US physician also working at the Mayo Clinic.

FURTHER READING

Owen W: Dysphagia. *BMJ* 323:850–853, 2001.

CASE 61 | ENLARGED KIDNEY **

INSTRUCTION

'Examine this gentleman's abdominal system.'

APPROACH

Expose the patient and begin with the hand (Case 43).

VITAL POINTS

Inspect

• Inspection is likely to be normal.

TOP TIP

☑ Demonstrate to the examiner that the mass is an enlarged kidney using the acronym **SPRUE** as used for hepato-/splenomegaly (see Cases 46 and 49).

• **S**ite of enlargement – from the costal margin towards the ipsilateral iliac fossa

• **P**ercussion note – resonant due to gas in the overlying colon

• **R**espiration movement – it descends

• **U**nique features – ballottable and bimanually palpable

• **E**dge – in most instances only the lower pole of the kidney is palpable. This is smooth and hemi-ovoid.

Palpate

• In advanced renal tumours, there may be supraclavicular lymphadenopathy

• Note the presence of a mass in the left or right loins or upper quadrants

• This mass can be ballotted between one hand on the anterior abdominal wall and the other behind the patient in the renal angle (Figs 2.38 and 2.39). It relies on the fact that the kidney is reducible into the loin.

Finish your examination here

? QUESTIONS

(a) What is the differential diagnosis for an enlarged kidney?

Congenital:

• Cystic disease (including polycystic kidney disease)

• Horseshoe kidney

• Hypertrophic single kidney

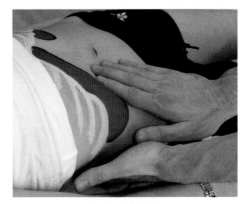

Figure 2.38 Ballotting the right kidney.

Table 2.6 Polycystic kidney disease

	Adult	Infantile
Inheritance	Autosomal dominant	Autosomal recessive
Incidence	1 in 500	1 in 5000–40 000
Genetics	Chromosomes 4, 16	6
Age of presentation	30s–50s	Perinatal
Pattern of presentation	Hypertension Haematuria Loin pain	Oligohydramnios Large liver and kidneys Chronic renal failure
Pattern of enlargement	Asymmetrical	Symmetrical
Liver involvement	Adult liver cysts common	Always congenital hepatic fibrosis Sometimes biliary ectasia
Other systemic involvement	Intracranial aneurysms Colonic diverticula Mitral regurgitation	None
Prognosis	Often require dialysis but good prognosis	All die by age 20, but often in neonatal period

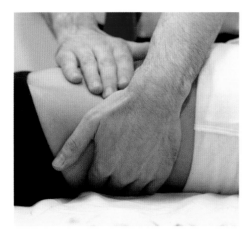

Figure 2.39   Ballotting the left kidney.

Acquired:
- Diseases specific to the kidney:
  - Solitary cysts
  - Tumours
  - Hydronephrosis
  - Pyonephrosis
  - Perinephric abscess
  - Renal vein thrombosis
- As part of systemic disease:
  - Diabetes
  - Amyloidosis
  - Systemic lupus erythematosus.

(b) What are the differences between infantile and adult polycystic kidney disease?
See Table 2.6.

(c) What is the normal mode of presentation of renal cell carcinomas?
- Usually occur in the over-50s, although it may affect younger patients. Indeed, it is the commonest cause of a renal mass in women of childbearing age.
- Classic presentation is a triad (Beck's triad) of:
  - Haematuria
  - Mass
  - Loin pain
- Other presentations:
  - Incidentally found on abdominal ultrasound or CT scans performed for another reason (very common)
  - Pyrexia of unknown origin
  - Anaemia of chronic disease
  - Polycythaemia (due to erythropoietin secretion by the tumour)
  - Raised erythrocyte sedimentation rate
  - Hypercalcaemia
  - Left-sided varicocele.

? ADVANCED QUESTIONS

(a) Simple cysts are found in 33% of patients by the age of 60. How should they be managed?

History and clinical examination:

- They usually present incidentally but occasionally with a renal mass or haematuria

Investigations:

- Urine cytology
- Blood tests would be expected to be normal
- A renal ultrasound scan shows a cyst with a smooth outline, sharply defined thin wall and no internal echoes (which imply solid components)
- Increasingly, CT and MRI are being used as they allow detailed characterisation of renal masses

Treatment:

- The major differential diagnoses would be with a renal tumour and adult polycystic kidney disease and if there is any doubt of a tumour, then the cyst fluid may be sent for cytological analysis.

(b) What radiological features would make you suspicious of an occult renal cell carcinoma?

More worrying features for a tumour would include:

- Thick or irregular wall
- Extensive calcification within the cavity or wall of the cyst
- Multilocular cysts.

FURTHER READING

Gladman MA, Macdonald D, Webster JJ, et al: Renal cell carcinoma in pregnancy. *J R Soc Med* 95:199–201, 2002.

Godley PA, Taylor M: Renal cell carcinoma. *Curr Opin Oncol* 13(3):199–203, 2001.

Tomson CR: Recent advances: nephrology. *BMJ* 320(7227):98–101, 2000.

www.pkdcure.org – website of the Polycystic Foundation, a worldwide organisation devoted to determining the cause and treatment for polycystic kidney disease.

CASE 62   COMMON SURGICAL SCARS   *

INSTRUCTION

'Inspect this patient's abdomen.' (Fig. 2.40)

APPROACH

Introduce yourself and expose the patient's abdomen, positioning the patient flat on the bed. Leave the external genitalia covered at this point to maintain dignity but expose the whole of the top half of the body down to the symphysis pubis. If the examiner indicates the patient should leave his / her shirt on, then expose from above the xiphisternum to the symphysis pubis.

VITAL POINTS

Inspect

Comment on the presence of any surgical scars (Fig. 2.41):

- Use the correct technical names for the scars where possible; if not, describe the anatomical position of the scar and indicate

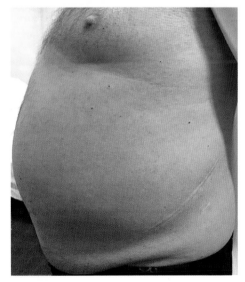

Figure 2.40   Abdominal scar.

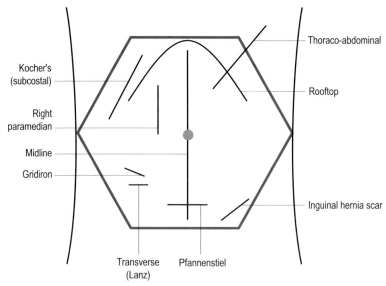

Figure 2.41 Common surgical scars. Remember to examine the flanks for the loin incision of a nephrectomy.

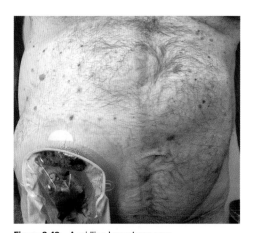

Figure 2.42 A midline laparotomy scar.

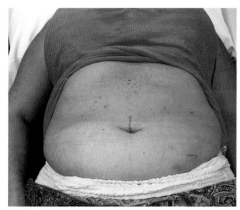

Figure 2.43 Laparoscopic surgical scars.

whether it looks well healed or recently formed

- You should not guess at the operation the patient underwent in order to produce the scar unless asked specifically to do so by the examiner
- Traditionally, major abdominal surgery has been performed via a midline laparotomy incision and this is still the most common scar to be revealed in examinations (Fig. 2.42).
- Increasingly, abdominal surgery is being performed via a laparoscopic approach, so inspect the umbilicus and iliac fossa with great care to avoid missing three to five small 5–10-mm scars from port-site insertion (Fig. 2.43).

TOP TIP

☑ When you see a scar on the abdomen, always think of the presence of an incisional hernia (see Case 47). From the end of the bed, ask the patient to raise the head off the bed and cough in order to demonstrate this. Similarly, be sure to check for port-site herniation in the small laparoscopic scars. Continue to examine each scar more carefully during the palpation section to rule out incisional herniae.

✓

Finish your examination here

❓ QUESTIONS

(a) Which operation do you think this patient may have had?

Although you should not voluntarily make a guess at which operation the patient may have had in order to produce the scar, in the short cases and OSCEs the examiner may ask you for an educated opinion.

There may be a few pointers:

- Is there evidence of a new or old stoma site or scar (from a colorectal operation)?
- Is there evidence of a small (5-mm) incision to one side of the scar (from a drain – this may have been due to a gastrointestinal operation)?
- In cases with laparoscopic port-site scars, is there evidence of extension of the umbilical wound or a separate, slightly longer wound

elsewhere on the abdomen? Such scars result from the wound used for extraction of the pathological specimen and the position and length can give clues to the procedure performed. For example, 2–4 cm at umbilicus or longitudinal midline epigastric suggest gallbladder / upper GI procedures, whilst 5–7 cm at umbilicus (Fig. 2.43) or located suprapubically suggest colorectal procedures.

- Are there also scars in the groins (perhaps iliofemoral-segment surgery in a patient who has also had an abdominal aortic aneurysm repaired through a midline incision)?
- Are there striae gravidarum (Pfannenstiel incision may have been for a Caesarean section)?

Herman Johannes Pfannenstiel (1862–1909). Gynaecologist from Breslau who described the popular slightly, curved suprapubic incision.

CASE 63 | BREAST EXAMINATION – GENERAL APPROACH *

INSTRUCTION

'Examine this lady's breasts.'

APPROACH

Before beginning this examination, irrespective of whether in a long case or short case, you must be accompanied by a chaperone and a nurse will often be available for this purpose in the examination. Increasingly in OSCE examinations, models wearing breast prostheses, containing pathological signs, are used rather than actual patients, for obvious reasons.

Expose the patient from the waist up and lie her at 45° on the couch.

VITAL POINTS

Inspect

Begin by asking the patient if she has noticed a lump in the breast and, if so, which breast it is in.

Stand away from the couch and look at the patient's breasts from the front.

- Ask the patient to lift both her hands above her head. This will stretch the skin and emphasise any tethering of a breast tumour to the skin
- Next, ask her to place both her hands on her hips, and while watching her breasts, ask her to press firmly into the hips with both hands. This emphasises any attachment of a breast tumour to the underlying pectoralis major muscle, which contracts with this manoeuvre, making it more obvious on visual inspection.

Move closer to the patient and look more carefully at the breasts:

- Inspect the nipple and areola (see Top Tip below)
- Inspect the rest of the breasts for:
  - Asymmetry in size or shape
  - Skin changes or subcutaneous nodules
  - Previous scars from excision of benign or malignant lumps.

THE SEVEN DS OF NIPPLE SIGNS

☑ When inspecting the nipple, or taking a history of nipple symptoms, look for:

- **D**iscoloration
- **D**ischarge
- **D**epression (often referred to as inversion)
- **D**eviation
- **D**isplacement
- **D**estruction
- (**D**uplication – unlikely in the exam).

- The location of the lump within the breast should be named according to the quadrant (upper outer, lower outer, upper inner, lower inner)
- Describe any lump as in Case 1, noting whether it is attached to the skin or the underlying muscle
- Palpate the five areas of lymph nodes in the axilla – medial, lateral, anterior, posterior and apical (Fig. 2.44) – palpating the left axilla with your right hand and vice versa
- Palpate the supraclavicular fossa for lymphadenopathy (Fig. 2.44).

Finish your examination here

Palpate

Ask the patient to position her hands in her lap. Ask her to tell you where the lump in the breast is first, but start by palpating the normal breast.

- Palpate systematically round the breast, using the tips of your fingers held together
- Retract the breast with the left hand and use the right hand to palpate each of the four quadrants
- Imagine the breast as a clock face and make sure that each area is palpated
- Pay particular attention to the axillary tail and underneath the nipple, where masses are frequently missed
- When palpating the abnormal breast, ensure that the area of abnormality that you have found is the same that the patient has noticed

Completion

Say that you would like to continue with:

- Percussing and auscultating the chest
- Palpating the abdomen for hepatomegaly
- Percussing the axial spine for tenderness
- Examining the lower abdomen and back for scars from flaps used for breast reconstruction – latissimus dorsi myocutaneous, transverse rectus abdominis muscle, deep inferior epigastric perforator, superficial inferior epigastric artery flaps (see Case 66).
- Completing a general physical examination to determine the patient's fitness for surgery.

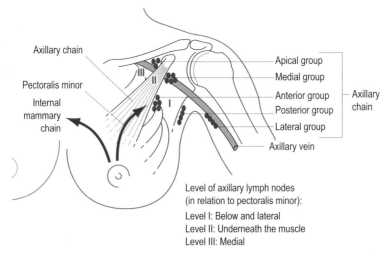

Level of axillary lymph nodes (in relation to pectoralis minor):

Level I: Below and lateral
Level II: Underneath the muscle
Level III: Medial

Figure 2.44 Lymph nodes and lymphatic drainage of the breast.

CASE 64 | BREAST LUMP *

INSTRUCTION
'Examine this lady's breasts.'

APPROACH
Expose the patient to the waist to expose the breasts and chest wall adequately.

VITAL POINTS

Inspect

- The lump may be tethered to the skin or underlying muscle
- There may be associated nipple changes, or changes to the skin of the breast
- There may be scars from previous surgery.

Palpate

As in Case 63, begin with the normal breast, examining with the patient's hands in her lap. When you have identified the lump, describe the lump in detail:

- Site (position): name the quadrant the lump is located within
- Size: measure the lump approximately
- Surface: smooth/irregular/nodular
- Edge: well/poorly defined
- Consistency: soft/firm/hard
- Tenderness
- Fluctuation
- Fixation: to skin or the underlying chest wall

Continue as in Case 63 by palpating the axilla and supraclavicular fossa and complete the examination as in Case 63.

Finish your examination here

? QUESTIONS

(a) How would you investigate this patient?

You must mention a triple assessment, which consists of:

- Clinical: history and physical examination
- Radiological: ultrasound or mammography, occasionally MRI
- Pathological: cytology (fine-needle aspiration) or histological (Tru-Cut biopsy).

(b) How would you classify breast disease?

Generally, disease of the breast is classified as follows:

Malignant disease:

- Ductal carcinoma (also referred to as cancer of no specific type), accounts for ~70% of cancers
- Lobular carcinoma, accounts for ~20% of cancers
- Other (mucinous, tubular, medullary), accounts for ~10% of cancers

Benign disease:

- Congenital abnormalities (supernumerary nipples, hypoplasia, etc.)
- Aberrations of normal development and involution (ANDI)
  - Fibroadenomas
  - Breast cysts
  - Sclerotic/fibrotic lesions
- Non-ANDI conditions:
  - Infective
  - Lipomas
  - Fat necrosis

Single lumps in the breast are most likely to be:

- Fibroadenomas
- Breast cysts
- Fat necrosis
- Breast cancer.

(c) What features of the lump would make you suspicious that it is a breast cancer?

- Surface: irregular or nodular
- Edge: poorly defined, with areas which are more like normal breast tissue in between more abnormal areas
- Consistency: breast tumours are usually firm, rather than hard
- Tenderness: usually non-tender
- Fluctuation: usually not fluctuant
- Fixation: to skin or the underlying chest wall
- Any involvement of the nipple in the lump or concurrent nipple changes

Also mention the presence of any lymphadenopathy, or features in the history or physical examination, that suggest disseminated disease.

? ADVANCED QUESTIONS

(a) What are the principles of local treatment for breast cancer?

- The aim of local treatment of breast cancer is to achieve long-term local disease control with the minimum local morbidity.
- For solitary breast cancers, survival outcomes from breast-conserving treatment (wide local excision) are equivalent to mastectomy.
- The major surgical factor influencing local recurrence is completeness of excision, and clear margins (≥1 mm) must be obtained when performing breast-conserving surgery. However, wider margins (>5 mm) do not achieve better local control rates than narrow margins.
- All patients who have wide local excision require radiotherapy, which reduces the rate of local recurrence and improves overall survival.

(b) What are the options for managing the axilla in patients with breast cancer?

- Lymph node status (local and regional) remains one of the strongest prognostic factors in breast cancer
- Historically, a complete axillary node dissection with removal of level I and II lymph nodes or even levels I–III was standard (Fig. 2.44), and while this provided excellent prognostication and local control, it was associated with significant morbidity in terms of lymphoedema and decreased range of movement of the shoulder.
- More recently, axillary sentinel node biopsy using blue dye or radioactive tracers (or both

together) has replaced this approach and allows stratification of patients into those with node-positive / negative.

- Currently, patients with a positive sentinel node biopsy result will usually undergo axillary clearance, although this is being increasingly challenged in certain situations.

(c) What adjuvant treatments are available for treatment for breast cancer?

- Adjuvant treatment after surgery significantly improves outcomes.
- Tamoxifen for 5 years remains the standard for premenopausal patients with oestrogen receptor-positive early breast cancer and an aromatase inhibitor (anastrozole and letrozole) for postmenopausal patients
- Chemotherapy reduces the risk of recurrence and death from breast cancer, particularly for oestrogen receptor-negative and/or HER-2-positive disease.
- Trastuzumab (Herceptin), in addition to adjuvant chemotherapy, confers a significant further benefit in patients with HER-2-positive disease.

FURTHER READING

Brennan M, Houssami N, French J: Management of benign breast conditions. Part 2 – breast lumps and lesions. *Aust Fam Physician* 34(4):253–255, 2005.

Drukker BH: Fibrocystic change of the breast. *Clin Obstet Gynecol* 37(4):903–915, 1994.

Houssami N, Cheung MN, Dixon JM: Fibroadenoma of the breast. *Med J Aust* 174(4):185–188, 2001.

CASE 65　POST-MASTECTOMY BREAST　*

INSTRUCTION

'Examine this lady's chest.' (Fig. 2.45)

APPROACH

Expose the patient and begin examining the remaining breast as in Case 63 and then move on to the chest wall at the site of mastectomy, if requested.

VITAL POINTS

Inspect

- Note the asymmetrical chest wall and describe the location of the scar
- Look at the surrounding skin and into the axilla, determining whether there has also been radiotherapy to the surrounding area
- Ask the patient to press her hands into her hips, ascertaining whether the pectoralis major remains underneath the mastectomy.

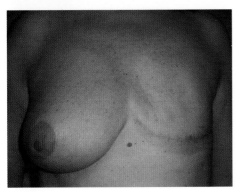

Figure 2.45   Post-mastectomy breast (from Dixon JM *Breast Surgery: A Companion to Specialist Surgical Practice*, 5th edn. Philadelphia, PA: Saunders, 2013, with permission).

Palpate

- It is likely that you would not have to continue to palpate the breast, but if the examiner wants you to continue, you should examine the remaining breast as in Case 63
- Palpate the axilla and supraclavicular fossa for lymphadenopathy.

Finish your examination here

Completion

Say that you would like to:
- Examine the abdomen, neck, lung fields and spine
- Examine the ipsilateral arm for lymphoedema.

? QUESTIONS

(a) What are the indications for mastectomy?

Modern oncological surgery involves breast conservation wherever possible and usually involves wide local excision and assessment of the axillary contents (sentinel node biopsy, axillary node sampling or clearance).

There are some occasions where mastectomy is still considered, although these indications are by no means absolute and are being increasingly challenged by surgical oncologists:

- Patient preference
- Clinical evidence of multifocal/multicentric disease

- Large lump in small breast tissue (depends on the size of the breast but often defined as a lump >4 cm)
- Large area (>4 cm) ductal carcinoma in situ
- Women with a strong family history of breast cancer or who are proven BRCA1 and BRCA2 mutation carriers

? ADVANCED QUESTIONS

(a) What different types of mastectomy can be performed?

- Simple mastectomy – removal of the breast alone

The following procedures are rarely performed now as survival benefit has not been demonstrated:

- Modified radical mastectomy (Patey) – removal of the breast, pectoralis minor and the axillary structures
- Radical mastectomy (Halsted mastectomy) – removal of the breast, pectoralis major and minor, and the axillary contents
- Extended radical mastectomy – as for the radical procedure, but also removing the internal mammary nodes (between the second and fourth anterior intercostal spaces).

The disadvantage with simple mastectomy, although least disfiguring, is that the axilla still needs to be managed following surgery (for instance, with radiotherapy), whereas the other types involve surgical dissection of the axillary nodes. Postoperative radiotherapy is more common for limited resections.

(b) How would you prepare a patient prior to breast surgery?

Physical preparation:

- Mark the side prior to anaesthetic
- Explanation of the procedure should include the use of a suction drain to close the cavity following surgery and decrease the risk of scar and haematoma formation
- An anaesthetised patch of skin in the axilla and the upper medial part of the arm will follow division of the intercostobrachial nerve (T1), which is divided as it emerges from the chest wall just posterior to the origin of the pectoralis minor muscle
- Anaesthetic work-up should include chest X-ray to exclude pulmonary metastasis

Psychological preparation:

- All patients should see the breast care nurse preoperatively and the reasons for mastectomy should be discussed fully

- The option of reconstructive surgery (see Case 66) should be discussed.

(c) When should the drains be removed post-surgery?

- Often surgeons place two drains, one in the axilla and one at the site of surgery within the breast tissue
- The drains are usually left for 3–5 days, or until the drainage volume is <50 mL in 1 day
- Patients can safely be sent home with drains in place and district nurse support, as otherwise they may spend a week in hospital.

William Stewart Halsted (1852–1922). First Professor of Surgery at Johns Hopkins Medical School, Baltimore, where Harvey Cushing was his assistant. He also introduced rubber gloves to surgery (made for him by the company Goodyear) and was one of the first to use regional anaesthesia with cocaine.

FURTHER READING

Eatock J: Counselling in primary care: past, present and future. *Br J Guidance Counselling* 28(2):161–173, 2000.

CASE 66 | BREAST RECONSTRUCTION *

INSTRUCTION

'Examine this lady's chest wall.'

APPROACH

Expose the patient as in Case 63.

VITAL POINTS

Inspect

- Note any asymmetry of the chest wall
- The reconstructed breast can be identified by the presence of surgical scars and by a different shape from the normal breast contour.

FLAP RECONSTRUCTION

- More extensive surgical scarring
- Scars extend over the back or abdominal wall
- Look at the patient's back and see the recess where the latissimus dorsi has been removed
- Ask the patient to lift her head off the bed (when lying flat) to see the recess in the rectus abdominis muscle.

IMPLANT RECONSTRUCTION

- Shape is rounder than a 'normal' breast
- Lie of the breast is usually higher
- A Becker implant may have a palpable subcutaneous filling port in the axilla.

Finish your examination here

TOP TIP

☑ Do not be embarrassed to ask the patient for permission to examine the reconstructed breast and the other breast. Do so with confidence. In this situation it is useful to inform the examiner of your findings on inspection prior to palpation.

❓ ADVANCED QUESTIONS

(a) What are the possible types of breast reconstruction surgery?

Timing:

- Immediate (advantages: single operation; preservation of/better-quality skin flaps)
- Delayed (allows increased patient decision time, avoidance of delay/detrimental effects of adjuvant therapy)

Technique:

- Tissue expansion reconstruction (implants)
  - Subcutaneous prosthesis
  - Submuscular implant
- Autologous tissue reconstruction (myocutaneous flaps)
  - Pedicled/free transverse rectus abdominis myocutaneous (TRAM) flap
  - Free deep inferior epigastric perforator (DIEP) flap: spares rectus muscle/destruction of abdominal wall
  - Free superficial inferior epigastric artery (SIEA) flap: vessel absent in one-third of patients
  - Latissimus dorsi (LD) flap.

Table 2.7   Using an implant

Advantages	Disadvantages
Technique simpler than flaps	Cosmetic result less satisfactory than using a flap
Place under the pectoralis muscles to reduce the incidence of contraction of the capsule	Requires plenty of available skin following surgery
Can be performed at the time of the mastectomy or at a later date	Lies above the natural inframammary fold, leaving the breast higher than the other one

Table 2.8   Myocutaneous flaps

Advantages	Disadvantages
Useful where remaining skin and muscle in short supply, e.g. following extensive surgery Cosmetic results can be very good Suitable for use post-mastectomy Suitable for salvage after local recurrence	May need to be performed in combination with plastic surgeon Greater blood loss Greater operating time and operative complications Use of rectus abdominis may be impossible if the patient has had previous abdominal surgery Late complications include flap necrosis and infection

(b) What are the advantages and disadvantages of using an implant?
See Table 2.7.

(c) What are the advantages and disadvantages of myocutaneous flaps?
See Table 2.8.

FURTHER READING

Cordeiro PG: Breast reconstruction after surgery for breast cancer. *N Engl J Med* 359(15):1590–1601, 2008.

Malata CM, McIntosh SA, Purushotham AD: Immediate breast reconstruction after mastectomy for cancer. *Br J Surg* 87(11):1455–1472, 2000.

Malyon AD, Husein M, Weiler-Mithoff EM: How many procedures to make a breast? *Br J Plast Surg* 54(3):227–231, 2001.

CASE 67   GYNAECOMASTIA *

INSTRUCTION

'Look at this gentleman's chest.' (Fig. 2.46)

APPROACH

Expose the patient as for the chest examination and position him at 45°.

VITAL POINTS

Inspect

Note the presence of unilateral or bilateral breast swellings. They may be simply small breast buds, or more significant amounts of breast tissue may be present.

Finish your examination here

Completion

Say that you would like to:

- Look for a cause of the gynaecomastia, including examination of the external genitalia, examining for clinical signs of thyroid dysfunction, and for signs of liver disease
- Ask the patient some directed questions, especially about the use of prescription or recreational drugs.

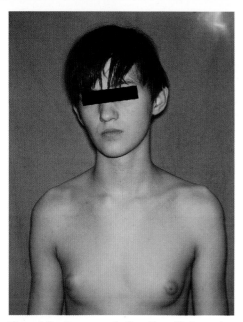

Figure 2.46 Gynaecomastia (from Moore KL, Persaud TVN, Torchia MG *Before We Are Born*, 8th edn. Philadelphia, PA: Saunders, 2011, with permission).

? QUESTIONS

(a) What are the causes of gynaecomastia?

Causes may be classified as the 3 **P**s:

Physiological:

- Particularly common at puberty, when the patient may have noticed unilateral or bilateral gynaecomastia – may enlarge to considerable size but usually disappear before adulthood

Pathological (due to relative hyperoestrogenism):

Decreased androgens:

- Reduced androgen production (i.e. hypogonadism)
  - Testicular atrophy (bilateral cryptorchidism; post-orchitis/bilateral torsion)
  - Klinefelter's syndrome
  - Hyperprolactinaemia
  - Renal failure
- Androgen resistance
  - Testicular feminisation

Increased oestrogens:

- Increased secretion
  - Testicular tumours
  - Lung carcinoma

- Increased peripheral aromatisation
  - Liver disease
  - Adrenal disease
  - Thyrotoxicosis

Potions (i.e. drugs):

- Recreational drugs: marijuana, amphetamines, diazepam
- Gastrointestinal drugs: cimetidine, ranitidine
- Cardiovascular drugs: digoxin, angiotensin-converting enzyme inhibitors (e.g. captopril, enalapril), spironolactone, nifedipine, verapamil
- Antibiotics: metronidazole, isoniazid, ketoconazole.

? ADVANCED QUESTIONS

(a) How might you investigate this patient?

The level of investigation depends very much on the clinical situation, and some patients may require no investigations at all. Possible useful investigations would include:

- Plasma α-fetoprotein and β-human chorionic gonadotrophin – raised levels may indicate a testicular tumour
- Testosterone and luteinising hormone levels to demonstrate hypogonadism
- Thyroid function tests.

(b) What would make you concerned the patient may have a breast cancer?

Male breast cancer is responsible for 1% of all cases of breast cancer in the UK. Suspicious features include:

- Older age
- Unilateral gynaecomastia
- Firm or hard nodules within the breast tissue (the texture is normally rubbery or soft)
- Remember to examine the axillary and supraclavicular fossae for lymphadenopathy.

If in doubt, the patient should undergo triple assessment (see Case 64), including imaging and pathological evaluation.

Fuller Albright (1900–1969). Professor of Medicine, Harvard Medical School, who contributed a huge amount to the study of metabolic diseases.

Harry Fitch Klinefelter Jr (1912–1990). Associate Professor of Medicine at Johns Hopkins University – the syndrome in its full form is known as Klinefelter–Reifenstein–Albright syndrome.

E.C. Reifenstein also worked with Albright. Reifenstein syndrome is male pseudohermaphroditism.

FURTHER READING

Neuman JF: Evaluation and treatment of gynecomastia. *Am Fam Physician* 55(5):1835–1844, 1849–1850, 1997.

CASE 68 | CHEST – POST-LOBECTOMY/ PNEUMONECTOMY *

INSTRUCTION

'Examine this gentleman's respiratory system.'

APPROACH

Position the patient and begin to examine the chest as in Case 59, beginning with the hands, but expect that the examiner may move you directly on to examining the chest wall.

VITAL POINTS

Inspect

- Note the lateral thoracotomy scar over the chest wall – the scar begins at the sternal end of the fifth or sixth intercostal space and curves posteriorly and upwards, ending midway between the spine of the scapula and the thoracic vertebral spines
- Scars at the sites of chest drains may be present
- Muscle bulk over the side of the scar may be reduced as parts of serratus anterior and latissimus dorsi may have been removed.

Palpate

- The trachea is deviated away from the side of surgery
- Expansion will be reduced over the side of surgery.

Percuss

- Percussion note over the side of surgery is hyper-resonant.

Auscultate

- Breath sounds are harsher over the side of the pneumonectomy.

Finish your examination here

? QUESTIONS

(a) What are the indications for lung resections?

- 90% of lung resections in the Western world are performed for non-small-cell lung carcinoma
- Other indications include:
  - Traumatic injury
  - Bronchiectasis
  - Chronic infection, including tuberculosis
  - Benign tumours (e.g. carcinoid)
  - Metastatic tumours.

(b) What are the types of lung resection?

- Lobectomy is the excision of a single lobe of the lung
- Pneumonectomy is the excision of an entire lung
- Non-anatomical resections are often performed for traumatic injury
- Sleeve resection is the resection of a lobe including its bronchial origin with re-anastomosis of the proximal and distal bronchus.

? ADVANCED QUESTIONS

(a) What is the operative mortality for lung resections?

A retrospective study looked at 442 patients who had undergone lobectomy and pneumonectomy over an 18-year period (see Further Reading). The operative mortality for lobectomy was 7% and for pneumonectomy 12%, but no difference in long-term survival was detected. Techniques such as sleeve lobectomy and bronchoplasty have been developed as a result of the high operative mortality of pneumonectomy. Risk of operative mortality is higher with:

- Higher American Society of Anesthesiologists score (preoperative morbidity)
- Age >70 years
- Poor respiratory function, especially FEV_1/FVC ratio of <55%.

FURTHER READING

Ferguson MK, Karrison T: Does pneumonectomy for lung cancer adversely influence long-term survival? *J Thorac Cardiovasc Surg* 119(3):440–448, 2000.

Groenendijk RP, Croiset van Uchelen FA, Mol SJ, et al: Factors related to outcome after pneumonectomy: retrospective study of 62 patients. *Eur J Surg* 165(3):193–197, 1999.

CASE 69 | MEDIAN STERNOTOMY *

INSTRUCTION

'Examine this gentleman's chest.' (Fig. 2.47)

APPROACH

Expose the patient to examine the chest as in Case 59.

VITAL POINTS

Inspect

- The median sternotomy scar runs from the suprasternal notch vertically in the midline to the xiphisternum

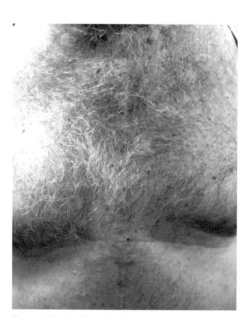

Figure 2.47 Median sternotomy.

- Subtotal median sternotomy involves an incision from the sternomanubrial junction to the fifth or sixth intercostal space.

Palpate

- Occasionally there is non-union of the two sides of the manubrium sternum, when a 'click' can be felt on palpation
- Unless there is comorbidity, the examiner wants you to pick up that the rest of the thoracic examination is likely to be normal.

Finish your examination here

? QUESTIONS

(a) What are the indications for median sternotomy?

- Emergency procedures, e.g. following penetrating chest trauma
- Cardiac surgery
- Resection of lung cancer.

There is some evidence that median sternotomy may be as efficient an approach to the lung as lateral thoracotomy (see Further Reading).

? ADVANCED QUESTIONS

(a) What are the principles of cardiopulmonary bypass?

- The aim of bypass is to provide a systemic circulation while the heart is stopped and emptied of blood (Fig. 2.48)
- Blood is drained by gravity from the right heart to a circuit where, after gas and temperature exchange, it is returned to the arterial side of the circulation

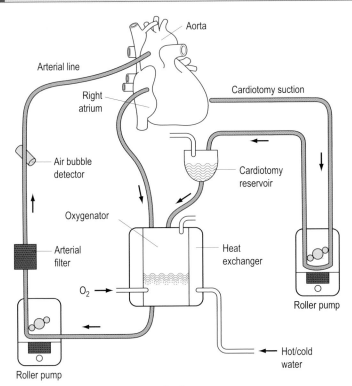

Figure 2.48 Components of a cardiopulmonary bypass circuit.

- The components of the perfusion circuit are:
  - An oxygenator: oxygen added and carbon dioxide removed from the blood
  - A heat exchanger: initially blood is cooled; later in the procedure it is warmed again
  - Cardiotomy suction: pericardial sump suckers return spilt blood to the circulation
  - Roller pump: returns blood to the aorta
  - Arterial line filter: removes debris and matter from the circulation.

(b) What are the major complications of bypass?

- Systemic activation of inflammatory mediators causes coagulopathy
- Cerebral damage due to ischaemia (1–2%)
- Microemboli, e.g. to kidneys, terminal arteries in limbs, retina.

FURTHER READING

Asaph JW, Handy JR Jr, Grunkemeier GL, et al: Median sternotomy versus thoracotomy to resect primary lung cancer: analysis of 815 cases. *Ann Thorac Surg* 70(2):373–379, 2000.

CASE 70 | TESTICULAR TUMOUR *

INSTRUCTION

'Examine this gentleman's scrotum.'

APPROACH

See Case 51.

VITAL POINTS

Inspect

The scrotum may look normal but often an enlarged testis is visible.

Palpate

The mass is:

- Usually inseparable from the testis
- Hard, irregular, nodular
- Non-tender
- Not transilluminable
- Distinct from the superficial inguinal ring (you can 'get above' the mass)

It may have an associated hydrocele and there may be some thickening of the spermatic cord due to malignant infiltration.

Finish your examination here

Completion

Say that you would like to:

- Examine the contralateral scrotum
- Continue to examine for abdominal lymphadenopathy
- Perform an examination of the abdomen (for hepatomegaly) and chest (for thoracic metastases).

? QUESTIONS

(a) What is the differential diagnosis?

- Testicular tumours can be mimicked by chronic or old infection leading to scarring, such as in orchitis or tuberculosis
- Occasionally a long-standing hydrocele may develop calcification and become harder, clinically similar to a tumour
- Tumours occasionally grow locally to become adherent to the inside of the scrotal skin; again, it is possible for a chronic hydrocele to mimic this, but the level of suspicion of a tumour would be high.

(b) How do testicular tumours usually present?

- The commonest presentation is a painless lump or a dull ache in one testis in a young man
- Occasionally there is a history of trauma accompanying the discovery of the mass
- 10% present with an acutely painful testis (which must be distinguished from a testicular torsion)
- If para-aortic nodes have become infiltrated with metastases, the patient may complain of back pain.

(c) How is a testicular tumour removed?

Through an inguinal approach, with early clamping of the testicular artery and vein within the spermatic cord before the testis is mobilised out of the scrotum – this prevents intraoperative seeding of tumour up the testicular vein.

? ADVANCED QUESTIONS

(a) What is the classification of testicular malignancies?

Almost all are seminomas or teratomas (Table 2.9); other types are:

- Embryonal carcinoma (arising from a very primitive germ cell)
- Choriocarcinoma
- Yolk sac tumour
- Leydig cell tumours – associated with gynaecomastia, but only 10% are malignant
- Sertoli cell tumours – also produce gynaecomastia
- Lymphoma – most commonly in patients who have generalised lymphoma elsewhere and is generally associated with a poor prognosis.

Table 2.9

	Teratoma	Seminoma
Age of presentation	20–30 years	30–40 years
Tumour markers	AFP and βhCG raised in 90%	Usually normal
Treatment of early disease	Chemotherapy (often only two cycles)	Radiotherapy to the para-aortic nodes + single dose of cisplatin
Treatment of advanced disease	Combination chemotherapy	Adjuvant chemotherapy, either single dose or in combination

AFP, α-fetoprotein; βhCG, β-human chorionic gonadotrophin.

Enrico Sertoli (1842–1910). Professor of Experimental Physiology, Milan.

Franz von Leydig (1821–1908). German histologist who first described the androgen-producing Leydig cell.

FURTHER READING

Dearnaley D, Huddart R, Horwich A: Regular review: managing testicular cancer. *BMJ* 322(7302):1583–1588, 2001.

Oliver RT: 2001 Testicular cancer. *Curr Opin Oncol* 13(3):191–198.

www.icr.ac.uk/everyman/about/testicular.html – guide to testicular self-examination for patients.

CASE 71   ENTEROCUTANEOUS FISTULA   *

INSTRUCTION

'Inspect this gentleman's abdomen and comment on what you can see.' (Fig. 2.49)

APPROACH

Expose the patient as in Case 43 and inspect the abdominal wall; do not begin with the hands, as you have been given a specific instruction to inspect the abdomen.

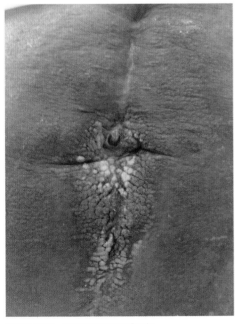

Figure 2.49   Enterocutaneous fistula.

VITAL POINTS

Inspect

Describe the appearance of the fistula:

- Site
- Size
- Discharge (fluid/solid/colour) – material may be bile or faeces
- Surrounding skin (may be damaged by irradiation, inflammatory bowel disease or chemical irritation from small intestine contents)

Describe the rest of the abdominal wall:

- Presence of recent scar; an anastomotic leak may have led to the fistula
- Previous surgery – especially for malignancy or inflammatory bowel disease
- Presence of a stoma, healed stoma or drain sites

Comment on any other 'clues' around the bed:

- General condition of the patient (anaemic, cachectic, etc.)
- Drips and parenteral nutrition
- Catheters/central venous pressure lines.

Finish your examination here

Completion

Say that you would like to:

- Examine the patient looking for an underlying aetiology (see below).

? QUESTIONS

(a) What is the definition of an enterocutaneous fistula?

- A fistula is an abnormal connection between two epithelial or endothelial surfaces
- An enterocutaneous fistula is an abnormal connection between the gastrointestinal tract and the skin.

(b) What is the aetiology of enterocutaneous fistulae?

Inflammation:

- Inflammatory bowel disease, especially Crohn's disease
- Diverticular disease
- Tuberculosis

Malignancy:

- Often following spontaneous rupture and abscess formation by the tumour

Radiotherapy:

- Pelvic irradiation can damage the intestine

Trauma:

- Penetrating wounds to the abdomen, especially involving the perforation of several separate loops of bowel with significant contamination and sepsis

Post-surgery:

- Anastomotic leak, often following primary anastomosis in contaminated conditions, e.g. sepsis or distal obstruction.

? ADVANCED QUESTIONS

(a) How may the anatomical locations of these fistulae be classified?

A high intestinal fistula involves the stomach, duodenum, jejunum or proximal ileum and results in high-volume fluid losses; a low fistula involves the distal ileum large intestine and fluid losses are lower in volume.

(b) What investigations are required?

Blood tests:

- Full blood count – anaemia may be caused by haemorrhage and sepsis raises white cell count
- Blood cultures should be taken prior to commencement of antibiotics
- Electrolytes, especially to check the patient is not severely hypokalaemic

- Inflammatory markers (C-reactive protein, erythrocyte sedimentation rate)
- Liver function tests – reduced albumin indicates malnutrition

Radiological investigations:

- Enhanced CT scanning with administration of oral contrast is the investigation of choice. This will (usually) reveal the site of the fistula within the bowel, whether there is distal progression of contrast beyond the fistula and whether there are any associated intra-abdominal collections or underlying pathology of the bowel
- A barium follow-through or enema (depending on the site) contrast study may provide additional information, but will not identify extraluminal collections
- A fistulogram is the injection of contrast material into the fistula opening in order to see (using screening) where the fistula connects to the bowel.

(c) What are the principles of treatment?

Early intervention to close fistulae should be avoided due to the high mortality due to sepsis, electrolyte imbalance and malnutrition. Therefore, non-operative therapy (see Top Tip, below) is favoured in the first instance, particularly as the majority will close spontaneously. In the absence of diseased bowel (inflammation/malignancy) or distal obstruction, the majority will close spontaneously within approximately 6 weeks. If it has not closed by 12 weeks, it is unlikely to do so and definitive surgery should be planned.

TOP TIP

☑ The acronym **SNAPP** summarises the principles of management of enterocutaneous fistulae:

- **S**epsis elimination: open or percutaneous drainage of collections; administration of appropriate antimicrobials
- **N**utritional resuscitation/optimisation: patients may be fluid- and electrolyte-depleted (losing litres of electrolyte-rich fluid through the fistula) and malnourished. Resuscite with intravenous fluid with supplementary potassium with careful monitoring and consideration for nutritional optimisation, which may involve parenteral administration
- **A**natomy: predominantly defined using radiological investigations (see above)
- **P**rotect surrounding skin from intestinal enzymes with stoma appliances
- **P**lan definitive surgery if remains unhealed

FURTHER READING

Berry SM, Fischer JE: Classification and pathophysiology of enterocutaneous fistulas. *Surg Clin North Am* 76(5):1009–1018, 1996.

Metcalf C: Enterocutaneous fistulae. *J Wound Care* 8(3):141–142, 1999.

CASE 72 | MOUTH SIGNS IN ABDOMINAL DISEASE *

INSTRUCTION

'Look inside this patient's mouth', or as part of 'Examine this gentleman's abdominal system.'

VITAL POINTS

Inspect

Abnormalities within the mouth can be grouped according to the appearances seen.

ABNORMAL PIGMENTATION

- Addison's disease: the mouth and lips are hyperpigmented
- Lichen planus: white lines and streaks inside the mouth
- Peutz–Jeghers disease: pigmented freckles around the lips and inside the mouth; associated with intestinal intussusception and gastrointestinal bleeding from colonic polyps. The patients have a higher incidence of concurrent gastrointestinal (stomach/pancreatic/colonic) and extragastrointestinal (breast/gonad) malignancy
- Hereditary telangiectasia (Rendu–Osler–Weber disease): multiple telangiectasia (clusters of dilated capillaries and venules) around the mouth and on the tongue and lips; associated with gastrointestinal bleeding due to arteriovenous malformations; a group of clustered autosomal-dominant conditions
- Acanthosis nigricans: black discoloration of the skin, associated with carcinoma of the stomach and oesophagus, lymphomas and with endocrine disorders (acromegaly, Cushing's, diabetes complicated by severe insulin resistance).

ULCERATION

- Aphthous ulcers are small, round and shallow, and have a shallow yellow base with surrounding erythema; they are common in childhood and are associated with infection and minor trauma to the oral cavity. In inflammatory bowel disease and coeliac disease, the ulcers tend to be more persistent and much larger; in Crohn's disease, the mouth takes on a 'cobblestone' appearance due to frequent ulceration, healing with some fibrosis
- Behçet's disease: a rare autoimmune disease most common in young men, causing a triad of genital and oral ulceration and anterior uveitis
- Herpes simplex: small vesicles with an erythematous base on the lips and inside of the mouth; diagnosed with scrapings of the base of the lesions and usually responsive to topical acyclovir.

LIP DISORDERS

- Angular stomatitis: chapping and splitting of the corners of the lips is normal, but can also occur in:
  - Herpes simplex and candidal infections
  - Iron, folate, vitamin B and C deficiencies.

INFECTIONS

- Herpes simplex causes both stomatitis and ulceration (see above)
- Oral candidiasis is the most common abnormality; it causes creamy white patches that may be rubbed off, and may be seen in:
  - Patients prescribed inhaled steroids for the treatment of asthma and chronic obstructive airways disease (the patient information leaflet advises patients to wash their mouths out after using these inhalers)
  - Oral antibiotic use
  - Immunocompromised patients, including those who are diabetic, and those on oral steroids.

Sir William Osler (1849–1919). Tremendously significant medical educator, who was Professor of Medicine at Johns Hopkins and Oxford Universities, and was responsible for the formation of the Association of Physicians of Great Britain and Northern Ireland, and for setting up full-time chairmen of medicine in London hospitals.

Thomas Addison (1793–1860). Physician at Guys Hospital, who was by reputation an excellent diagnostician and lecturer. Known as the founder of endocrinology.

Halushi Behçet (1889–1948). Turkish dermatologist.

Harald Jos Jeghers. Professor of Medicine, New Jersey College of Medicine and Dentistry, Jersey City.

Frederick Parkes Weber (1863–1962). London physician.

John Law Augustine Peutz (1886–1957). Dutch physician; Chief of Internal Medicine, St John's Hospital, The Hague.

Henry Jules Louis Marie Rendu (1844–1902). Parisian physician.

Harvey Williams Cushing (1869–1939). 'The founder of neurosurgery' and Professor of Surgery, Harvard.

CASE 73 | EPIGASTRIC HERNIA *

INSTRUCTION

'Examine this gentleman's abdomen.'

APPROACH

Expose the patient and begin to examine as for Case 43.

VITAL POINTS

Inspect

- When you ask the patient to lift his head off the bed, a lump may appear in the epigastric region, in the midline
- Ask him to cough and see if this lump becomes more prominent in the abdominal wall.

Palpate

- Palpate the area of the hernia carefully
- It can be very difficult to find the hernia; ask the patient to help by again lifting his head off the bed and coughing
- Try to identify the borders of the defect and the size of the neck.

TOP TIP

☑ If there is no scar but there is a longitudinal bulging of the abdominal wall in the midline when the patient lifts his head off the bed or coughs, consider *divarication of the recti.*

Finish your examination here

Completion

Say that you would like to:

- Complete the rest of the abdominal examination.

? QUESTIONS

(a) What is an epigastric hernia?

An abnormal protrusion of abdominal contents (usually extraperitoneal fat, but occasionally peritoneal contents) through a defect in the linea alba, usually halfway between the xiphoid process and umbilicus.

(b) What symptoms might the patient have complained of at presentation?

The symptoms are commonly confused with other upper gastrointestinal pathologies and include:

- Epigastric pain, which may increase after meals
- May be acutely painful after physical exercise
- Nausea and early satiety
- Reflux and non-ulcer dyspepsia.

? ADVANCED QUESTIONS

(a) How would you treat this patient?

Non-surgical:

The same principles as when managing an incisional hernia (see Case 47) would apply. The patient may present with non-specific upper gastrointestinal symptoms; it is particularly important that other causes are considered and ruled out; possible investigations would include:

- Liver function tests and a biliary tree ultrasound scan
- *Helicobacter pylori* serology and upper gastrointestinal endoscopy

Surgical:

- The principles of surgery are that the sac is excised completely or inverted, and the defect in the linea alba repaired
- The fat contained within the hernia can be excised or reduced

- The site of the defect should be marked with the patient lying supine preoperatively, as it may not be possible to find when the patient is anaesthetised.

FURTHER READING

Coats RD, Helikson MA, Burd RS: Presentation and management of epigastric hernias in children. *J Pediatr Surg* 35(12):1754–1756, 2001.

www.surgerydoor.co.uk – patient-centred information on how to prepare for over a hundred common operations.

CASE 74 | FEMORAL HERNIA *

INSTRUCTION

'Examine this lady's groin.' (Fig. 2.50)

APPROACH

Expose the patient as for the inguinal hernia examination (see Case 42), remembering to examine her lying down if she is presented on a couch, and standing up if she is sitting in a chair (see Top Tips boxes in Case 42).

VITAL POINTS

These cases are seen only infrequently in the clinical examination as they are often repaired surgically due to the risk of complication. It is important to know the essential differences from an inguinal hernia and the differential diagnosis of a lump in the groin.

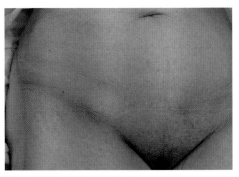

Figure 2.50 Right femoral hernia.

Inspect

- There may be a marble-shaped lump in the groin
- There may be a scar from previous surgery.

Palpate

- Identify the anterior superior iliac spine and the pubic tubercle, demonstrating the inguinal ligament between the two (see Case 42)
- Femoral herniae are found below the inguinal ligament (Fig. 2.51) – compared with inguinal herniae, which lie above (Fig. 2.2)
- Palpate the femoral pulse – the lump lies medial to the pulse (Fig. 2.52)
- Ask the patient to cough – femoral herniae usually do not have a cough impulse
- Ask the patient if she can push the lump back – femoral herniae are usually irreducible
- Ask if there is any pain and palpate the lump for the characteristic features of a femoral hernia:
  - Shape: usually round
  - Surface: smooth
  - Edge: well defined
  - Consistency: firm
  - Temperature: same as surrounding skin
  - Tenderness: may or may not be tender
  - Transilluminability: not transilluminable
  - Pulsatility: not pulsatile
  - Compressibility: not compressible
  - Fluctuance: not fluctuant.

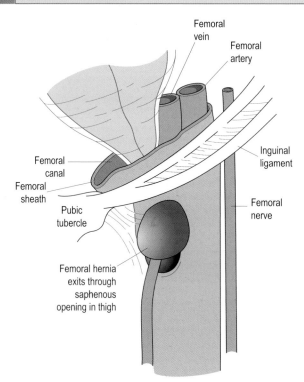

Figure 2.51 Femoral hernia.

Femoral
vein

Femoral
artery

Inguinal
ligament

Femoral
canal

Femoral
sheath

Femoral
nerve

Pubic
tubercle

Femoral hernia
exits through
saphenous
opening in thigh

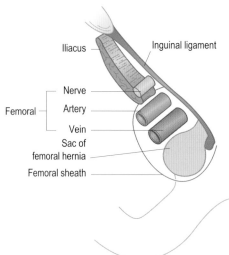

Iliacus

Inguinal ligament

Nerve

Femoral — Artery

Vein

Sac of
femoral hernia

Femoral sheath

Figure 2.52 NAVY acronym for arrangement of femoral structures (**N**erve, **A**rtery, **V**ein, **Y**-fronts).

Finish your examination here

Completion

Say that you would like to:

- Examine the contralateral groin for herniae.

Table 2.10

Inguinal hernia	Femoral hernia
Above the inguinal ligament	Below the inguinal ligament
Usually reducible	Usually not reducible
M:F – 6:1	M:F – 1:2 (but note inguinal herniae are still commoner in women than femoral herniae)
Risk of strangulation low	Risk of strangulation high
Cough impulse present	Cough impulse usually absent

? QUESTIONS

(a) How can you tell this lump is a femoral hernia (rather than an inguinal hernia)?
See Table 2.10.

(b) What is the differential diagnosis for a femoral hernia?

Skin and soft-tissue masses:

- Sebaceous cyst
- Lipoma
- Sarcoma

Vascular masses:

- Saphena varix
- Femoral aneurysm
- Inguinal lymphadenopathy

Other herniae:

- Inguinal hernia
- Obturator hernia (rarely actually palpable)

Others:

- Psoas bursa
- Ectopic testis.

Use the acronym **L-SHAPE** (see Case 42) to help remember these causes:

- **L**ymph node/**L**ipoma of the cord
- **S**aphenovarix/**S**kin lesions (sebaceous cyst/lipoma, etc.)
- **H**ernia: inguinal/femoral
- **A**neurysmal dilatation of the femoral artery
- **P**soas abscess/bursa
- **E**ctopic/undescended testis.

? ADVANCED QUESTIONS

(a) What are the surgical options for management of a femoral hernia?

The surgical principles are:

- Reduction of the contents of the sac
- Excision of the sac
- Repair of the defect – taking care not to narrow the femoral vein while tightening up the femoral canal (Fig. 2.1)

Possible surgical techniques are:

- Low approach (Lockwood) (easiest and most commonly used for elective repair):
  - An incision is made directly over the hernia, below the medial half of the inguinal ligament
  - The sac is ligated and the femoral canal closed with non-absorbable sutures or a plug
  - Best option for elective procedures but risk of narrowing the femoral vein when closing the femoral canal

- Transinguinal (Lotheissen) repair:
  - The posterior wall of the inguinal canal is opened to access the femoral canal from above
  - Best approach if the nature of the hernia is uncertain as inguinal hernias can also be repaired
  - Recurrent inguinal hernias are common
- High approach (McEvedy):
  - Involves a transverse incision above the inguinal ligament and dissection to expose the preperitoneal space
  - Conversion to a Pfannenstiel incision allows repair of bilateral hernia
  - Useful for repair in the emergency setting as it allows inspection of the peritoneal contents (bowel) with easy conversion to laparotomy if bowel resection is necessary
  - The femoral canal can be closed from above without breaching the peritoneum.
- Laparoscopic approach – increasingly, femoral hernias are being addressed via the transabdominal preperitoneal (TAPP) repair or totally extraperitoneal (TEP) repair with placement of synthetic mesh across the femoral (and inguinal) hernia orifices.

FURTHER READING

Chammary VL: Femoral hernia: intestinal obstruction is an unrecognised source of morbidity and mortality. *Br J Surg* 80(2):230–232, 1993.

Cheek CM, Black NA, Devlin HB, et al: Groin hernia surgery: a systematic review. *Ann R Coll Surg Engl* 80(Suppl 1):S1–S80, 1998 (meta-analysis of results from hernia surgery in the UK).

www.nlm.nih.gov/medlineplus/ency/article/001136.htm#treatment – patient-focused discussion of the causes and treatments of femoral hernia.

CASE 75 | DIGITAL RECTAL EXAMINATION *

INSTRUCTION

'Perform a digital rectal examination on this patient.'

APPROACH

Clearly, you will not be asked to perform a digital rectal examination (DRE) on a patient in an examination; neither should you attempt to. However, DRE simulators are widely available and are increasingly being used in examinations. Additionally, you should be competent performing this important exam in everyday clinical practice, so the description that follows in the remainder of this case will focus on the 'real-life' clinical scenario. These principles should be extrapolated to DRE simulators in exam situations.

TOP TIP

☑ Assemble everything you need *before* you begin exposing / examining the patient and have within easy reach as you start the examination. Essential items include: a light source (see below); non-sterile examination gloves; lubricating jelly (preferably sachets rather than a tube); and soft tissues to wipe away excess lubricant at the end of the exam.

You should only perform this examination if a chaperone is present and state this in simulated situations in exams. Assemble the essential items (see above); in simulated scenarios in the exam you should state what is required to perform the exam. Building rapport is crucial in this (and other) intimate examinations. Introduce yourself, explain the procedure and obtain consent to proceed. As detailed below, the inspection phase is extremely important and nearly always comprised / completely omitted in the clinical scenario. With this in mind, you should always ensure that you have additional lighting available when performing the examination; especially behind drawn curtains at the bedside. Ideally, a mobile examination light positioned at the foot-end of the patient will help ensure that you will not miss important signs during the inspection stage of the examination; at the very least, ask your chaperone to shine a bright torch if a mobile light is not available.

The preferred position for examination is the left lateral position and not the 'bent-over' or 'all-fours' position that is often adopted in the USA. As always, stand and examine from the right side of the bed. Elevate the bed to a suitable height to optimise your comfort during the examination. Ask the patient to remove all lower garments beneath the waist, whilst you cover the patient with a sheet or blanket. Next, ask the patient to roll away from you to lie on his / her left side on the bed and to bring the knees up towards the chest. Whilst keeping the hips flexed, ask the patient to move the feet forward so that you have good access to the perineum and anus (Fig. 2.53). Only at this point are you ready to uncover the lower half of the patient, exposing the perineum.

TOP TIP

☑ As with most clinical examinations, refrain from touching / moving the patient to position / expose him or her, unless it is quite obvious that help is required or requested. Instead, concentrate on providing clear, explicit instruction about which garments need to be removed and how you would like the patient to position him/herself. Otherwise, you may end up wrestling with, rather than helping, the patient.

☑ Correct positioning of the patient is critical in maximising patient comfort and clinical information obtained by the clinician. Ask the patient to roll away from you to lie on his / her left side on the bed and to shuffle the bottom towards you / the edge of the bed whilst moving the head away from you / the edge towards the other side of the bed. The aim is for the patient to end up laying at an angle to the long axis of the bed.

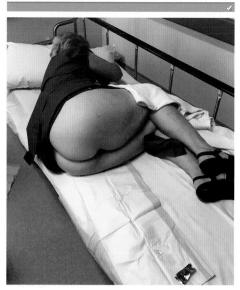

Figure 2.53 Patient position for digital rectal examination.

VITAL POINTS

TOP TIP

THE RULE OF THREES APPLIES TO DIGITAL RECTAL EXAMINATION (DRE)

☑ There are three components to the examination – the first two of which are often suboptimally performed or even completely omitted. As with all clinical examinations, DRE begins with inspection and palpation:

- Part 1: Inspection of the perineum and perianal region
- Part 2: Palpation of the perineum and perianal region
- Part 3: Digital examination of the anorectum

☑ There are also three components to each of these three parts (see below).

Inspect

Part 1 involves very careful examination of the anus and perineum and is often performed suboptimally. You will need to part the buttocks gently to facilitate thorough inspection of the perianal region, particularly in men and obese patients. With a gloved hand on each buttock, very gently but deliberately 'walk' from the buttocks towards the anal canal so that each hand is positioned on either side of the anal canal and gently part the buttocks.

Abnormalities may be very subtle, emphasising the need for adequate lighting. There are three important components to inspection, all beginning with **S**:

- **S**kin: assess the perineal / perianal skin, noting the presence of erythema (abscess formation / sepsis); excoriation (from irritation from scratching or mucus / faecal leakage); and other dermatoses
- **S**igns of proctological abnormalities: is there evidence of skin tags (Fig. 2.54), external haemorrhoids (Fig. 2.55), fissures (Fig. 2.56), external openings of fistulae (Fig. 2.57); when all are present be suspicious of Crohn's disease (Fig. 2.58). Also note evidence of scars from previous anal surgery.
- **S**tate of the anus: the anal canal is normally closed at rest, and a patulous anus usually indicates gross neuromuscular dysfunction.

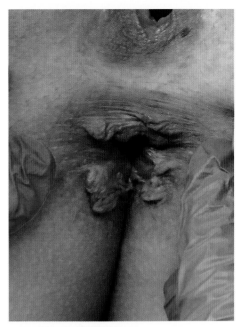

Figure 2.54   Perianal skin tags.

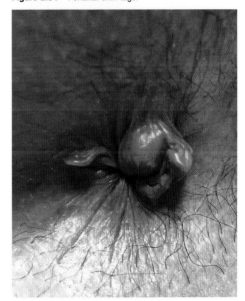

Figure 2.55   External haemorrhoids.

TOP TIP

☑ Abnormalities are described anatomically according to the clock face, where 12 o'clock is anterior towards the scrotum in men or vaginal fourchette in women and 6 o'clock is posterior towards the coccyx. Naturally, when the patient is in the left lateral position, the clock face is 'rotated' 90°, meaning that 9 o'clock is the position pointing towards the ceiling and 12 o'clock is actually in line with the patient's legs towards the feet (Figure 2.59).

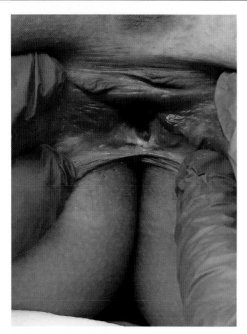

Figure 2.56   Anal fissure.

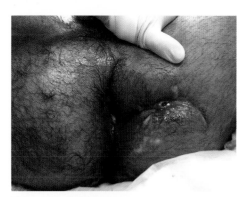

Figure 2.57   Fistula-in-ano.

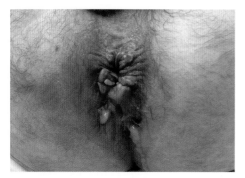

Figure 2.58   Perianal Crohn's disease.

In specific clinical scenarios (e.g. suspected cauda equina syndrome), formal neurological examination of saddle sensation in the sacral dermatomes should be formally evaluated and the anocutaneous reflex tested by stroking the perianal skin with a cotton bud in each quadrant.

DIGITAL PALPATION

Part 2 involves gentle digital palpation of the perineum and perianal region and is often overlooked. As with examination of the abdomen, it is important to evaluate the perineum and perianal region for tenderness by performing systematic digital palpation. There are three components to this part of the examination. Palpation of the:

- Ischiorectal region: apply gentle digital pressure with your index finger, beginning laterally at each ischial tuberosity and working systematically towards the perianal region to determine whether there is any tenderness, suggestive of an underlying ischiorectal abscess
- Perianal region: again, apply gentle digital pressure with your index finger in systematic fashion in the four quadrants immediately surrounding the anus to determine whether there is any tenderness, suggestive of a perianal abscess
- Anus: position each index finger of both hands close to the anal verge on either side anteriorly and gently roll your fingers apart to flatten / separate the folds created by the corrugator (cutis ani) muscle and forwards to evert the anal mucosa to allow inspection of the anal verge and the distal anal canal just inside the anus (Fig. 2.59). Repeat the same manoeuvre posteriorly at 6 o'clock to exclude a posterior fissure.

TOP TIP

☑ Do *not* apply any lubrication to your finger or the patient until inspection / palpation is complete, otherwise your hands will be too slippery to achieve adequate separation of the buttocks / anal canal in the above manoeuvres.

☑ However, if do you identify perineal / perianal abnormalities, the application of lubricant to the gloved index finger and skin allows more informative evaluation of the tissues. This is especially true when evaluating a fistula-in-ano, when a lubricated finger will be able to detect the fistula tract running subcutaneously towards the anal verge as a 'thickened cord-like' structure.

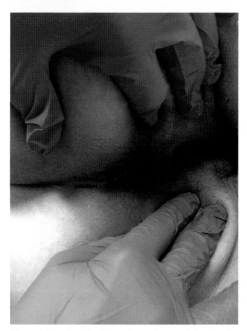

Figure 2.59   Examination of the anal verge / distal anal canal for anal fissures.

DIGITAL EXAMINATION

Part 3 involves digitation of the anal canal and rectum and is the part of the examination that most doctors are familiar with. Indeed, most begin the DRE at this point having omitted the preceding two stages, frequently resulting in failure to detect important pathology / signs.

TOP TIP

☑ You must move slowly during all parts of the digital rectal examination, especially the internal digital examination. Communication is crucial and get used to talking your patients through each part of the examination, explaining what to expect next rather than leaving them to be surprised by the rapid, unexpected insertion of your finger into their anal canal!

☑ Considering the anatomy of the anal canal and rectum is crucial to ensure gentle and effective conduct of the digital component of the examination. Of particular importance is consideration of the direction of the structures to be examined:

- The anal canal is directed from the anus towards the umbilicus
- The anal canal joins the distal rectum at a 90° angle – the anorectal junction to protect continence
- The rectum follows the curvature of the sacrum

Consequently, once gently inserted, the examining finger is first directed towards the umbilicus, followed by an abrupt 90° direction change posteriorly towards the patient's sacrum to allow examination of the rectum.

If not already applied during digital palpation of the perineum / perianal region, ensure that you apply adequate amounts of lubricating jelly to the gloved index finger of your right hand and to the anus itself. Whilst retracting the patient's right buttock with your left hand, hold your right index finger gently against the anus for a second or two, so that you avoid taking the patient by surprise and causing the patient to contract the anal sphincter involuntarily. Direct your finger towards the patient's umbilicus. Once again there are three objectives during this part of the examination:

- Anal canal: take time to feel slowly and circumferentially inside the anal canal, along its full length. The anal canal is approximately 3–5 cm long, but is shorter in females than males. It should be smooth with no palpable lesions / irregularities. Pause to feel the U-shaped ring of muscle posterior-laterally formed by the puborectalis 'sling', before proceeding above it to the rectum
- Rectal mucosa: the aim is to detect any masses of the rectum, specifically of the rectal mucosa. Systematically and carefully examine the entire surface of the rectal mucosa that is within reach for abnormalities. Usually, only the lowest few centimetres of the rectum, 6–8 cm from the anal verge, are within reach. Be careful to ensure that you have adequately reached and examined the rectum. In certain situations, such as patients with large, obese buttocks and / or men with long anal canals, it will not be possible to reach the actual rectum, particularly if you have short fingers. Documenting this situation is important, as a rectal examination has *not* been performed. Detection of mucosal abnormalities demands further visual evaluation with rigid / flexible sigmoidoscopy / colonoscopy. The presence of faeces / blood should be noted by inspecting the examining finger after withdrawal.
- Pelvic organs: finally, focus on palpating the pelvic structures through the rectal wall. Anteriorly, the prostate in men and the cervix / uterus in women are palpable and should be examined for abnormalities, especially irregularities in the surface of these structures. Slightly more laterally,

enlarged ovaries will be palpable in women. Finish by examining posteriorly to ensure there are no pre-sacral masses.

Finish your examination here

Completion

Say that you would like to:

- Perform a procto-sigmoidoscopic examination if you detect any abnormalities during the DRE.

? QUESTIONS

(a) Can anal fissures be seen on inspection of the anus?

Anal fissures are small tears in the mucosa that lines the anal canal and usually affect the lower third anteriorly or posteriorly (in other locations, there is increased suspicion that they are secondary to pathological processes, e.g. Crohn's disease / infection with herpes simplex virus). Consequently, they do not occur on the perianal skin. As the anus is closed at rest, it is not usually possible to observe the anal mucosa and thus identify fissures. However, gentle separation of the anus will allow inspection of the distal anal canal and identification of fissures. Additionally, the presence of a sentinel pile on inspection raises the possibility that it is 'guarding' (sentinel: from the Latin – a guard) a fissure within the anal canal. Failure to perform this manoeuvre will result in missing a fissure-in-ano.

(b) Are haemorrhoids palpable on DRE?

Haemorrhoids are abnormal vascular structures arising from the anal canal and represent pathological dilatation of the physiological vascular cushions that contribute to the maintenance of continence. When they arise above the dentate line (demarcating the transition from glandular, columnar epithelium of the rectum to squamous epithelium of the anal canal) they are known as internal haemorrhoids and below, external haemorrhoids.

Uncomplicated haemorrhoids are not palpable during digital examination, as they will be emptied of blood under the pressure generated by insertion of a finger into the anal canal. However, if they are complicated by thrombosis and / or prolapse they may be detectable. Similarly, prolapsed external haemorrhoids are visible on inspection of the perianal region (Fig. 2.55) (see part 1 of the DRE, above).

Haemorrhoids are most reliably detected during proctoscopy.

CASE 76 ORTHOPAEDIC HISTORY TAKING – GENERAL APPROACH ***

INSTRUCTION

'Ask this patient some questions about her painful hip.'

APPROACH

In orthopaedics, the key elements of history taking are:

- Pain
- Loss of function
- Stiffness
- Deformity
- Swelling.

VITAL POINTS

Introduction

- Ask the patient's age
- Ask her occupation
- Ask about hand dominance (for upper-limb cases)
- Ask which joints are symptomatic.

Pain

- Site: remembering that superficial pain tends to be recognised at the site but pain may be referred, so pain from the hip may radiate to the groin, anterior thigh, knee or shin
- Intensity: such as a pain severity score, where the patient allocates a mark out of 10 for the pain
- Frequency: early-morning pain is a hallmark of inflammation; pain that is relieved at night and by rest is often mechanical in nature; night pain is a very important symptom, as it indicates severe pain and may also raise suspicion of an underlying malignant process
- Analgesic requirements.

Loss of function

- Impact on patient's life, e.g. activities of daily living, work, sleep, sporting activities.

Lower limb (general):

- Going to the shops
- Use of walking aids, e.g. walking stick(s), Zimmer frame, crutches

- Walking distance (ask the patient how long or far she can walk before stopping because of her specific joint problem)
- Use of stairs

Upper limb (general):

- Feeding, washing, dressing, brushing hair, writing

Specific to the spine:

- History of injury
- Radiation of pain – particularly looking for dermatomal distribution
- Associated neurological symptoms (e.g. numbness or paraesthesia) and their distribution – the two nerve roots most commonly involved in lumbar disc prolapse are shown in Table 3.1.
- Sphincter disturbance – bladder and bowel symptoms secondary to cauda equina compression (unlikely to be present in patients used for examination purposes)

Specific to the hip:

- Assess the stiffness and pain arising from the hip joint
- Ask specifically about ability to:
  - Care for her feet/pedicure
  - Get in and out of the bath
  - Get in and out of a car

Specific to the knee:

- Locking of the knee is an intermittent inability to extend the knee fully and suggests a mechanical block – 'Does your knee ever get stuck when you are trying to straighten it?'
- Giving way – a sign of a patellofemoral problem, loose body, meniscal flap tear or ligamentous laxity – 'Does your knee ever give way when you walk?'

Specific to the feet:

- Ask the patient about back pain (pain on the sole of the foot may be due to an L5/S1 disc prolapse)
- Pins and needles may be due to lumbar spine pathology, nerve entrapment (such as tarsal tunnel syndrome, which is caused by a posterior tibial nerve palsy) or peripheral neuropathy
- Pain present when the patient is barefoot is suggestive of metatarsalgia

Table 3.1

Prolapsed disc	Involved nerve root	Distribution of sensory symptoms	Distribution of motor signs	Involved reflexes
L4/L5	L5	Lateral aspect of the leg and dorsum of the foot	Weakness of big-toe extension and ankle dorsiflexion	None
L5/S1	S1	Lateral aspect of the foot and heel	Weakness of ankle plantarflexion and foot eversion	Ankle jerk

- Ask about the patient's shoes – does she have to have special footwear?

Stiffness

- Distinguish between early-morning stiffness (suggestive of an inflammatory condition) and stiffness following activity (suggestive of a mechanical condition).

Deformity

- As fixed deformities develop, patients (or their friends or family) may notice a change in shape of their spine or lower limbs.

Swelling

- May be noticed by patients in superficial joints (such as the hip and ankle)
- Enquire as to whether the swelling is permanent or transient (e.g. following injury)
- Is there an inflammatory component, e.g. erythema?

Past medical history

- This essentially refers to fitness for surgery/ contraindications to anaesthesia and the presence of other underlying diseases
- A rapid family history and allergies check can also be performed here.

CASE 77 | OSTEOARTHRITIS OF THE HIP ***

INSTRUCTION

'Examine this gentleman's right hip.'

APPROACH

- Expose the patient's legs but allow him to keep his underwear on. However, if the patient has long shorts on, be sure to lift them in the area of the lateral thigh to check for scars.
- This examination should be divided clearly into:
  - Examining with the patient standing
  - Watching the patient walk
  - Examining with the patient supine.

VITAL POINTS

Examining with the patient standing (looking from the front, then the side and finally the back)

- Comment on the presence of any walking aids

- Look at the hip for scars or sinuses – look particularly for lateral and posterior scars, which are the two most common surgical approaches to the hip
- Look for muscle wasting (particularly the gluteal muscles)
- Look from the side at the patient's posture – increased lumbar lordosis may indicate a fixed flexion deformity at the hip
- Look from the back at the spine – scoliosis may indicate a fixed adduction deformity
- Turn the patient back to face you and perform the Trendelenburg test with the patient standing. It can help to ask the patient to mirror your actions in order to explain what the patient needs to do.

Trendelenburg test (Fig. 3.1)

Ask the patient to stand on his good leg and flex the other leg at the knee as you face him and place your hands on his pelvis, while he places his hands on your shoulders (this allows you to feel what happens to the patient's pelvis

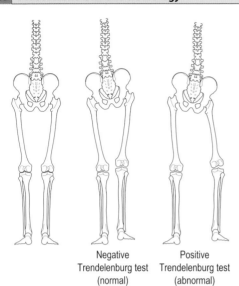

Negative   Positive
Trendelenburg test   Trendelenburg test
(normal)   (abnormal)

Figure 3.1 Trendelenburg test.

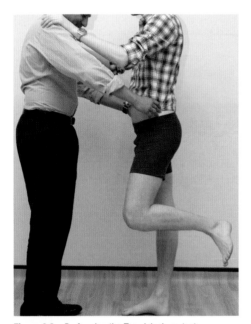

Figure 3.2 Performing the Trendelenburg test.

during the test and how the patient responds with respect to weight transfer). This manoeuvre is then repeated on the bad leg. The test is positive if the pelvis on the unsupported side (i.e. the side where the knee is flexed) sags down (Fig. 3.2). A positive Trendelenburg test typically occurs in patients with hip abductor weakness – this can be due to chronic hip pain, multiple surgeries, underlying structural abnormalities such as developmental

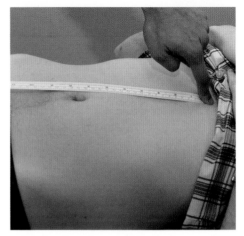

Figure 3.3 Measuring apparent leg length from a fixed midline bony point (the xiphisternum).

hip dysplasia, or neuromuscular diseases such as polio.

A positive Trendelenburg lurch may be also seen in the patient – he throws the upper part of his body over the affected hip in order to compensate for his loss of balance due to the pelvic dip on the contralateral side.

Watching the patient walk

- Begin by asking the patient to stand in front of you
- Watch the patient walk (see Case 94) – ask him to walk away from you and then back towards you; look specifically for:
  - A Trendelenburg gait, due to abductor weakness (Fig. 3.1) – characterised by the presence of a sideways lurch of the trunk to bring the patient's body weight over the affected limb
  - An antalgic gait (due to pain) – decreased stance phase and increased swing phase.

Examining with the patient lying down

- Ask the patient to lie on the couch
- Measure the real and apparent leg lengths using a tape measure – this is a difficult concept but you may be asked about it in the examination
- In both cases, the 'good' leg should be measured first, then the abnormal leg, comparing one side with the other
- The apparent leg length is measured from the xiphisternum (a fixed midline bony point) (Fig. 3.3) to the medial malleolus (Fig. 3.4),

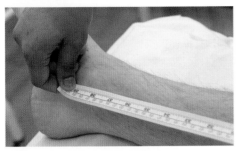

Figure 3.4 Measuring apparent leg length to a fixed bony point (the medial malleolus).

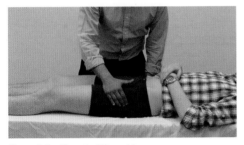

Figure 3.5 'Squaring' the pelvis.

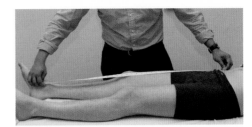

Figure 3.6 Measuring real leg length.

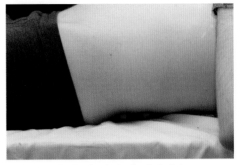

Figure 3.7 Feeling for the lumbar lordosis in Thomas' test.

while the patient is lying supine with the legs parallel. With a fixed adduction deformity of the hip, the apparent leg length will be shorter on the affected side, while with a fixed abduction deformity, the apparent leg length will be greater (remembering that you are measuring from the leg to a fixed midline point)

- Now ensure that the patient is 'square' on the couch; in other words, that he is lying with his pelvis at 90° to the body's long axis (Fig. 3.5). If you are unable to square the pelvis, 'correct' the deformity by placing the normal leg in the same position as the abnormal leg. The real leg length is measured from the anterior superior iliac spine to the medial malleolus of the ipsilateral ankle (Fig. 3.6). If the measurement is different between the two legs, it is due to a 'real' difference in the length of the bones. Real leg length discrepancies can be:
  - In the femur, either above the greater trochanter (i.e. in the hip joint) or below it
  - Above or below the knee
- A quicker screen for leg length discrepancy (and one we would recommend for the clinical examination) is Galeazzi's test. Flex both knees to 90°, ensure the heels are together and assess the position of the tibial tuberosities. If the tibial tuberosity of the shorter leg lies distal and inferior when

looking from the side, the tibia is shorter. If it lies proximal and inferior, the femur is shorter.

Palpate

- With the patient still supine, feel over the greater trochanter for any tenderness (trochanteric bursitis)
- Remember that the joint itself is deep and that the femoral head can only be palpated with deep pressure over the midpoint of the inguinal ligament (see Case 42) – this may be uncomfortable for the patient and usually does not add further information.

Thomas' test for fixed flexion deformity

- This measures a loss of extension at the hip (fixed flexion deformity)
- Begin by placing one hand in the small of the patient's back (Fig. 3.7), feeling for the lumbar lordosis and assisting him to flex his good hip as far as possible, feeling for flattening of the lumbar lordosis (Fig. 3.8)
- Maintain flexion in one hip (ask the patient to hold on to the knee) while asking the patient to flex the other hip as far as possible (Fig. 3.9) and then to extend it. By

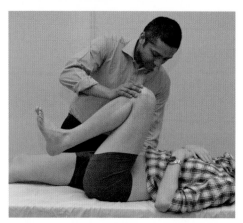

Figure 3.8 Flexing the good hip while feeling for obliteration of the lumbar lordosis.

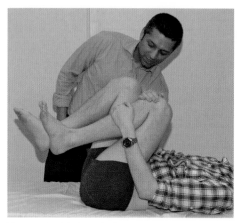

Figure 3.9 Ask the patient to hold on to the good hip while flexing the affected hip.

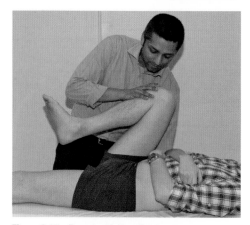

Figure 3.10 Repeat with the other leg.

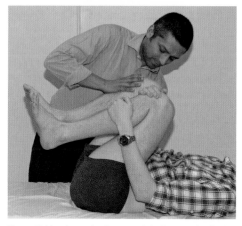

Figure 3.11 Assessing how much further passive flexion can be obtained from the affected hip.

maintaining the flexion of the other hip, the lumbar lordosis is obliterated
- In the presence of any fixed flexion deformity, there will be a point at which further extension ceases and the residual flexion (i.e. fixed flexion) can be measured from the horizontal
- Repeat with the other leg (Fig. 3.10)
- These movements can also be combined with measuring range of movement of the hips in a 'cycling' manoeuvre and passive and active flexion can also be assessed by asking the patient to flex the hip actively as much as possible and then assessing how much further flexion is possible passively (Figs 3.8–3.11). Figure 3.12 diagrammatically summarises Thomas' test.

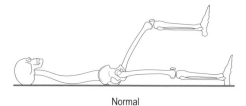

Normal

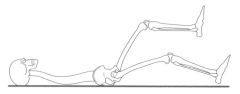

Positive Thomas test:
fixed flexion deformity in right hip

Figure 3.12 Thomas' test.

Movements of the hip

Carefully watch the patient's face at all times during this examination and be sure to ask the patient to tell you if there is any discomfort before attempting any passive joint movements.

- Assess each muscle group in turn, remembering that the movements of the hip are flexion/extension, abduction/adduction and internal/external rotation (Table 3.2)
- Flexion has already been assessed during Thomas' test
- Extension can only be assessed by turning the patient prone (as this is time consuming, say that you would assess the patient prone normally and the examiner will often let you move on to testing other movements)
- Ask the patient to straighten the leg and, with the hip fully extended, measure abduction and adduction. Detect any tilting of the pelvis by placing one hand on one of the anterior superior iliac spines (it is best simply to feel the spine which is furthest away from the hip being assessed) (Figs 3.13 and 3.14)
- Bring the hip back to 90° of flexion, at right angles to the couch. Keeping the knees flexed, measure internal and external rotation (Figs 3.15 and 3.16)
- You can also measure internal and external rotation with the knee in extension by comparing movements of the patella (Figs 3.17 and 3.18).

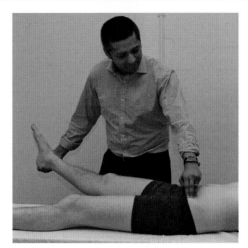

Figure 3.13 Testing hip abduction.

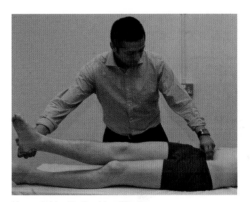

Figure 3.14 Testing hip adduction.

Table 3.2 Movements of the hip

Hip movement	Muscle group	Expected movement
Flexion	Iliopsoas, rectus femoris, tensor fasciae latae, quadriceps	140°
Extension	Gluteus maximus and hamstrings	10°
Abduction	Gluteus medius and minimus	45°
Adduction	Adductors (longus, brevis, magnus)	30°
Internal rotation	Gluteus medius, minimus, iliopsoas	40°
External rotation	Gluteus maximus	40°

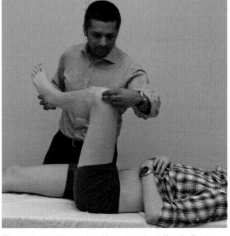

Figure 3.15 Measuring hip external rotation in flexion.

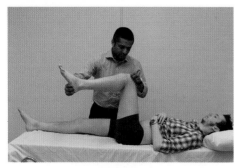

Figure 3.16 Measuring hip internal rotation in flexion.

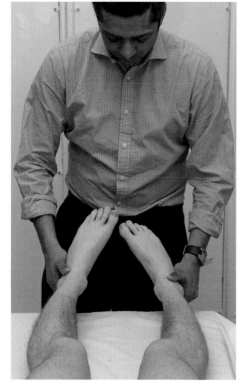

Figure 3.17 Measuring hip internal rotation in extension.

Finish your examination here

Completion

Say that you would like to:

• Examine the back and knee (the joints above and below the hip, as pain in one joint may be referred to the next)
• Examine the neurology of the limb

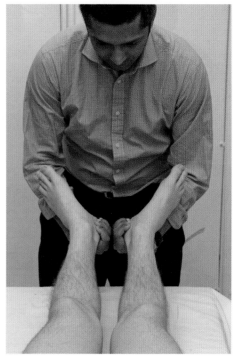

Figure 3.18 Measuring hip external rotation in extension.

• Examine the vascular supply of the limb
• Offer to help the patient dress.

? QUESTIONS

(a) How should this patient be investigated?

There is no specific laboratory test for osteoarthritis – usually the diagnosis is made with a combination of clinical features and X-ray appearances. However, tests are performed to exclude other systemic diseases that may cause hip pain, particularly rheumatological disorders:

Blood tests include:

• Haematological: full blood count, erythrocyte sedimentation rate
• Biochemical: baseline renal and liver function, particularly if long-term non-steroidal anti-inflammatory medication is being considered. C-reactive protein can help rule out inflammation or infection
• Immunological: rheumatoid factor, antinuclear antibody.

Radiological tests used are plain anteroposterior and lateral X-rays of the hip and pelvis.

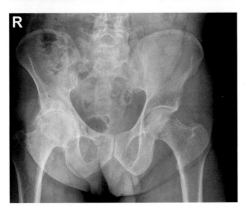

Figure 3.19 Anteroposterior pelvis X-ray showing right hip osteoarthritis.

(b) What are the X-ray features of osteoarthritis of the hip?

Use the mnemonic **LOSS** to remember these X-ray features (Fig. 3.19):

- **L**oss of the joint space
- **O**steophyte formation
- **S**ubchondral sclerosis
- **S**ubchondral cysts.

(c) What are the treatment options?

This is a 'classic' examination question that should be answered in a clearly structured way.

Non-surgical options would include:

- Lifestyle modifications: diet and exercise are important, including weight loss if appropriate, and patients may need referral to appropriate services
- Physiotherapy: some patients will respond to personalised exercise regimens that will improve their symptoms and may delay the need for a total hip replacement
- Occupational therapy: fitting of suitable devices to aid mobility (such as walking sticks, frames, etc.) and, more importantly, practical advice on how to use them
- Analgesic therapy: using the pain ladder (see Case 120), beginning with paracetamol and non-steroidal anti-inflammatories

Surgical options include:

- Osteotomy
- Arthroplasty (i.e. hip resurfacing or hip replacement)
- Arthrodesis

The US National Institute of Health concluded in 1994 that the indications for total hip replacement are:

- Severe pain or disability that is not substantially relieved by an extended course of non-surgical management
- Rest pain or pain with movement
- Instability
- Loss of mobility.

? ADVANCED QUESTIONS

(a) What are the complications of total hip replacement?

Complications can be divided into intraoperative, immediate (within 24 h), early (within 30 days) and late (later than 30 days). Specific complications include:

Intraoperative:

- Fracture of the acetabulum or femur

Immediate:

- Dislocation (due to malalignment of the prosthetic components)

Early:

- Deep vein thrombosis (DVT) and pulmonary embolus
- Sciatic nerve palsy (more common in the posterior surgical approach to the hip joint)
- Infection
- Fat embolism syndrome

Late:

- Infection
- Loosening (septic or aseptic)
- Heterotopic ossification
- Leg-length discrepancy
- Periprosthetic fractures
- Thigh pain.

(b) How do you prevent postoperative DVT following a total hip replacement?

DVT is the commonest complication following total hip replacement, with a peak incidence at 5–10 days postoperatively.

Prevention is impossible but measures that can be taken are classified according to:

- Preoperative: thromboembolic deterrent (TED) stockings fitted preoperatively
- Perioperative: TED stockings, minimising the length of surgery, using compression boots and foot pumps
- Postoperative: low-dose or low-molecular-weight heparin can reduce the incidence of

DVT; early mobilisation of patients with the help of physiotherapists.

Ricardo Galeazzi (1856–1952). Italian surgeon at the Instituto de Rachitici in Milan, known for his extensive work on congenital dislocation of the hip.

Hugh Owen Thomas (1834–1891). General practitioner in Liverpool who founded orthopaedic services in the city and also designed a range of splints, as he believed in the power of complete rest to heal fractures – many of these were used in the First World War.

Friedrich Trendelenburg (1844–1924). Professor of Surgery, Bonn and Leipzig, Germany.

FURTHER READING

http://orthoinfo.aaos.org/ topic.cfm?topic=A00213 – information for patients on osteoarthritis of the hip.

Nelson AE, Allen KD, Golightly YM, et al: A systematic review of recommendations and guidelines for the management of osteoarthritis: The chronic osteoarthritis management initiative of the U.S. Bone and Joint Initiative. *Semin Arthritis Rheum* 43(6):701–712, 2014.

Zhang W, Moskowitz RW, Nuki G, et al: OARSI recommendations for the management of hip and knee osteoarthritis, Part II: OARSI evidence-based, expert consensus guidelines. *Osteoarthritis Cartilage* 16(2):137–162, 2008.

CASE 78 | OSTEOARTHRITIS OF THE KNEE ***

INSTRUCTION

'Examine this lady's right knee.'

APPROACH

Adequately expose both lower limbs, keeping the lady's underwear on (patients in exams will often be wearing appropriate clothing, such as shorts).

VITAL POINTS

Inspect with the patient standing (front and back)

- Comment on the presence of any walking aids
- Shape:
  - Alignment – is the knee in varus or valgus? (You can measure intermalleolar distance if the examiner asks you to quantify this.) Is there fixed flexion or hyperextension present? Look particularly for varus and fixed flexion deformities in patients with osteoarthritis
  - Is there obvious quadriceps wasting?
- Scars – look particularly for:
  - Arthroscopic portal scars (see Case 91)
  - Meniscectomy scars (see Case 91)
  - Total or unicondylar knee replacement scars – midline longitudinal incision
- Swellings – especially popliteal fossa, e.g. Baker's cyst (see Case 96).

Gait (see Case 94)

- Antalgic: if the knee is painful – seen in osteoarthritis
- Stiff-knee gait: pelvis rises to allow the leg clearance during the swing phase – seen in severe osteoarthritis
- Instability (thrust) gait: may be mechanical or neuropathic.

Ask the patient to lie down on the couch

Measure

- Quadriceps wasting – measure thigh circumference at a set distance (e.g. 15 cm) above the tibial tuberosity (fixed bony point) and compare with the opposite side (Fig. 3.20).

Feel

- Temperature – using the dorsum of the hand from the proximal thigh to the distal leg
- Tenderness – start with the knee in extension and feel around the margins of the patella:
  - Grind test – move patella up and down while pressing it gently against the femur – painful grating is indicative of patellofemoral compartment pathology, e.g. patellofemoral osteoarthritis (PFOA)

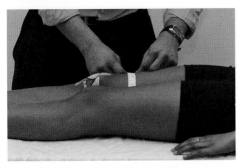

Figure 3.20 Measuring quadriceps wasting.

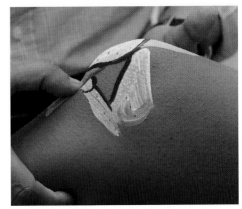

Figure 3.22 Palpating the patellar ligament.

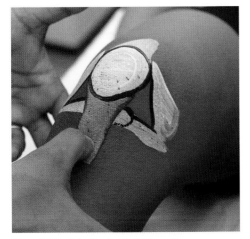

Figure 3.21 Palpating the tibial tuberosity.

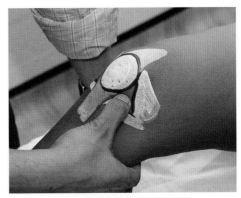

Figure 3.23 Palpating the medial joint line.

- Clarke's test – press the patella backwards and distally on to the patellofemoral groove, and ask the patient to contract his quadriceps muscle gently – pain at this point is indicative of patellofemoral compartment pathology, e.g. PFOA
- Note that the two tests described above can be very painful and may have to be omitted in your exam routine
- Next flex the knee to 90° and ensure the foot is flat on the couch:
  - Feel the tibial tuberosity (Fig. 3.21), patellar ligament (Fig. 3.22), medial joint line (Fig. 3.23) and lateral joint line (Fig. 3.24) of the knee – there may be tenderness of the joint line of involved compartments in osteoarthritis)
  - Feel the posterior aspect of the knee for any popliteal fossa swellings (Fig. 3.25) (see Case 96)
- Effusion:
  - Patellar hollow test (for very small quantities of fluid) – as the normal knee is

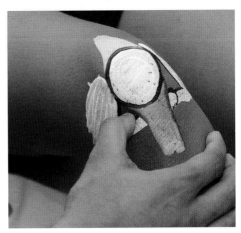

Figure 3.24 Palpating the lateral joint line.

flexed, a hollow appears medial to the patella (Fig. 3.26) and disappears with further flexion – with intra-articular fluid, the hollow fills and disappears at lesser angles of flexion – you may even notice

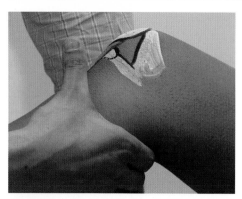

Figure 3.25 Palpating the posterior aspect of the knee for popliteal swellings.

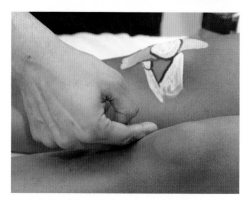

Figure 3.27 Patellar swipe test: emptying the medial aspect of the knee.

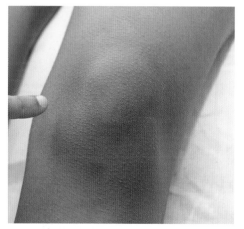

Figure 3.26 Patellar hollow test.

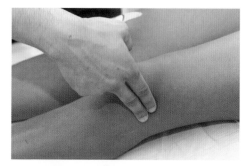

Figure 3.28 Patellar swipe test: swiping across the lateral aspect of the knee.

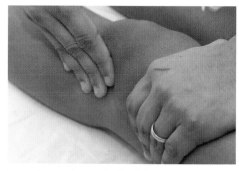

Figure 3.29 Cross-fluctuation test.

that the hollows have disappeared altogether compared with the normal knee
- Bulge test (for small quantities of fluid) – empty the medial compartment by pressing on that side of the joint (Fig. 3.27), then sharply swipe across the lateral aspect of the knee (Fig. 3.28) and observe for a ripple or bulge to appear on the medial aspect of the knee
- Cross-fluctuation (for moderate quantities of fluid) – use your left hand to compress and empty the suprapatellar pouch (Fig. 3.29), and with your right hand, empty the medial side of the knee by sweeping the back of the hand up the medial side, then sweep down the lateral side and observe the fluid impulse transmitted across the joint
- Patellar tap (for large amounts of fluid) – use the index finger of your right hand to

push the patella sharply downwards – the patella can be felt to hit the femoral condyles and to bounce off.

Move

- Extension – ask the patient to press her thigh into the couch and note any presence of hyperextension (if no hyperextension, the range of movement is 0° extension) and then ask her to lift her leg straight up in the air (Fig. 3.30), looking for an extensor lag due to weak quadriceps – a lag exists if there is loss of extension, but this can be passively corrected (Fig. 3.31); if this cannot be passively corrected, then there is a fixed flexion deformity

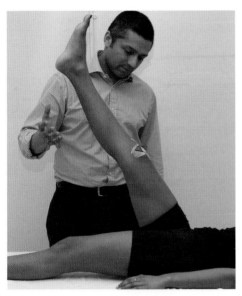

Figure 3.30   Assessing for extensor lag.

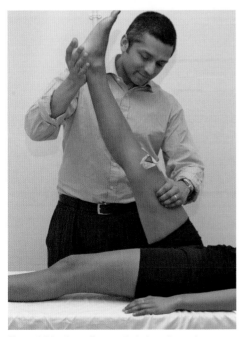

Figure 3.31   Correcting passively for extensor lag.

- Flexion – normally the knee flexes until the calf meets the hamstring – this is around 140° – during this movement, place your hand over the patella and joint lines, noting any clicks or crepitus (Fig. 3.32)
- You may elicit a fixed flexion deformity and decreased flexion in patients with osteoarthritis – the movements may also be painful, so it is important to be very gentle.

Special tests

This is part of the routine knee examination and should be carried out in the exam unless the examiner stops you. In patients with osteoarthritis, the most common finding with these tests is a degenerate meniscal tear, which may give you a positive McMurray's test.

- Cruciate ligaments (ensure that the quadriceps and hamstrings are relaxed):
    - Posterior sag – flex both knees to 90°, keeping the feet flat on the couch, and look across at the anterior profile of both knees – if there is a 'drop back' or sag of the upper end of the tibia, or the upper end can be gently pushed back, this indicates a tear of the posterior cruciate ligament (PCL) (the 'sag sign')
    - Anterior drawer – flex the knee to 90°, ensure the hamstrings are relaxed and use both hands to pull the upper end of the tibia forwards (= anterior drawer) (Fig. 3.33). A positive test indicates an

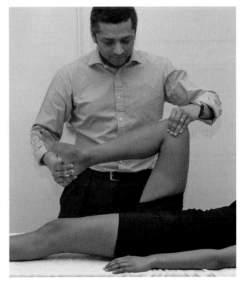

Figure 3.32   Palpating for joint line crepitus.

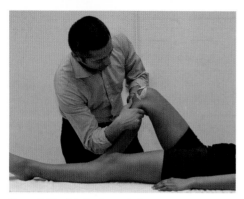

Figure 3.33 Anterior drawer test.

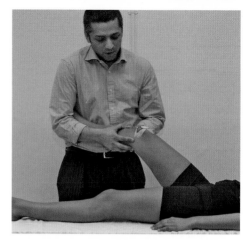

Figure 3.34 Standard test for collateral ligament laxity.

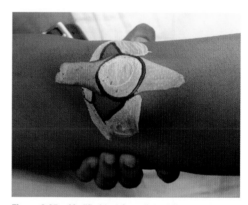

Figure 3.35 Modified test for collateral ligament laxity.

anterior cruciate ligament (ACL) injury. The test can be graded according to the distance forward that the tibia moves (1+=0–5 mm, 2+=6–10 mm, 3+=11–15 mm and 4+=>15 mm) and according to the feel of the endpoint of the movement (firm = ACL intact, marginal or soft). Note that a positive posterior sag can give you a false-positive anterior drawer test, which is why it is important to look for a posterior sag first

- Posterior drawer – performed in a similar manner to the anterior drawer test, except that the upper end of the tibia is pushed backwards. A positive test is indicative of a PCL injury. It is graded in a similar manner to the anterior drawer test
- Lachman test (most sensitive for ACL injury) – flex the knee to 30° and, holding the distal thigh firmly with one hand, lift the proximal tibia forward with your other hand with its thumb on the anteromedial joint line. If you find this difficult, either because you have small hands or the patient has big thighs, an alternative method is to flex the patient's knee over your thigh, press down on the distal thigh of the patient with one hand and lift the proximal tibia forward with the other. The test can be graded according to the distance forward that the tibia moves and according to the feel of the endpoint of the movement, as in the anterior drawer test
- Collateral ligaments:
  - Tuck the patient's foot under your arm and flex the knee to 20–30°, then apply valgus and varus stresses to the knee alternately while feeling the joint line for opening (Fig. 3.34). This may be difficult,

as this manoeuvre often results in rotation at the hip rather than true stress testing of the knee. Alternatively, you can perform this test by using one hand to hold the knee from beneath, feeling the joint lines (Fig. 3.35), and the other to hold the heel, although this does require more strength. Opening of the medial joint line on valgus stress testing signifies a medial collateral ligament injury, while opening of the lateral joint line on varus stress testing signifies a lateral collateral ligament injury. You can also perform this test by placing your flexed knee on the examination couch and resting the patient's knee over it, which flexes the knee to 30° without you needing to hold it. You can then apply the valgus and varus stress

- Repeat the varus and valgus stress test with the knee in full extension. Instability in extension signifies a combined collateral and cruciate ligament injury

- Menisci:
  - McMurray's test – this test, if done accurately, can help to differentiate between medial and lateral meniscal tears, but often does not add much information to your clinical examination. Flex the knee maximally, and grasp the knee with one hand and the foot with the other. To test the medial meniscus, palpate the posteromedial joint line and externally rotate and valgus stress the leg and, for the lateral meniscus, palpate the posterolateral joint line and internally rotate and varus stress the leg. Now slowly extend the knee and feel for a palpable click, which is indicative of a meniscal tear. Pain during the test is also suggestive of a meniscal tear
  - A click that is palpable from moving from full flexion to 90° flexion is suggestive of a posterior tear of the meniscus, while a click that is palpable moving from 90° flexion to full extension is suggestive of a middle or anterior tear of the meniscus
  - Modified McMurray's test – this is far easier to perform in a surgical exam. Flex the knee maximally, palpating both medial and lateral joint lines, then bring the knee slowly into extension, rotating internally and externally and feeling for a click (Fig. 3.36). Although not specific to either meniscus, this is the simplest and quickest way to assess the menisci rapidly.

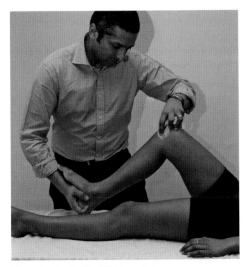

Figure 3.36 Modified McMurray's test.

Finish your examination here

Completion

Say that you would like to:

- Examine the hip and ankle (the joints above and below the knee joint)
- Assess the neurovascular status of the limb
- Ask the patient some questions to ascertain how much the problem affects her life, particularly activities of daily living, the presence of night pain and mobility.

? QUESTIONS

(a) What are the X-ray changes of osteoarthritis of the knee?

Remember the mnemonic **LOSS** for radiological features of osteoarthritis (Fig. 3.37):

- **L**oss of the joint space
- **O**steophyte formation
- **S**ubchondral sclerosis
- **S**ubchondral cysts.

More specifically, ensure that the X-rays have been taken with the patient standing and bearing weight, so that even small degrees of articular cartilage thinning can be seen. The tibiofemoral joint space is diminished (usually medial compartment) and the lateral X-ray may show patellofemoral osteoarthritis.

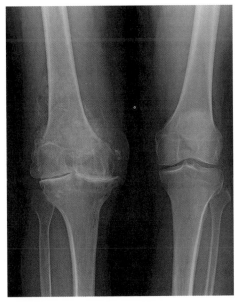

Figure 3.37 Anteroposterior X-ray of both knees showing severe right-knee osteoarthritis.

(b) How do you treat osteoarthritis of the knee?

Non-surgical:

- Lifestyle modifications – diet and exercise are important, including weight loss if appropriate, and patients may need referral to appropriate services
- Physiotherapy – many patients will respond to personalised exercise regimens that will improve their symptoms and may delay for many years the need for a knee replacement. Strengthening the quadriceps muscles is very important
- Occupational therapy – fitting of suitable devices to aid mobility (such as walking sticks, frames, etc.) and, more importantly, practical advice on how to use them. Even a simple elastic support may help, probably by improving proprioception in an unstable knee
- Medical therapy – using the pain ladder (see Case 120), beginning with paracetamol and non-steroidal anti-inflammatories
- Intra-articular steroid injections – may provide temporary relief, but repeated injections may lead to progressive cartilage and bone destruction
- Viscosupplementation – intra-articular injections of hyaluronic acid may provide benefit

Surgical options include:

- Arthroscopic debridement and washout – may give temporary relief and are of use in younger patients as a temporising procedure before subsequent arthroplasty; degenerate meniscal tears and osteophytes can be trimmed; more recently, the evidence for arthroscopic debridement and washout has been shown to be poor
- Patellectomy – indicated in rare cases where osteoarthritis is confined to the patellofemoral joint; may result in decreased extensor mechanism power, and if total knee replacement is needed later, results in less predictable pain relief
- Realignment osteotomy – useful particularly in younger patients (under 50 years) with medial compartment osteoarthritis, in whom a high tibial valgus osteotomy redistributes weight to the lateral side of the joint
- Unicompartmental or total knee arthroplasty (i.e. knee replacement) – indicated in older patients with progressive joint destruction. If the disease is confined to one compartment, a unicompartmental knee replacement can be performed as an alternative to osteotomy.
- Arthrodesis – indicated if there is a strong contraindication to arthroplasty (e.g. previous sepsis) or as a salvage procedure for a failed arthroplasty.

? QUESTION

(a) What are the complications of a total knee replacement?

Intraoperative:

- Fracture of the tibia or femur

Immediate:

- Vascular injuries – superficial femoral, popliteal and genicular vessels

Early:

- Deep vein thrombosis and pulmonary embolus
- Peroneal nerve palsy (1%)
- Infection
- Fat embolism syndrome

Late:

- Infection
- Loosening (septic or aseptic)
- Patellar instability/fractures/disruption of extensor mechanism
- Periprosthetic fractures.

? ADVANCED QUESTIONS

(a) Rheumatoid arthritis is another disease that can affect the knee. What do you know of the clinical features of rheumatoid arthritis of the knee?

Stage 1 – proliferative:

- Palpable effusions and thickened synovium, but stable joint
- Posterior capsule at risk of rupture
- Acute rupture of Baker's cysts (see Case 96)

Stage 2 – destructive:

- Increasing instability of the knee joint
- Marked muscle wasting
- Some loss of flexion and extension

Stage 3 – reparative:

- Severe pain and instability – there may be marked stiffness or severe instability

- Most common deformities are fixed flexion and valgus
- Instability manifests as increased anteroposterior glide and lateral wobble.

(b) What are the surgical options for rheumatoid arthritis of the knee?

- Synovectomy and debridement – for failed medical treatment. This procedure can be performed arthroscopically and involves removing the articular pannus and cartilage
- Supracondylar osteotomy – useful if the knee is stable and pain-free but can be complicated by valgus and flexion deformity
- Total knee arthroplasty – for advanced joint destruction.

FURTHER READING

American Academy of Orthopedic Surgeons guidelines:

Non-surgical management – http://www.aaos.org/research/guidelines/TreatmentofOsteoarthritisoftheKneeGuideline.pdf.

Surgical management – http://www.aaos.org/uploadedFiles/PreProduction/Quality/Guidelines_and_Reviews/SMOAK%20CPG__12.4.15.pdf.

National Clinical Guideline Centre (UK): *Osteoarthritis: Care and Management in Adults*. Editors:. London: National Institute for Health and Care Excellence (UK), 2014. http://www.ncbi.nlm.nih.gov/pubmedhealth/PMH0068962/.

CASE 79 | DUPUYTREN'S CONTRACTURE ***

INSTRUCTION

'Examine this patient's hands (Fig. 3.38).'

APPROACH

Expose to elbows and ask the patient to place his hands palm upwards on a pillow (if available).

VITAL POINTS

Look

- Describe any tethering or pitting of the skin on the palmar aspect of the hand, and also note the appearance of any visible cords

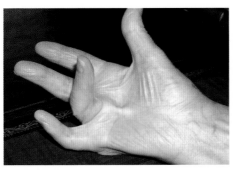

Figure 3.38 Dupuytren's contracture (from Young C, Gladman M: *Examination Surgery*. Chatsworth, NSW, Australia: Churchill Livingstone, 2013, with permission).

- Look for scars from previous surgery
- Describe any flexion deformities at the metacarpophalangeal and proximal interphalangeal joints (MCPJ and PIPJ) of the involved fingers
- Look for involvement of the thumb and the first web space (a sign of more aggressive disease)
- Ask the patient to turn his hands over to look for Garrod's pads (thickening of the subcutaneous tissues) over the PIPJ.

Feel

- Palpate the swelling, particularly noting its fixation to skin
- Does the other palm have similar thickening?

Move

- Assess the range of motion in the involved fingers
- Note the presence of fixed deformities by passively moving the involved joints.

TOP TIP

✅ Asking the patient to lay the involved hand flat against a hard surface, e.g. a table may facilitate assessment of the deformities and allow you to judge the extent to which they are fixed (table-top test).

Finish your examination here

Completion

Say that you would like to:

- Enquire about causes and associations (see below)
- Assess the patient's function, e.g. writing and dressing
- Look for other features of diffuse fibromatosis.

? QUESTIONS

(a) What is your differential diagnosis?

The differential diagnosis includes:

- Skin contracture – look for scar from previous wound
- Tendon contracture – thickened area, which moves on passive flexion of involved finger
- Congenital contracture of the little finger – affects PIPJ
- Ulnar nerve palsy – ring and little fingers are hyperextended at MCPJ and flexed at PIPJ.

(b) What conditions are associated with Dupuytren's contracture?

We have found the following mnemonic helpful to remember the associations – **DEAFEST PAIL**:

- **D**iabetes mellitus
- **E**pilepsy
- **A**ge (positive correlation)
- **F**amily history (autosomal-dominant)/ fibromatoses*
- **E**pileptic medication (e.g. phenobarbital)
- **S**moking
- **T**rauma and heavy manual labour
- **P**eyronie's disease (fibrosis of the corpus cavernosum – seen in 3% of patients with Dupuytren's)
- **A**IDS
- **I**diopathic (most common)
- **L**iver disease (secondary to alcohol).

*A group of disorders characterised by diffuse fibrosis, which include such diverse conditions as desmoid tumours, Reidel's thyroiditis, retroperitoneal fibrosis and Ledderhose disease (fibrosis of the plantar aponeurosis – seen in 5% of patients with Dupuytren's).

(c) What are the surgical options available?

Operative management is considered when MCPJ or PIPJ contracture exceeds 30°:

- Fasciotomy – for prominent bands (note that medical treatment for contractures can be achieved by *Clostridium histolyticum* collagenase injection, although the long-term safety and recurrence rate of this procedure require further assessment
- Partial fasciectomy (with Z-plasty to lengthen wound) – in conjunction with postoperative physiotherapy (early active flexion range-of-motion exercises for grip strength) and night-time splintage in extension
- Dermofasciectomy (with full-thickness skin grafting) – associated with the lowest risk of recurrence
- Arthrodesis/amputation – for late presentations and repeated recurrences.

? ADVANCED QUESTIONS

(a) What is the underlying pathophysiology of the condition?

The condition has been attributed to the presence of oxygen free radicals, trauma to the palmar fascia, aberrant immune responses with altered antigen presentation, or to interactions between these mechanisms. The presence of immune cells and related phenomena in affected tissue suggests that it may be immune-related. Mechanically, digital contracture is caused by myofibroblasts in the palmar fascia; however, the exact origin of this cell type remains unknown.

The process of chronic inflammation is thought to be essential to the subsequent fibrosis (see Further reading).

Baron Guillaume Dupuytren (1777–1835). Surgeon in Chief, Hôtel-Dieu, Paris. He described the condition as 'permanent retraction of the fingers' and was also surgeon to Louis XVIII and Charles X during the restoration of the Bourbon monarchy. He was a cold, rude, ambitious and arrogant man, earning him the epithet 'the Napoleon of surgery'. He died following a stroke and was described as 'first among surgeons; last among men'.

Sir A. E. Garrod (1857–1936). English physician, St Bartholomew's Hospital, London, later succeeding William Osler as Regius Professor at Oxford.

G. Ledderhose (1855–1925). German surgeon.

François Gigot de la Peyronie (1678–1747). French surgeon.

FURTHER READING

Rayan GM: Dupuytren disease: Anatomy, pathology, presentation, and treatment. *J Bone Joint Surg Am* 89(1):189–198, 2007.

Shih B, Bayat A: Scientific understanding and clinical management of Dupuytren disease. *Nat Rev Rheumatol* 6(12):715–726, 2010.

www.patient.co.uk/showdoc/23068725/ – patient-centred information.

CASE 80 　 CARPAL TUNNEL SYNDROME 　 ★★★

INSTRUCTION

'This lady is complaining of a tingling sensation in the thumb and index fingers of the right hand. Examine her hands and tell me what you think the diagnosis is.'

APPROACH

Expose to elbows and ask the patient to place her hands palm upwards on a pillow (if available).

VITAL POINTS

The clues are in the instruction. The examiner is expecting you to perform a directed neurological assessment of the hands. He is leading you towards to the diagnosis with his question, but is interested in seeing how you approach the task.

Look

- Wasting of the thenar muscles (in advanced cases)
- Scar from previous surgery over the transverse carpal ligament.

Sensory assessment

Test light touch over the palmar aspects of the thumb, index and middle fingers of the involved hand – deficiency implies median-nerve involvement. Compare this with the other fingers, proceeding to other sensory modalities such as pain only if the examiner wishes you to.

TOP TIP

✅ The autonomous sensory areas of the hand (i.e. only one nerve always supplies this area) are as follows:

Median nerve – distal phalanges of index and middle fingers

Ulnar nerve – middle and distal phalanges of little finger

Radial nerve – over first dorsal interosseus muscle between first and second metacarpals (but usually there is no autonomous zone)

✅ Testing these three areas confirms restriction of pathology to one nerve only.

Motor assessment

Test the power of muscles innervated by the median nerve (**LOAF**) (Fig. 3.39):

- **L**ateral two lumbricals – difficult to test
- **O**pponens pollicis – oppose the patient's thumb and little finger and ask her to stop you pulling the fingers apart
- **A**bductor pollicis brevis – place dorsum of hand on a flat surface and ask the patient to lift her thumb to the ceiling against resistance, feeling the thenar eminence for the power of abductor pollicis brevis
- **F**lexor pollicis brevis – not an autonomous muscle (innervation varies).

Test only for abductor pollicis brevis in the exam.

TOP TIP

✅ The autonomous motor supply of the hand is:

Median nerve – abductor pollicis brevis (as above)

Ulnar nerve – palmar interossei (adduction of the fingers)

Radial nerve – metacarpophalangeal extensors (extension of the fingers at the knuckles).

Finish your examination here

Completion

Say that you would like to perform the following special tests:

- Tinel's sign – tapping over the median nerve at the wrist reproduces tingling sensation in the distribution of the nerve

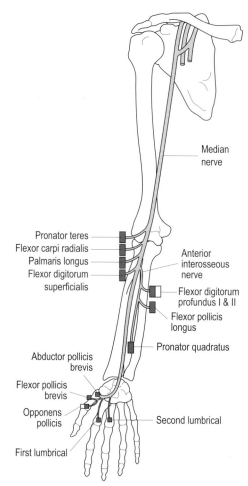

Pronator teres
Flexor carpi radialis
Palmaris longus
Flexor digitorum
superficialis

Median
nerve

Anterior
interosseous
nerve

Flexor digitorum
profundus I & II

Flexor pollicis
longus

Pronator quadratus

Abductor pollicis
brevis

Flexor pollicis
brevis

Opponens
pollicis

Second lumbrical

First lumbrical

Figure 3.39   Muscles supplied by the median nerve.

- Phalen's test – maximal flexion of the wrist for 1 min exacerbates symptoms which are promptly relieved when flexion is discontinued
- Flexion compression test (also known as Duran's test) – maximal flexion of wrist and direct digital compression of the median nerve at the wrist reproduces symptoms (if symptoms appear within 20 s, sensitivity = 82% and specificity = 99%).

Assess the effect of the symptoms on the patient's quality of life, e.g. symptoms are usually worse at night and first thing in the morning – sleep quality may be affected.

Look for underlying causes and associations (see below).

(a) What are the causes of carpal tunnel syndrome?

The most common cause is idiopathic. The other causes can be classified as follows:

- Anatomical abnormalities:
  - Bone – previous wrist fractures, e.g. Colles' fracture, acromegaly
  - Soft tissues – lipomas, ganglia
- Physiological abnormalities:
  - Inflammatory conditions – rheumatoid arthritis, gout
  - Alterations of fluid balance – pregnancy, menopause, hypothyroidism, obesity, amyloidosis, renal failure
- Neuropathic conditions – diabetes mellitus, alcoholism.

(b) Name one investigation you might perform before offering this lady treatment

Nerve conduction studies:

- Symptoms of carpal tunnel syndrome can be mimicked by higher (more proximal) lesions of the median nerve. These high lesions are characterised by loss of sensation over the thenar eminence due to involvement of the palmar cutaneous branch, and loss of the relevant forearm flexors (especially flexor pollicis longus)
- Symptoms may also be due to cervical nerve root lesions (e.g. secondary to a cervical disc herniation) or thoracic outlet syndrome
- Nerve conduction studies also assist in determining the severity of the lesion.

(c) How would you treat this lady?

- Non-surgical – removal of underlying causes, splinting of the wrist in a neutral position (especially at night time) and local steroid injections just proximal to the carpal tunnel
- Surgical – carpal tunnel decompression (division of the flexor retinaculum under tourniquet control) can be performed either as an open or endoscopic procedure.

(d) What complications would you warn this lady about if you were offering her surgery?

- Scar formation – high-risk area for keloid or hypertrophic scars
- Scar tenderness – can occur in up to 40% of patients
- Wound infection
- Nerve injury – palmar cutaneous branch of the median nerve (which lies superficial to

the retinaculum) and the motor branch to the thenar muscles (which usually leaves the radial side of the median nerve towards the distal extent of the standard incision). The risk of nerve injury is decreased if the skin incision is made on the ulnar side of the palmar crease
- Failure to relieve symptoms – if the retinaculum is incompletely divided.

? ADVANCED QUESTIONS

(a) What are the boundaries of the carpal tunnel?
- Ulnar aspect: pisiform (where flexor carpi ulnaris attaches) and hook of hamate
- Radial aspect: scaphoid and trapezium
- Volar aspect: transverse carpal ligament.

(b) Where else is the median nerve likely to be compressed?

The following causes are rare:
- Pronator syndrome – compression of the median nerve by the ligament of Struthers (fibrous band arising from the medial epicondyle of the humerus that passes medially and upwards to attach to a supratrochlear spur on the lower anterior humerus), pronator teres muscle or the proximal arch of the flexor digitorum superficialis
- Anterior interosseous syndrome – entrapment of the anterior interosseous branch of the median nerve, usually at the origin of the deep head of pronator teres. The nerve supplies flexor pollicis longus, pronator

quadratus and the radial side of flexor digitorum profundus, leading to loss of precise pinch (inability to make the 'OK sign'), but there are no sensory signs.

(c) What is the pathophysiology underlying carpal tunnel syndrome (or any compression syndrome)?

The primary change is thought to be vascular in origin. Pressure on the nerve results in blood-flow obstruction in the vasa nervorum, resulting in venous congestion and oedema. With time, fibroblast proliferation occurs in the nerve, leading to inefficiency of cell transport mechanisms and the sodium pump, resulting in impairment of nerve conduction.

> *George S. Phalen (1911–1998).* American orthopaedic surgeon who worked at the Cleveland Clinic in Ohio.
> *Jules Tinel (1879–1952).* French neurologist.

FURTHER READING

American Academy of Orthopedic Surgeons guidelines:

Diagnosis – http://www.aaos.org/research/guidelines/CTS_guideline.pdf.

Treatment – http://www.aaos.org/research/guidelines/CTSTreatmentGuideline.pdf.

Verdugo RJ, Salinas RA, Castillo JL, et al: Surgical versus non-surgical treatment for carpal tunnel syndrome. *Cochrane Database Syst Rev* 4:CD001552, 2008.

www.patient.co.uk/showdoc/23068696/ – guide to carpal tunnel syndrome for patients.

CASE 81 | RHEUMATOID HANDS ***

INSTRUCTION

'Examine this lady's hands.' (Fig. 3.40)

APPROACH

Expose the hands and the forearms to the elbows (to examine for rheumatoid nodules later in the case) and place on a white pillow or blanket, palm upwards.

VITAL POINTS

Almost all the clinical signs are elicited on inspection alone.

Look

Wrist:
- Radial deviation of the wrist
- Volar subluxation of the wrist joint
- Piano-key sign – subluxation of the radioulnar joint causes the head of the ulna to pop up on the dorsum of the wrist where it can be jogged up and down

Thumb:
- The 'Z-thumb' appearance, with flexion of the interphalangeal joint and hyperextension of the metacarpophalangeal joint (MCPJ)

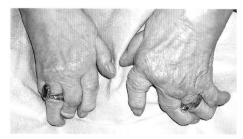

Figure 3.40 Rheumatoid hands.

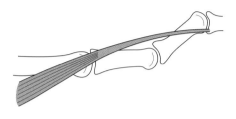

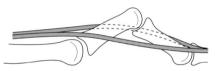

Figure 3.41 Swan neck (above) and boutonnière (below) deformities of the rheumatoid hand.

Palm:

- The presence of palmar erythema

Fingers:

- Ulnar deviation of the fingers, involving the more lateral digits in more advanced cases
- MCPJ volar subluxation, most commonly over the index and middle fingers
- Swelling of the proximal interphalangeal joints (PIPJ)
- Swan neck deformity (flexion of the distal interphalangeal joint [DIPJ] and hyperextension of the PIPJ) (Fig. 3.41)
- Boutonnière deformity (hyperextension of the DIPJ and flexion of the PIPJ) (Fig. 3.41)

Dorsum:

- Wasting of the interossei, best seen in the first dorsal web space.

Palpate

- Palpate over any swollen joints to detect the warmth and tenderness of acutely inflamed joints
- Finally palpate the elbows (over the subcutaneous border of the ulna) for

rheumatoid nodules – present in 25% of patients, especially in active seropositive disease. You may also find rheumatoid nodules at other pressure areas, e.g. the pulps of the fingers and the radial side of the index finger.

Sensory and motor assessment

See the section under carpal tunnel syndrome (Case 80) – the median nerve may be involved in rheumatoid arthritis if carpal tunnel syndrome is a complication.

Functional assessment

Ask the patient to perform simple tests such as unbuttoning a shirt and writing with a pen, in order to assess the function of the hands, and determine the need for specific treatments.

Finish your examination here

Completion

Say that you would like to:

- Ask the patient what other joints in the body are affected by rheumatoid arthritis
- Examine the rest of the patient for other features of rheumatoid arthritis (see below)
- Ask the patient how the condition affects her life.

? QUESTIONS

(a) What are the extra-articular manifestations of rheumatoid arthritis?

Ophthalmic:

- Episcleritis
- Scleritis
- Keratoconjuctivitis sicca

Respiratory:

- Pleural effusions
- Pulmonary fibrosis

Cardiac:

- Pericarditis

Reticuloendothelial:

- Lymphadenopathy
- Splenomegaly
- Felty's syndrome (see Case 49)

Neurological:

- Multifocal neuropathies
- Carpal tunnel syndrome

Vascular:

- Vasculitis.

(b) What investigations can be used to confirm the diagnosis of rheumatoid arthritis?

Blood tests:

- Haematological
  - Anaemia of chronic disease (due to decreased production of red blood cells, increased destruction of red cells or ineffective erythropoiesis)
  - Raised erythrocyte sedimentation rate
- Immunological
  - Rheumatoid factor is positive in 75%
  - Anti-CCP antibody is positive in approximately 77%
  - HLA-DR3/DR4 is present in approximately one-third of patients
  - Antinuclear antibody is raised in 30%
- X-rays (see below).

(c) What are the treatment options for rheumatoid arthritis?

Non-surgical (hand therapy/physiotherapy):

- Splinting (static and dynamic)
- Active hand and wrist exercises
- Household aids and personal aids (orthoses)

Injections:

- Local injections of corticosteroid and local anaesthetic for persistent synovitis of a few joints or tendon sheaths

Pharmacological:

- According to National Institute for Health and Care Excellence guidelines, in people with newly diagnosed active rheumatoid arthritis, a combination of disease-modifying antirheumatic drugs (DMARDs, including methotrexate and at least one other, such as gold, plus short-term glucocorticoids) is offered as first-line treatment as soon as possible, ideally within 3 months of the onset of persistent symptoms. Anti-inflammatory drugs such as non-steroidal anti-inflammatory drugs may also be used for short periods.
- Newer (but more expensive and injectable) biologics include antitumour necrosis factor-α drugs such as etanercept, and infliximab and interleukin-1 inhibitors such as anakinra – these are being used more commonly for cases which are resistant to the above

medications; this must be done under strict specialist involvement. They are best used in the context of a long-term clinical study

Surgical:

- Operative options include soft-tissue procedures (e.g. synovectomy, carpal tunnel decompression and tendon repairs/transfers) and bone/joint procedures (e.g. arthrodesis and arthroplasty). You would not be expected to know the details of these procedures for finals or the MRCS.

❓ ADVANCED QUESTIONS

(a) What are the clinical stages of rheumatoid arthritis of the hand?

- Stage 1 – proliferative: synovitis of the joints (swelling of MCPJ and PIPJ) and of tendon sheaths (flexor and extensor tenosynovitis, the former leading to carpal tunnel syndrome)
- Stage 2 – destructive: joint and tendon erosions, e.g. drop finger and mallet thumb due to extensor tendon ruptures, radial deviation of the wrist and ulnar deviation of the fingers
- Stage 3 – reparative: leading to established deformities such as marked ulnar deviation of the fingers, volar dislocation of the MCPJs, and multiple swan-neck and boutonnière deformities.

(b) What are the radiological stages of rheumatoid arthritis?

- Stage 1 – soft-tissue swelling and periarticular osteoporosis
- Stage 2 – joint space narrowing and small periarticular erosions (most common at MCPJs and styloid process of the ulna)
- Stage 3 – marked articular destruction, seen most commonly at MCPJs, PIPJs and wrist joints.

FURTHER READING

http://www.arthritisresearchuk.org/arthritis-information/conditions/rheumatoid-arthritis.aspx – patient information on rheumatoid arthritis from Arthritis Research UK.

https://www.nice.org.uk/guidance/cg79 – guidelines from the National Institute for Health and Care Excellence.

Longo UG, Petrillo S, Denaro V: Current concepts in the management of rheumatoid hand. *Int J Rheumatol* 2015:648073, 2015.

CASE 82 | OSTEOARTHRITIS IN THE HANDS ***

INSTRUCTION

'Examine this gentleman's hands.'

APPROACH

Expose the hands and the forearms to the elbows and place on a white pillow or blanket, palm upwards.

VITAL POINTS

Almost all the clinical signs are elicited on inspection alone.

Look

- The distal interphalangeal joints (DIPJs) are swollen (Heberden's nodes) and may be fixed in flexion
- Bouchard's nodes are bony swellings at the proximal interphalangeal joints (PIPJs) in osteoarthritis
- 'Square hand' appearance – see below.

Palpate

- Continue to test active and passive movements of the affected joints to define degree of reduction of movement.

Functional assessment

Ask the patient to perform simple tests, such as unbuttoning a shirt, in order to assess the function of the hands.

Finish your examination here

Completion

Say that you would like to:

- Examine other joints for arthritis. In comparison with rheumatoid arthritis, the hips, lumbar spine and knees are more commonly affected than the hands.

? QUESTIONS

(a) Which joints in the hands are most frequently affected by osteoarthritis?

- DIPJs (Heberden's nodes)
- PIPJs (Bouchard's nodes) – these are strongly associated with polyarticular osteoarthritis, i.e. arthritis at other joints in the body, including carpometacarpal arthritis
- Carpometacarpal joint of the thumb – which sometimes leads to the 'square hand' or 'metacarpal bossing' appearance.

(b) What are the treatment options for osteoarthritis of the hands?

Non-surgical:

- Physiotherapy may help to maintain functional ability, and especially with thumb involvement, splints may also be used
- Pain relief (using analgesic ladder – Case 120): paracetamol, aspirin or other non-steroidal anti-inflammatory drugs for symptomatic relief

Surgical:

- Joint arthrodesis, and in the case of thumb carpometacarpal joint involvement, trapeziectomy can be performed with tendinous interpositional graft (from flexor carpi radialis)
- Arthroplasty (with the Swanson silicone trapezium implant) has largely been abandoned due to the problems of dislocation and silicone-induced synovitis
- Heberden's and Bouchard's nodes rarely require surgical management, but sometimes an arthrodesis is required if the joint becomes unstable or very painful.

C.J. Bouchard (1837–1925). French physician who was also one of the initial physicians to describe spider naevi.

William Heberden (1710–1801) also described angina, chickenpox and night blindness. 'Heberden disease' is another name for angina pectoris. He was physician to King George III and attended to Dr Johnson during his last illness.

FURTHER READING

Van Heest AE, Kallemeier P: Thumb carpal metacarpal arthritis. *J Am Acad Orthop Surg* 16(3):140–151, 2008.

www.medicinenet.com/script/main/art.asp?articlekey=20167 – information for patients.

CASE 83 │ ULNAR NERVE LESIONS ★★★

INSTRUCTION

'Examine this gentleman's left hand.' (Fig. 3.42)

APPROACH

Within surgical short cases, the likely reason for weakness of the hand will be a specific neurological lesion of the median, ulnar or radial nerves. Beginning with the Top Tips (see Case 80) will allow the candidate to get swiftly to the diagnosis without wasting time.

Expose to elbows and ask the patient to place his hands palm upwards on a pillow (if available).

VITAL POINTS

Inspect

- Note the claw hand appearance, with paralysis of lumbricals and interossei, and unopposed action of the long flexors and extensors, causing flexed, deformed little and ring fingers (see difference between high and low lesions below) (see Fig. 3.42 with low lesion and scar at level of wrist)

- Examine the palm, noting the wasting of the hypothenar eminence (all muscles here are supplied by the ulnar nerve) (Fig. 3.43)

- Ask the patient to turn his hands over and observe the guttering between the metacarpals as the interossei are wasted (best seen in the first dorsal webspace) (note the hand in Fig. 3.42 has no obvious wasting).

Sensory assessment

- Test the autonomous area (see Case 80) over the middle and distal phalanges of the little finger.

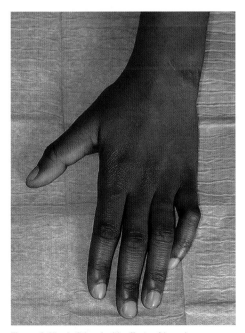

Figure 3.42   Left hand with effects of low ulnar nerve lesion.

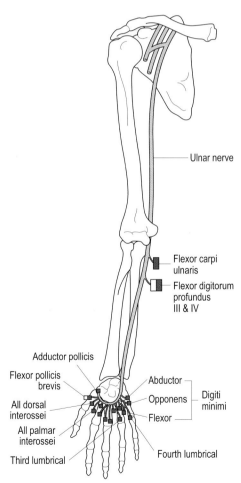

Figure 3.43   Muscles supplied by the ulnar nerve.

Motor assessment

- Test the palmar interossei (which adduct the fingers) by asking the patient to hold a piece of paper between two fingers while you attempt to pull it away – you have now tested the autonomous motor supply (see Case 80)
- Continue to test the dorsal interossei (which abduct the fingers) by asking the patient to spread his fingers and prevent you from pushing them together
- Assess for weakness of flexor digitorum profundus to the ring and little fingers (see Case 89).

Special tests

- Froment's sign: this test is based on the fact that adductor pollicis is supplied by the ulnar nerve, and if there is an ulnar nerve palsy, the only way to adduct the thumb is by using flexor pollicis longus to compensate (this muscle is supplied by the median nerve). Ask the patient to hold a piece of paper between the thumb and radial aspect of the index finger and, as you pull this piece of paper away from the patient, observe the thumb – you will see the distal phalanx flex if the patient is using flexor pollicis longus to hold the piece of paper
- Elbow flexion test: with the elbow fully flexed, the patient will complain of numbness and tingling in the ring and little fingers, often within 1 min – this test may be quite uncomfortable for the patient, and therefore you are better off describing it first to the examiner.

TOP TIP

☑ When examining the peripheral nerves of the upper limb, begin at the hand and move proximally. Continue examining one nerve in its entirety before moving on to the next nerve, by which time the examiner will usually have stopped you. This allows a precise definition of the anatomical location of the nerve lesion described.

Finish your examination here

Completion

Say that you would like to:

- Examine the neck and all the other peripheral nerves of the affected limb.

? QUESTIONS

(a) What causes of ulnar nerve palsies do you know?

The causes can be divided up according to broad aetiological categories:

- Anatomical: cubital tunnel syndrome at the elbow (due to repeated elbow flexion leading to traction injury ± recurrent subluxation of the nerve within the tunnel)
- Trauma: anywhere along the course of the nerve, e.g. supracondylar fractures and dislocations of the elbow (also late sequelae of trauma can lead to ulnar nerve palsy, e.g. cubitus valgus deformity at the elbow)
- Degenerative arthritis: with compressing proliferative synovitis and osteophytes, or loose bodies
- Rare causes: compression from tight fascia or ligaments, tumour masses, aneurysms, vascular thromboses or anomalous muscles (e.g. anconeus epitrochlearis).

(b) How do you clinically differentiate between a high and a low ulnar nerve lesion?

Low lesions (below elbow) (Fig. 3.43):

- More marked clawing as flexor digitorum profundus to ring and little fingers still functioning

High lesions (above elbow):

- Paralysis of flexor digitorum profundus to ring and little fingers leads to less marked clawing of these fingers as the flexion component of the clawing is less prominent – this is known as the 'ulnar paradox'
- Decreased sensation over ulnar border of the hand
- Otherwise as for low lesion.

? ADVANCED QUESTIONS

(a) How do you treat ulnar nerve palsies?

Non-surgical:

- For patients with mild, intermittent symptoms and no significant neurological deficits – avoid repetitive flexion–extension motions and prolonged elbow flexion, and use of night splintage with the elbow in extension

Surgical:

- For patients with persistent, significant symptoms or neurological deficit, surgical options include:
  - Ulnar nerve decompression (decompression of the roof of the cubital tunnel at the elbow)
  - Ulnar nerve anterior transposition ± subcutaneous or submuscular transposition
  - Medial epicondylectomy.

Jules Froment (1878–1946). Neurologist and Professor of Clinical Medicine, Lyons, France.

FURTHER READING

Chimenti PC, Hammert WC: Ulnar neuropathy at the elbow: an evidence-based algorithm. *Hand Clin* 29(3):435–442, 2013.

Elhassan B, Steinmann SP: Entrapment neuropathy of the ulnar nerve. *J Am Acad Orthop Surg* 15(11):672–681, 2007.

Toussaint CP, Zager EL: What's new in common upper extremity entrapment neuropathies. *Neurosurg Clin N Am* 19(4): 573–581, 2008.

CASE 84 | HALLUX VALGUS   ***

INSTRUCTION

'Examine this lady's feet.' (Fig. 3.44)

APPROACH

Expose both ankles and feet and begin by describing any obvious deformities. You should position yourself either sitting on a chair facing the patient or kneeling on the ground opposite her.

VITAL POINTS

Look

- Unilateral or bilateral?
- Estimate degree of valgus of the big toe
- Is there rotation (pronation) of the big toe (nail faces medially)?
- Is there a bunion present? A bunion is a prominence of the medial aspect of the first metatarsal head with or without an overlying bursa
- Are there visible signs of inflammation of the bursa, e.g. erythema?
- Is there an overridden, hammered or retracted second toe (see Case 85)?
- Look at the soles of the feet – are there any callosities present? Are the metatarsal heads prominent?

Feel

- Is there any inflammation of the bunion, e.g. warmth, tenderness?
- Localise any areas of tenderness, e.g. osteoarthritis of the first metatarsophalangeal joint (MTPJ).

Move

- Assess range of movement of the first MTPJ, including noting the presence of any hypermobility (indicating instability).

Finish your examination here

Completion

Say that you would like to:

- Assess the range of motion of the other toe joints
- Watch the patient walk (gait) – this allows inspection of the heel and ankle from the back, again noting any gross deformities

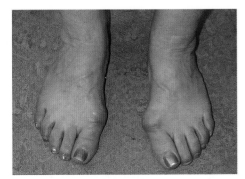

Figure 3.44   Bilateral hallux valgus.

- Examine her shoes – abnormalities of weightbearing will be reflected in the pattern of wear
- Ask her questions to assess the effect of the condition on her life.

? QUESTIONS

(a) Name one investigation you would perform in order to assess the condition further

Plain weightbearing X-rays in order to assess:

- Degree of valgus deformity
- First/second intermetatarsal angle (IMA) and distal metatarsal articular angle (Fig. 3.45)
- Presence of osteoarthritis of the first MTPJ.

(b) What do you know of the aetiology of hallux valgus?

- Essentially unknown
- Strong familial trait
- Increased incidence in people who wear

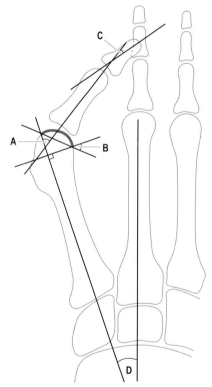

Figure 3.45 Important radiological angles in hallux valgus: A, hallux valgus angle; B, distal metatarsal articulation angle; C, interphalangeal angle; D, intermetatarsal angle.

enclosed footwear; rarely seen in those who have never worn shoes
- Associated with rheumatoid arthritis
- Secondary to metatarsus primus varus in younger age groups, which itself may be congenital or secondary to loss of muscle tone with age.

(c) What treatment options are available in hallux valgus?

Non-surgical:

- Appropriate footwear, e.g. wide shoe with soft upper, wide toe box and protective padding over prominences (follow the patient up after a couple of months in order to examine the footwear and note wear patterns)
- Physiotherapy

Surgical:

Several options are available, depending on the wishes of the patient, her level of activity and the state of her peripheral vascular system. These include:

- Bunionectomy
- First metatarsal realignment osteotomy
- Excision arthroplasty (Keller's procedure) – essentially a proximal hemiphalangectomy
- Fusion – for degenerative joint disease or for instability.

? ADVANCED QUESTION

(a) How would you decide which surgical techniques to use in a specific patient?

If the examiner moves you on to specific surgical options (very unlikely), a rough outline of treatment can be given, although decisions are tailored to the individual.

Arthritic joint:

- In an active patient – first MTP arthrodesis or prosthetic arthroplasty
- In a low-demand elderly patient – Keller's procedure (becoming less popular)

Non-arthritic joint:

- IMA <15°, e.g. Chevron or scarf osteotomy
- IMA >15°, e.g. scarf osteotomy.

Colonel William Keller (1874–1959). Director of Professional Services of the American Expeditionary Forces during the First World War. He first devised the procedure in Manila during the Philippine War.

FURTHER READING

Hecht PJ, Lin TJ: Hallux valgus. *Med Clin North Am* 98(2):227–232, 2014.

www.bofas.org.uk/PublicArea/PatientAdvice/
Halluxvalgusbunion/tabid/101/Default.aspx –
information for patients.

CASE 85 | HAMMER TOES ***

INSTRUCTION

'Examine this man's toes.' (Fig. 3.46)

APPROACH

Expose both ankles and feet by removing socks and shoes, and begin by describing any obvious deformities.

VITAL POINTS

Look

- Affects the lesser toes, most commonly the second toe
- May be associated with hallux valgus
- Flexion deformity at the proximal interphalangeal joint (PIPJ) of the involved toe(s) – this is the major deformity to note
- The distal interphalangeal joint (DIPJ) can be in any position, but extension is most common (Fig. 3.46)
- Neutral or extension at the metatarsophalangeal joint (MTPJ), although hammer toe deformities are primarily confined to the interphalangeal joints (compared with claw toes; see Case 87 and Fig. 3.47)
- Note any associated callosities.

Feel

- Any tenderness of the affected toe(s).

Move

- Note whether deformity is fixed or mobile.

Finish your examination here

Completion

Say that you would like to:
- Watch the patient walk
- Examine her shoes
- Ask her questions to assess the effect of the condition on her life.

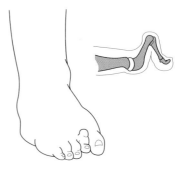

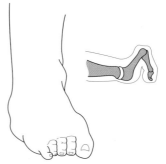

Figure 3.47 Hammer toe (top) and claw toes (bottom).

Figure 3.46 Hammer toes.

? QUESTIONS

(a) What is the aetiology of hammer toes?

- Imbalance between intrinsic (lumbricals and interossei) and extrinsic (long flexors and extensors) muscles of the lesser toes
- More common in:
  - Females than males
  - The elderly
  - Patients with rheumatoid arthritis.

(b) How would you treat this lady's condition?

Non-surgical:

- Appropriate footwear, e.g. high, wide toe boxes and semirigid longitudinal arch supports with metatarsal pads to distribute plantar pressure evenly

Surgical:

- Mobile deformity: consider flexor-to-extensor tendon transfer (split flexor digitorum longus transfer to the extensor hood – Girdlestone–Taylor procedure)
- Fixed deformity: consider:
  - Resection of the proximal phalangeal head and neck with possible flexor and extensor release
  - Proximal phalangectomy
  - PIPJ arthrodesis
- Painful callosities: consider terminal phalangectomy.

> *Gathorne Robert Girdlestone (1881–1950).* First Professor of Orthopaedic Surgery in Britain (at Oxford).

FURTHER READING

Shirzad K, Kiesau CD, DeOrio JK, et al: Lesser toe deformities. *J Am Acad Orthop Surg* 19(8):505–514, 2011.

www.patient.co.uk/showdoc/40002322/ – information for patients.

CASE 86 | MALLET TOES ★★★

INSTRUCTION

'Have a look at this lady's right foot.' (Fig. 3.48)

APPROACH

Expose both ankles and feet by removing the patient's socks and shoes, and begin by describing any obvious deformities.

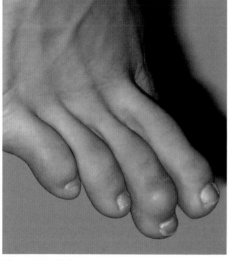

Figure 3.48   Mallet middle toe.

VITAL POINTS

Look

- Affects the lesser toes, commonly the second and third toe
- Flexion deformity at the distal interphalangeal joint (DIPJ) of the involved toe(s)
- No proximal interphalangeal joint (PIPJ) or metatarsophalangeal joint (MTPJ) involvement
- Note any associated callosities.

Feel

- Any tenderness of the affected toe(s).

Move

- Note whether deformity is fixed or mobile.

Finish your examination here

Completion

Say that you would like to:

- Watch the patient walk
- Examine her shoes

- Ask her questions to assess the effect of the condition on her life.

(a) What is the aetiology of mallet toes?

- As with hammer toes, imbalance between intrinsic (lumbricals and interossei) and extrinsic (long flexors and extensors) muscles of the lesser toes
- More common in females than males, the elderly and patients with rheumatoid arthritis and diabetics with peripheral neuropathy.

(b) How would you treat this lady's condition?

Non-surgical:

- Appropriate footwear: usually unhelpful

Surgical:

- Mobile deformity: consider flexor digitorum longus tenotomy (if extensor digitorum longus tendon intact)
- Fixed deformity: consider:
  - Flexor tenotomy with resection of the middle phalangeal head and neck
  - Fusion of the DIPJ
  - Amputation of distal half of distal phalanx to include nail and matrix.

FURTHER READING

Shirzad K, Kiesau CD, DeOrio JK, et al: Lesser toe deformities. *J Am Acad Orthop Surg* 19(8):505–514, 2011.

www.patient.co.uk/showdoc/40002322/ – information for patients.

CASE 87 ｜ CLAW TOES ***

INSTRUCTION

'Examine this lady's right foot.' (Fig. 3.49)

APPROACH

Expose both ankles and feet (by removing the patient's socks and shoes) and begin by describing any obvious deformities.

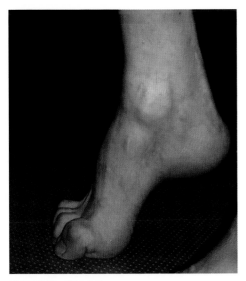

Figure 3.49 Claw toes.

VITAL POINTS

Look

- Affects the lesser toes – frequently all four involved – but may also involve the hallux
- May be bilateral
- Flexion deformity at the proximal interphalangeal joint (PIPJ) and distal interphalangeal joint (DIPJ) (see Fig. 3.49)
- Involves the metatarsophalangeal joint (MTPJ) – note MTPJ hyperextension
- Note any associated callosities – plantar to the metatarsal heads and dorsal to the PIPJs.

Feel

- Any tenderness of the affected toe(s).

Move

- Note whether deformity is fixed or mobile.

Finish your examination here

Completion

Say that you would like to:

- Watch the patient walk
- Examine her shoes

- Ask her questions to assess the effect of the condition on her life.

? QUESTIONS

(a) What is the aetiology of claw toes?

- As with hammer and mallet toes, imbalance between intrinsic (lumbricals and interossei) and extrinsic (long flexors and extensors) muscles of the lesser toes
- More common in females than males, the elderly and patients with rheumatoid arthritis
- May be secondary to neurological disorders such as peripheral neuropathy (diabetes, Charcot–Marie–Tooth disease), lower motor neurone disease (poliomyelitis) and upper motor neurone disease (cerebral palsy, multiple sclerosis, stroke).

(b) How would you treat this lady's condition?

Non-surgical:

- Appropriate footwear, e.g. high, wide toe boxes and semirigid longitudinal arch supports with metatarsal pads to distribute plantar pressure evenly

Surgical:

- Mobile deformity: consider flexor-to-extensor tendon transfer (see Case 85)

- Fixed deformity: consider:
  - Resection of the proximal phalangeal head and neck with possible flexor and extensor release
  - Extensor tenotomy for contractures of the MTPJ
  - Resection of the metatarsal heads of the lesser toes.

> Jean-Martin Charcot (1825–1893). See Charcot's joints (Case 105).
>
> Pierre Marie (1853–1940). Professor of Pathological Anatomy and Clinical Neurology, Salpêtrière Hospital, Paris.
>
> Howard Henry Tooth (1856–1926). English physician and neurologist.
>
> Charcot–Marie–Tooth syndrome (peroneal muscular atrophy) presents in puberty or early adult life and causes progressive weakness of the peroneal muscles, the foot and toe dorsiflexors, the plantar flexors and the intrinsic muscles of the foot, leading to claw toes, and varus and cavus deformities of the forefoot and hindfoot. It may also affect the median and ulnar nerves.

FURTHER READING

Shirzad K, Kiesau CD, DeOrio JK, et al: Lesser toe deformities. *J Am Acad Orthop Surg* 19(8):505–514, 2011.

www.patient.co.uk/showdoc/40002322/ – information for patients.

CASE 88 | MALLET FINGER ***

INSTRUCTION

'Examine this gentleman's right hand.' (Fig. 3.50)

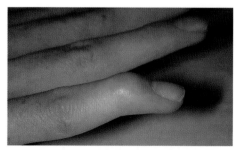

Figure 3.50 Mallet little finger.

APPROACH

Expose the patient as for any hand examination, asking him to place his hands palms upwards on a white pillow.

VITAL POINTS

Look

- Note the flexion deformity of the distal phalanx of the little finger.

Move

- Test for active movement of the finger – the terminal phalanx cannot be actively extended

- On passive movement of the joint, the digit can be moved back into the normal position (unless chronic).

Finish your examination here

? QUESTIONS

(a) What is the aetiology of mallet finger?

There has been damage (usually division) of the extensor tendon to the terminal phalanx of the finger involved. This may occur if a flake of bone is avulsed from the base of the distal phalanx (thus the term baseball finger, as this avulsion may occur in catching a ball).

Interestingly, note that in rheumatoid arthritis, rupture of the central slip of the extensor tendon more proximally leads to the classic boutonnière deformity (see Case 81).

(b) How is mallet finger managed when presenting acutely?

The finger should be X-rayed to exclude a fracture. The finger should be splinted for 6 weeks with the distal interphalangeal joint in extension in a mallet splint to allow reattachment of the tendon. If the avulsed flake of bone is greater than a third of the width of the joint space on the lateral X-ray, it should be repositioned with a fine Kirschner (K) wire or other internal fixation device.

> *Martin Kirschner (1879–1942).* A pupil of Trendelenburg who became Professor of Surgery in Heidelberg, Germany.

FURTHER READING

Cheung JP, Fung B, Ip WY: Review on mallet finger treatment. *Hand Surg* 17(3):439–447, 2012.

www.bssh.ac.uk/patients/commonhand conditions/malletfingerinjury – information for patients.

CASE 89 | TRIGGER FINGER **

INSTRUCTION

'Examine this gentleman's hand.'

APPROACH

Expose the patient as for any hand examination, asking him to place his hands palms upwards on a white pillow.

VITAL POINTS

Look

Note flexion of one or more of the fingers. However, the finger does not necessarily have to be fixed in flexion the whole time for it to be triggering. Trigger finger most frequently affects the middle or ring fingers.

Feel

Ask the patient if there is any pain and then palpate carefully over the palm proximal to the finger involved, as there may be a small nodule overlying the flexor tendon sheath as it enters the digit. The nodule is usually approximately at the level of the proximal transverse palmar crease.

Move

Test for active movement of the finger and note that, on gentle forced extension of the finger, there may be a characteristic snap as the distal finger passes the obstruction.

TOP TIP

EXAMINATION OF THE FLEXOR TENDONS OF THE HAND

☑ Place the patient's hand flat on a hard surface with the palms facing upwards.

- Flexor digitorum profunda tendon is tested by active flexion of the distal interphalangeal joint, with the proximal interphalangeal joint fixed in full extension
- Flexor digitorum superficialis tendon is tested by active flexion of the proximal interphalangeal joint when the examiner fixes the other fingers in full extension.

Finish your examination here

? QUESTIONS

(a) What is the aetiology of trigger finger?

Trigger finger is caused by fibrosis and thickening of the flexor tendon sheath as the tendon enters the digit. It may be idiopathic, or may follow trauma or some unusual activity. Occasionally it can be congenital and present in children, where it is most common in the thumb. The other name for this condition is stenosing tenovaginitis. A similar triggering may occur in rheumatoid arthritis, when other signs of rheumatoid arthritis of the hands would be expected.

(b) How is trigger finger treated?

If a nodule is present over the flexor tendon sheath then a steroid injection may be of benefit but often a tendon release, by incising the sheath, is required.

FURTHER READING

Giugale JM, Fowler JR: Trigger finger: adult and pediatric treatment strategies. *Orthop Clin North Am* 46(4):561–569, 2015.

CASE 90 | INGROWING TOENAIL **

INSTRUCTION

'Look at this gentleman's foot and tell me what you would do about his problem.' (Fig. 3.51)

APPROACH

Expose both feet for comparison.

VITAL POINTS

Inspect

- Most commonly affects the lateral aspect of the great toenail
- Lateral aspect of the nail seen to be digging into the substance of the toe
- Look for signs of inflammation such as swelling and erythema

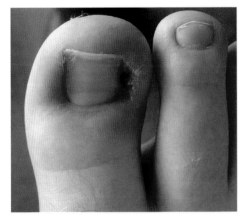

Figure 3.51   Ingrown toenail.

- Look for evidence of serous or purulent discharge.

TOP TIP

☑ If this diagnosis is obvious, tell the examiner immediately what is wrong and move on to discuss the treatment options.

Finish your examination here

? QUESTIONS

(a) What treatments are available for ingrowing toenails?

Non-surgical:

Good nail care, with the help of a chiropodist, trimming nail transversely, using cotton wool packs to lift up the nail and keeping the foot clean and dry.

Surgical options:

- Simple nail avulsion
  - Best treatment for acutely infected toes, as nail-bed treatment carries the risk of osteomyelitis in the presence of infection; recurrence and regrowth are common
  - When combined with the use of phenol, recurrence is less common, but this increases the risk of postoperative infection
- Wedge excision
  - Excision of the involved aspect (lateral or medial) of the nail and nail bed with a wedge of the nail fold down to the periosteum of the phalanx distal to the joint

- Zadek's procedure
  - Total excision of the nail bed, including the germinal matrix.

(b) What are the complications of ingrowing toenail surgery?

- Wound infection
- Regrowth
- Osteomyelitis and septic arthritis.

FURTHER READING

Heidelbaugh JJ, Lee H: Management of the ingrown toenail. *Am Fam Physician* 79(4):303–308, 2009.

http://www.bofas.org.uk/Patient-Information/Ingrowing-toenail – information for patients.

Rounding C, Bloomfield S: Surgical treatments for ingrowing toenails. *Cochrane Database Syst Rev* (2):CD001541, 2005.

CASE 91 | LIGAMENTOUS AND CARTILAGINOUS KNEE LESIONS **

INSTRUCTION

'Examine this gentleman's right knee.'

APPROACH

Proceed with the routine knee examination (see Case 78).

VITAL POINTS

Inspect standing (front and back)

- Scars – look particularly for:
  - Arthroscopic portal scars: anteromedial and anterolateral scars found in the triangle between the patellar tendon, tibial plateau and femoral condyle
  - Meniscectomy scars: transverse/oblique scar over anteromedial aspect of knee joint for open medial meniscectomy and transverse/oblique scar over anterolateral aspect of knee for open lateral meniscectomy
- Valgus or varus deformity of the knee: may be secondary to an old meniscectomy resulting in secondary osteoarthritis.

Gait

- Antalgic – if the knee is painful, e.g. secondary to a meniscal tear or recent injury.

Measure

- Quadriceps wasting may be demonstrated (see Case 78).

Feel (lying supine)

- Tenderness
  - Medial joint line – indicates likely medial meniscal tear or osteochondral defect
  - Lateral joint line – indicates likely lateral meniscal tear or osteochondral defect
- Effusion – may be a sympathetic effusion secondary to a cruciate ligament or meniscal injury.

Move

- Block to extension = locked knee (indicates meniscal, cruciate or osteochondral injury).

Special tests

- Cruciate ligaments
  - Posterior sag – posterior cruciate ligament (PCL) injury
  - Anterior drawer – anterior cruciate ligament (ACL) injury
  - Posterior drawer – PCL injury
  - Positive Lachman test (most sensitive) – ACL injury
- Collateral ligaments
  - Medial joint line opens up on stress testing – medial collateral ligament (MCL) injury
  - Lateral joint line opens up on stress testing – lateral collateral ligament (LCL) injury
- Menisci
  - Positive modified McMurray's test – medial or lateral meniscal tear.

Finish your examination here

Completion

Say that you would like to:

- Examine the hip and ankle (the joints above and below the knee joint)
- Assess the neurovascular status of the limb
- Ask the patient some questions to ascertain how much the problem affects his life, e.g. work, sports.

? QUESTIONS

(a) Cruciate ligament injuries are one cause of haemarthrosis of the knee. What other causes can you think of?

- Primary spontaneous haemarthrosis:
  - Occurs without trauma
  - May be secondary to disorders of coagulation or vascular malformations
- Secondary haemarthrosis:
  - Secondary to trauma
  - 80% are due to ACL injury
  - 10% are secondary to patellar dislocation
  - 10% follow tears in the peripheral third of the menisci (where the meniscus is vascularised), capsular tears and osteochondral or osteophyte fractures.

(b) What factors in the history point to an ACL injury?

- Most commonly associated with valgus/external rotation, hyperextension, deceleration and rotational movements
- Patient hears a 'pop' or feels something tear in >50% of cases
- Inability to continue sport or activity
- Effusion (haemarthrosis) developing within 4–6 h.

(c) What are the problems associated with ACL rupture?

Abnormal knee movements occur leading to:

- Meniscal tears
- Collateral ligament injury
- Progressive premature osteoarthritis.

(d) How do you treat a meniscal tear?

Treatment depends on age, chronicity of injury, activity requirements and location, type and length of tear, but there are options available.

- Non-surgical: no intervention; treat symptomatically

- Surgical:
  - Arthroscopic or open
  - Partial meniscectomy
  - Meniscal repair
  - Meniscal transplant and meniscal replacement (novel, unproven techniques).

? ADVANCED QUESTIONS

(a) What do you know of the anatomy of the menisci?

Medial meniscus:

- Semicircular
- Anterior horn attaches to the anterior intercondylar fascia of the tibia anterior to the ACL tibial insertion
- Posterior horn attaches posteriorly to the intercondylar fascia between the PCL tibial insertion and the posterior insertion of the lateral meniscus
- Bound to the joint capsule peripherally
- Bound to the femur and tibia at its midportion by the deep medial collateral ligament

Lateral meniscus:

- Nearly circular
- Covers a greater area of the tibial articular surface than the medial meniscus
- Anterior horn attaches to the tibial eminence behind the ACL tibial insertion
- Posterior horn attaches behind the tibial eminence anterior to the posterior edge of the medial meniscus
- Loosely attached to its respective tibial plateau by a capsular apron known as the coronary ligament
- Medial and lateral menisci are connected to each other anteriorly via the transverse ligament.

(b) What do you know of the anatomy of the cruciate ligaments?

Anterior cruciate ligament:

- Intracapsular
- Originates from the medial aspect of the lateral femoral condyle
- Inserts into the anterolateral aspect of the medial tibial plateau
- Stops tibia moving forward (anteriorly) in relation to the femur (and also resists tibial rotation and varus–valgus angulation)
- Consists of two bundles, the anteromedial (tight in flexion) and posterolateral (tight in extension) bands

Posterior cruciate ligament:

- Intra-articular but extrasynovial
- Broad origin forming a semicircle on the lateral aspect of the medial femoral condyle
- Inserts in a depression 1 cm inferior to the articular surface on the posterolateral aspect between the medial and lateral tibial plateaus
- Stops tibia moving backwards (posteriorly) in relation to the femur
- Consists of two functional components, the anterolateral group (tight in flexion) and the anteromedial group (tight in extension).

(c) How do you treat ACL ruptures?

Non-surgical: intensive physiotherapy

- Re-education of quadriceps and hamstrings; note that the hamstrings restrict the amount of forward movement of the tibia in relation to the femur
- The results of physiotherapy may be predicted by Noyes' rule of thirds – a third will compensate and pursue normal recreational sports, a third will reduce sporting activities with avoidance of jumping and pivoting exercises, and a third will do poorly and develop instability with sporting and activities of daily living, thus needing early surgery

Surgical:

- Intra-articular reconstruction: commonly autologous hamstring tendon or bone–patellar tendon–bone graft
- Extra-articular reconstruction: e.g. MacIntosh tenodesis
- Combination of both of the above.

(d) What are the causes of a locked knee?

Causes can be classified by age.

Childhood:

- Discoid meniscus
- Pathology in the hip
- Osteochondritis dissecans

Adolescent:

- Meniscal tear
- Cruciate ligament injury
- Osteochondritis dissecans
- Synovial chondromatosis

Adult:

- Meniscal tear
- Cruciate ligament injury
- Loose body
- Osteochondral fracture
- Synovial chondromatosis

Elderly:

- Meniscal tears
- Loose body
- Intra-articular tumour (rare).

FURTHER READING

http://www.aaos.org/research/guidelines/ACLGuidelineFINAL.pdf – American Academy of Orthopaedic Surgeons management guidelines.

Shea KG, Carey JL: Management of anterior cruciate ligament injuries: evidence-based guideline. *J Am Acad Orthop Surg* 23(5):e1–e5, 2015.

CASE 92 RADIAL NERVE LESIONS ★★

INSTRUCTION

'This gentleman is complaining of weakness of his right hand. Have a look at his hands and tell me what you think the problem may be.'

APPROACH

Within surgical short cases, the likely reason for weakness of the hand will be a specific neurological lesion, of the median, ulnar or radial nerves. Beginning with the Top Tips (see Case 80) will allow you to get swiftly to the diagnosis without wasting time.

Expose to elbows and ask the patient to place his hands palm upwards on a pillow (if available). To observe wrist drop, ask him to keep his hands out in front of him, palms downward.

VITAL POINTS

Inspect

- There is unlikely to be any wasting of the hand muscles, but the hand is held with the wrist and fingers flexed (drop wrist)
- If the radial nerve has been damaged at the origin in the brachial plexus the whole arm is deformed (as in Erb's palsy; see Case 102).

Sensory assessment

- Note the loss of sensation over the first dorsal interosseus web space, which is on the dorsum of the hand between the thumb and index finger
- Test also for sensory loss over the dorsal aspect of the forearm.

Motor assessment

- Begin with the metacarpophalangeal extensors (Top Tip, Case 80) and note that extension is lost (muscles supplied by the radial nerve are shown in Fig. 3.52)
- Fix the metacarpophalangeal joint extensors and demonstrate that extension at the proximal interphalangeal joint is preserved, as the lumbricals and interossei are supplied

by the median (lateral two lumbricals) and ulnar (rest of the muscles) nerves
- Finally, test triceps (extension of the elbow) to demonstrate weakness in high radial nerve lesions.

TOP TIP

☑ When examining the peripheral nerves of the upper limb, begin at the hand and move proximally. Continue examining one nerve in its entirety before moving on to the next nerve, by which time the examiner will usually have stopped you. This allows a precise definition of the anatomical location of the nerve lesion described.

Finish your examination here

Completion

Say that you would like to:

- Examine the neck and all the other peripheral nerves of the affected limb.

? QUESTIONS

(a) What are the likely causes of a radial nerve lesion?

High lesions:

- Occur at the level of the brachial plexus, usually due to crutches or Saturday-night palsy (secondary to falling asleep with arm leaning over the top of a chair, thus compressing the radial nerve in the axilla – usually secondary to a state of alcoholic stupor!)
- This causes loss of extension of the elbow, wrist drop and loss of sensation over the first dorsal interosseus web space

Middle lesions:

- Occur in the spiral groove of the humerus, usually as a result of a fracture of the middle third of the humerus, sometimes secondary to the use of a tourniquet
- In some instances the elbow is preserved, as the supply to the elbow leaves the main trunk of the nerve before it enters the groove

Low lesions:

- These occur at the elbow, due to local wounds, surgery or fracture/dislocations
- Only the posterior interosseus branch of the nerve is involved and sensation is preserved. The only lesion will be loss of extension at the metacarpophalangeal joint.

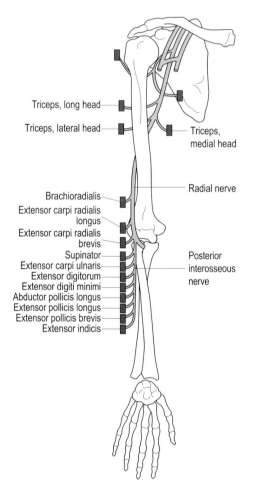

Triceps, long head
Triceps, lateral head
Triceps, medial head

Brachioradialis
Extensor carpi radialis longus
Extensor carpi radialis brevis
Supinator
Extensor carpi ulnaris
Extensor digitorum
Extensor digiti minimi
Abductor pollicis longus
Extensor pollicis longus
Extensor pollicis brevis
Extensor indicis

Radial nerve

Posterior interosseous nerve

Figure 3.52 Muscles supplied by the radial nerve.

? ADVANCED QUESTIONS

(a) What is Wartenberg's syndrome?

Compression of the sensory component of the radial nerve as it exits from under brachioradialis at the wrist. This is an unusual situation where an even more distal lesion can actually cause sensory loss over the first dorsal interosseus.

FURTHER READING

Toussaint CP, Zager EL: What's new in common upper extremity entrapment neuropathies. *Neurosurg Clin N Am* 19(4):573–581, 2008.

CASE 93 | EXAMINATION OF THE SHOULDER **

INSTRUCTION

'Examine this lady's right shoulder. She complains of pain during movement.'

Note

The three most common pathologies of the shoulder that you may encounter in the exam are rotator cuff tears, impingement syndrome and frozen shoulder (adhesive capsulitis). The latter two appear less commonly as they can be very painful.

APPROACH

You need to be able to see both shoulder joints – ask the patient to undress down to her bra (or suitable top) to be able to see both shoulders (you may wish to ask for a chaperone). Male patients should be asked to take off their shirt to expose both upper limbs adequately.

VITAL POINTS

Look (from front and behind)

- Skin – scars, sinuses
- Symmetry – looking particularly for wasting of:
  - Deltoid: loss of contour of shoulder
  - Supraspinatus: look at the muscle bulk above the spine of the scapula from behind
  - Infraspinatus: look at the muscle bulk below the spine of the scapula from behind
- Shape, looking particularly for:
  - Prominent sternoclavicular joint (SCJ) – due to subluxation or osteoarthritis
  - Clavicular deformity – due to old fracture
  - Prominent acromioclavicular joint (ACJ) – due to subluxation.

Feel

- Skin: increased temperature
- Bones and joints – systematically work your way laterally starting at the SCJ, feeling for tenderness:
  - SCJ
  - Clavicle
  - ACJ
  - Acromion
  - Humeral head
  - Greater tuberosity
  - Coracoid (Fig. 3.53)
  - Spine of the scapula (Fig. 3.54)
- Tendons:
  - Long head of biceps – can be palpated for tenderness anteriorly in the bicipital groove as the shoulder is internally and externally rotated
  - Supraspinatus – can be palpated just under the anterior edge of the acromion as the shoulder is held in extension.

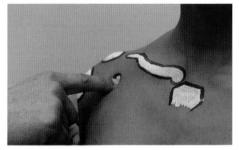

Figure 3.53 Palpating the coracoid.

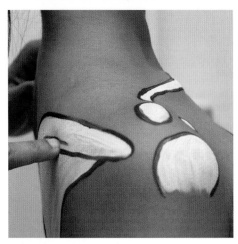

Figure 3.54 Palpating the spine of the scapula.

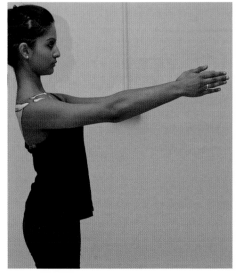

Figure 3.55 Assessing forward flexion of the shoulder.

Move

Stand opposite the patient and ask her to imitate you in order to test active movements. Normal ranges of movement are:

- Forward flexion to 165° – 'Lift both your arms forwards' (Fig. 3.55)
- Abduction to 180° (of which the first 90° is glenohumeral, although scapulothoracic movement starts at 30–40° abduction) – 'Lift both your arms up to the side' (Fig. 3.56)
  - If there is difficulty initiating abduction or the humeral head rises up, consider rotator cuff tear

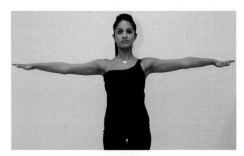

Figure 3.56 Assessing abduction of the shoulder.

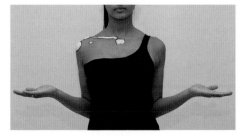

Figure 3.57 Assessing external rotation of the shoulder.

- If there is a painful arc from 60 to 120°, think of rotator cuff tendinitis (also known as impingement syndrome) or a minor rotator cuff tear
- If there is a painful arc from 140 to 180°, i.e. a painful high arc, think of osteoarthritis of the ACJ
- External rotation to 60° (with the elbow flexed to 90° and tucked into the side of the body) (Fig. 3.57)
  - This movement is most commonly affected in frozen shoulder
- Internal rotation measured as thumb reaching mid-thoracic level (T6) – 'put your hand behind your back and reach up as far as you can' (Fig. 3.58).

You can then test the passive range of the same movements, but prevent scapulothoracic movement by anchoring the scapula (press firmly down on top of the shoulder with one hand).

This is followed by testing for power, particularly of:

- Deltoid: test abduction against resistance (Fig. 3.59) – an axillary nerve palsy can result in decreased deltoid power, with loss of sensation in the 'regimental badge' (British) area of skin of the shoulder
- Serratus anterior: pushing against a wall may demonstrate winging of the scapula

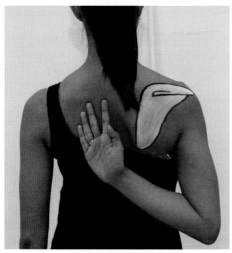

Figure 3.58   Assessing internal rotation of the shoulder.

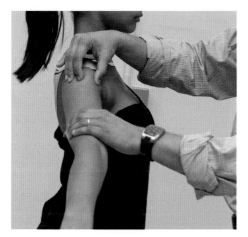

Figure 3.59   Testing the power of deltoid.

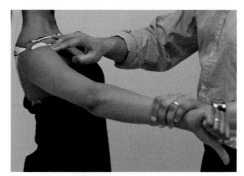

Figure 3.60   Testing the power of supraspinatus.

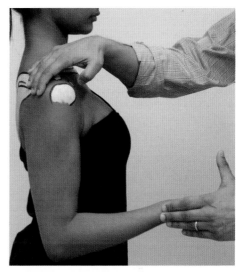

Figure 3.61   Testing the power of the external rotators (infraspinatus/teres minor).

secondary to a long thoracic nerve palsy (see Case 106).

• Subscapularis (internal rotator).

Special tests

You can test each muscle of the rotator cuff (see the mnemonic) individually for pain (in rotator cuff tendinitis) and weakness (in rotator cuff tears):

• Supraspinatus: resisted abduction with arm in maximum internal rotation with 20° abduction and 20° flexion (Fig. 3.60) – if torn, the patient cannot initiate abduction

• Infraspinatus/teres minor: resisted external rotation with elbow flexed to 90° (Fig. 3.61)

• Subscapularis: the most sensitive test is Gerber's lift-off test, where the shoulder is internally rotated with the arm behind the back and the hand is resisted from being lifted off posteriorly (Fig. 3.62); resisted internal rotation can be tested with the elbow flexed to 90°, but this does not isolate subscapularis.

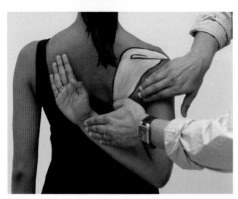

Figure 3.62 Testing the power of subscapularis.

If you have time, you can also test specifically for biceps tendon pathology:

- Resisted elbow flexion with forearm in neutral rotation: biceps bulge if the long head is ruptured ('Popeye' bulge)
- Speed's test: resisted forward flexion of the shoulder with the elbow extended and the forearm supinated
- Yergason's test: resisted supination with the elbow flexed to 90°.

Finish your examination here

Completion

Say that you would like to:

- Examine the neck (joint above) and elbow (joint below)
- Assess the neurovascular status of the limb
- Ask the patient some questions to assess how the condition affects her life.

? QUESTIONS

(a) What are the causes of a painful shoulder?

These can be divided up into:

- Tendon (rotator cuff) disorders:
  - Tendinitis
  - Rupture
  - Frozen shoulder
- Joint disorders:
  - Glenohumeral arthritis
  - Acromioclavicular arthritis
- Referred pain:
  - Cervical spondylosis
  - Cardiac ischaemia
  - Mediastinal pathology

- Instability:
  - Dislocation
  - Subluxation
- Bone lesions:
  - Infection
  - Neoplasms
- Nerve lesions
  - Suprascapular nerve entrapment.

(b) What is the aetiology of rotator cuff impingement?

- Repetitive rubbing of rotator cuff tendons under the coracoacromial arch (the coracoacromial ligament forms the roof of this arch and runs between the coracoid process anteriorly and the anterior third of the acromion posteriorly)
- The greatest amount of wear occurs in the 'impingement position' – abduction, slight flexion and internal rotation
- Site of impingement: 'critical area' of decreased vascularity in the supraspinatus tendon about 1 cm proximal to its insertion into the greater tuberosity
- Contributing factors to impingement:
  - Bone: osteoarthritic thickening of ACJ; osteophytes anterior edge of acromion
  - Tendon: rotator cuff swelling (in inflammatory disorders such as rheumatoid arthritis and gout)
  - Bursa: subacromial bursitis (in inflammatory disorders as above).

(c) How do you treat impingement syndrome?

Non-surgical:

- Eliminate aggravating activity/avoid 'impingement position'
- Physiotherapy
- Short courses of analgesia, e.g. non-steroidal anti-inflammatory drugs
- Subacromial corticosteroid injections for pain relief

Surgical:

- Open or arthroscopic subacromial decompression.

(d) How do you treat rotator cuff tears?

Non-surgical:

- Physiotherapy to improve overall shoulder muscle strength

Surgical:

- Open, mini-open or arthroscopic cuff repair (if amenable to repair) ± subacromial decompression

- Open, mini-open or arthroscopic cuff debridement or partial repair ± subacromial decompression.

? ADVANCED QUESTIONS

(a) What are the causes of a frozen shoulder?

Primary frozen shoulder (adhesive capsulitis):

- Often idiopathic
- Strong associations with diabetes and Dupuytren's contracture
- Global contracture of the shoulder joint, but maximally in the rotator interval area and around the coracohumeral ligament
- Histologically, the contracture is made of a dense collagen matrix, with numerous fibroblasts and myofibroblasts – this active fibroblast and myofibroblast proliferation is similar to the histology of Dupuytren's contracture (see Case 79)
- The frozen shoulder may remain 'frozen' due to slow remodelling as a result of high levels of tissue inhibitors of metalloproteinases, which inhibit matrix metalloproteinases

Secondary frozen shoulder:

- Intrinsic causes:
  - Chronic rotator cuff injuries
  - Post-traumatic scarring following fractures around the shoulder, e.g. surgical neck or tuberosity fractures
- Extrinsic causes (painful disorders leading to decreased movements of the shoulder):
  - Referred pain from cervical radiculopathy
  - Post-hand, wrist or elbow surgery

- Post-breast surgery (especially when axillary node dissection has been performed)
- Post-myocardial infarct.

(b) How do you treat a frozen shoulder?

Non-surgical:

- Pain relief – analgesic ladder (see Case 120), interscalene blocks
- Physiotherapy – especially pendulum exercises
- Manipulation under anaesthesia and steroid/local anaesthetic injections – once acute pain has settled

Surgical:

- Surgery has an ill-defined role
- Reserved for prolonged and disabling restriction
  - Hydrodilatation
- Open or arthroscopic rotator interval, coracohumeral ligament release and excision of the coracoacromial ligament.

FURTHER READING

http://orthoinfo.aaos.org/topic.cfm?topic=a00065 – patient information website on shoulder pain.

http://www.aaos.org/research/guidelines/RCP_guideline.pdf – American Academy of Orthopaedic Surgeons information on rotator cuff problems

http://www.nismat.org/clinicians/physical-exam/evaluation-of-the-shoulder – how to examine the shoulder.

Uppal HS, Evans JP, Smith C: Frozen shoulder: A systematic review of therapeutic options. *World J Orthop* 6(2):263–268, 2015.

CASE 94 | GAIT **

INSTRUCTION

'This gentleman has an abnormal gait. Watch him walk and tell me what you make of it.'

APPROACH

This is a potentially difficult case, as often the different abnormal gaits can be problematic to distinguish.

Expose the patient's lower limb, keeping his underwear on but ask him to remove his socks and shoes.

VITAL POINTS

Inspect

- Ask the patient to walk towards a given point at the other side of the room and then back towards you
- Note if he has difficulty in initiating movement or other signs of Parkinson's disease (unlikely in a surgical exam)
- Look to see if the patient grimaces as if with pain (does he have an antalgic gait?).

Table 3.3

Type of gait	Description	Reason for abnormality
Antalgic	Decreased stance and increased swing phase	Pain
Trendelenburg (see Case 77)	Hip dips instead of rising when foot is lifted off floor, shoulders also lurch to opposite side	Abductor weakness
Parkinsonian	Small shuffling steps (=festinant gait)	Parkinson's disease
Broad-based	Reels, lurches to one side	Cerebellar lesions
Short-leg	Ipsilateral hip drops when weight is on short leg	Previous fracture or congenital shortening
High-stepping	Foot lands flat or on ball instead of on heel, with foot 'slapping' to the ground	Foot drop – inability to dorsiflex the foot secondary to damage to L5 (which supplies extensor hallucis longus, extensor digitorum longus and tibialis anterior) – this is most commonly due to common peroneal nerve palsy (e.g. trauma to fibular head, tight casts) or sciatic nerve palsy (e.g. gunshot wounds, posterior hip dislocations, posterior approach during surgery to the hip joint)
Spastic	Jerky, feet in equinus, hips adducted ('scissoring')	Likely to be an upper motor neurone cause such as cord compression, multiple sclerosis or cerebral palsy

Finish your examination here

Completion

Say that you would like to:

- Examine the back and hip joints, including performing a Trendelenburg test (see Case 77)
- Measure the leg lengths (in short-leg gait) (see Case 77)
- Examine the lower-limb neurology, looking specifically for foot drop (see below).

? QUESTIONS

(a) What are the phases of gait?

Four phases make up the gait:

- Heel strike (more correctly known as initial contact)

- Stance, when foot is on the ground and the centre of gravity of the body moves forward
- Toe off, as the foot begins to lift off the ground from the heel forward
- Swing, as the foot moves forward while the contralateral foot supports the weight of the body.

(b) What are the common abnormalities of gait?

Table 3.3 summarises the various abnormalities you would be expected to know about.

FURTHER READING

Devinney S, Prieskorn D: Neuromuscular examination of the foot and ankle. *Foot Ankle Clin* 5(2):213–233, 2000.

CASE 95 | OSTEOCHONDROMA **

INSTRUCTION

'Examine this lump and tell me your diagnosis.' (Fig. 3.63)

APPROACH

Expose the relevant area – note that osteochondromas are adjacent to the

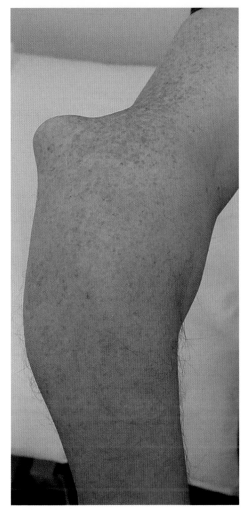

Figure 3.63 Osteochondroma arising from near the elbow joint.

epiphyseal line in the diaphyseal side of the bone and that they are most commonly found around the knee joint (lower end of the femur or upper end of the tibia) but can occur anywhere on the body.

Examine as for lumps (see Case 2).

VITAL POINTS

Inspect

- Hemispherical lump
- Solitary or multiple (the latter may be part of hereditary multiple exostoses).

Palpate

- Smooth surface
- Narrow or wide base
- Osteochondromas point away from the joint
- May be bony-hard in consistency or firm if there is an overlying bursa
- Move the adjacent joint while palpating the lump and assess the relationship with adjacent muscle and tendons, and degree of interference with joint movement.

? QUESTIONS

(a) What is an osteochondroma?

- Lump of cancellous bone with a covering of cortical bone and a cartilaginous cap
- They originate from the separation of small pieces of physeal cartilage from the main cartilaginous physis – these small pieces escape remodelling and carry on growing and ossifying
- Usually start to grow rapidly in adolescence.

? ADVANCED QUESTIONS

(a) What is multiple hereditary osteochondromatosis?

- An autosomal-dominant condition, characterised by multiple osteochondromas, particularly in the limb bones (previously known as diaphyseal aclasis)
- All bones that ossify in cartilage can be affected, except the spine and skull
- It is thought to be a failure of growth-plate remodelling
- There is a small incidence of sarcomatous change.

(b) What is the surgical treatment?

The osteochondroma should be excised if symptomatic (such as pressure symptoms or cosmesis) or if it increases in size or becomes more painful (suspicion of malignancy).

FURTHER READING

Hakim DN, Pelly T, Kulendran M, et al: Benign tumours of the bone: A review. *J Bone Oncol* 4(2):37–41, 2015.

CASE 96 | POPLITEAL FOSSA SWELLINGS **

INSTRUCTION

'Examine this gentleman's right knee.'

APPROACH

Approach as for knee examination (see Case 78).

VITAL POINTS

You should aim to elicit features of a lump (see Case 2). The vital points are outlined below.

Look from behind and from the side (with the patient standing)

- Visible swelling in the popliteal fossa (proceed with the following routine, leaving 'gait' and 'measure' until you have fully described this swelling)
- Skin involvement – sebaceous cyst.

Palpate from behind

- Pulsatile (swelling overlying popliteal artery) or expansile (popliteal artery aneurysm)
- Fluctuant (cystic swelling)
- Compressible (saphena varix of the saphenopopliteal junction)
- Transilluminable (cystic swelling).

Finish your examination here

Completion

Say that you would like to:

- Continue with the rest of the knee examination (the examiner may allow you to proceed if there are further signs to elicit, e.g. osteoarthritis of the knee)
- Perform a neurological and peripheral vascular examination, including the peripheral pulses
- Examine the joint above (the hip) and the joint below (the ankle).

? QUESTIONS

(a) What is your differential diagnosis?

- Skin and subcutaneous tissues – lipoma (see Case 3), sebaceous cyst (see Case 4)

- Artery – popliteal artery aneurysm (see Case 119)
- Vein – saphena varix (at the saphenopopliteal junction; see Case 111), deep vein thrombosis
- Nerve – neuroma (e.g. tibial nerve)
- Enlarged bursae, e.g. associated with semimembranosus and medial head of gastrocnemius medially and with popliteus and lateral head of gastrocnemius laterally (Fig. 3.64)
- Cysts – Baker's cyst (associated with degenerative changes in the knee joint) and popliteal cyst (enlargement of the popliteal bursa but the knee joint is normal).

(b) What is a Baker's cyst?

- Described by Baker as a posterior herniation of the capsule of the knee joint
- Leads to escape of synovial fluid into one of the posterior bursae, stiffness and knee swelling
- Often associated with degenerative knee joint disease
- Diagnosis is confirmed by ultrasound examination – identification of fluid between the semimembranosus and medial gastrocnemius tendons in communication with a posterior knee cyst indicates Baker's cyst with 100% accuracy
- Aspiration is possible, although recurrence is common

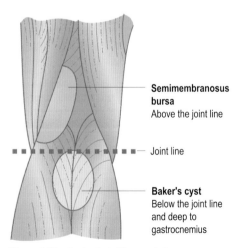

Semimembranosus bursa
Above the joint line

Joint line

Baker's cyst
Below the joint line and deep to gastrocnemius

Figure 3.64 Anatomical difference between a semimembranosus bursa and a Baker's cyst.

- Important to rule out deep vein thrombosis, but the two can coexist.

(c) What is a popliteal cyst?

- Usually located on the medial side of popliteal fossa, just distal to the flexion crease of the knee, under the medial head of gastrocnemius
- Found in children and young adults (in adults, may be associated with pathology in the knee)
- Twice as common in boys compared to girls
- Usually unilateral
- Becomes more prominent when knee extended and disappears in flexion
- Firm and can be transilluminated
- If the cyst is not found in the medial part of the popliteal fossa or has a solid component (on ultrasound), rule out tumour with a CT or MRI scan
- Cysts can be aspirated and sent for cytology, if the patient (or the child's parents) is concerned, or surgically excised (with a high rate of recurrence)
- Although spontaneous remission is not to be expected in all cases, asymptomatic popliteal cysts in children can be treated non-surgically with good results.

? ADVANCED QUESTIONS

(a) What are the boundaries of the popliteal fossa?

- Superomedial: semimembranosus and semitendinosus tendons
- Superolateral: biceps tendon
- Inferomedial: medial head of gastrocnemius
- Inferolateral: lateral head of gastrocnemius
- Roof: fascia lata
- Floor: (from proximal to distal) popliteal surface of the femur, capsule of the knee joint and popliteus muscle covered by its fascia.

William Morrant Baker (1839–1896). English surgeon, St Bartholomew's Hospital, London. Private assistant to Sir James Paget.

FURTHER READING

Frush TJ, Noyes FR: Baker's cyst: diagnostic and surgical considerations. *Sports Health* 7(4):359–365, 2015.

Herman AM, Marzo JM: Popliteal cysts: a current review. *Orthopedics* 37(8):e678–e684, 2014.

CASE 97 | HALLUX RIGIDUS ★★

INSTRUCTION

'Examine this gentleman's right foot.'

APPROACH

Expose both ankles and feet and begin by describing any obvious deformities.

VITAL POINTS

Look (and ask)

- Likely to be unremarkable – if you notice no abnormalities on initial inspection, ask the patient where exactly the problem is, in order to focus your examination on the big toe (this will stop you wasting time examining all the joints of the foot)
  - There may be swelling of the first metatarsophalangeal joint (MTPJ)
- Note that he is likely to be complaining of pain in the right big toe on

weightbearing, particularly during the push-off phase of gait.

Feel

- First MTPJ tenderness, particularly on the dorsal surface
- Unilateral versus bilateral involvement.

Move

- Limited first MTPJ dorsiflexion
- May be associated with crepitus (see below).

Finish your examination here

Completion

Say that you would like to:

- Watch the patient walk
- Examine his shoes

- Ask him questions to assess the effect of the condition on his life.

❓ QUESTIONS

(a) What is hallux rigidus?

- Painful loss of motion (particularly dorsiflexion) of the first MTPJ secondary to degenerative joint disease
- May be due to bony degeneration, which can be either primary, as in osteoarthritis, or secondary to degenerative conditions, such as gout
- May be due to capsular damage and contraction.

(b) What are the radiological changes associated with hallux rigidus?

- Initially normal
- Degenerative osteoarthritic changes seen later, particularly joint space narrowing and marginal osteophytes (especially dorsally and laterally).

(c) How would you treat this condition?

Non-surgical:

- Appropriate footwear, e.g. stiff-soled shoes to limit dorsiflexion of the first MTPJ or rocker-bottom soles
- During acute exacerbations – use of non-steroidal anti-inflammatories or intra-articular steroid injections for temporary relief – this is technically difficult if the space between the joints has narrowed

Surgical:

- Early disease (good range of movement and little loss of joint space) – cheilectomy (excision of dorsal segment of metatarsal head)
- Advanced disease – consider Silastic interposition arthroplasty or, most commonly, arthrodesis.

❓ ADVANCED QUESTIONS

(a) What other diagnosis should you be aware of when managing a patient with hallux rigidus?

- Diffuse joint osteoarthritis – characterised by tenderness of the sesamoid bones and more crepitus than in hallux rigidus.

(b) What is the optimal position for fusion of the MTPJ during arthrodesis?

The position of fusion should be tailored to the individual, but generally:

- 10–15° of dorsiflexion (with respect to the floor)
- 15° of valgus
- Neutral rotation.

FURTHER READING

Hamid KS, Parekh SG: Clinical presentation and management of hallux rigidus. *Foot Ankle Clin* 20(3):391–399, 2015.

www.bofas.org.uk/Patient-Information/Hallux-rigidus – information for patients.

CASE 98 | CASTS **

INSTRUCTION

Patients with casts can easily be recruited for the clinical examination. Be prepared to describe casts and to discuss their advantages and complications.

Description of the cast

- Plaster of Paris or newer cast material (see below)
- Complete or incomplete (the latter is also known as a slab, or backslab)
- Positioning of the cast, such as above or below the joint. Remember that ideally the joints above and below the fracture should

be immobilised in order to prevent displacement of the fracture

- Special casts, such as patellar tendon-bearing (Sarmiento) casts that allow movement of the knee while controlling the rotation of tibial fractures
- Has functional cast bracing been used? These are casts with hinges attached to allow some movement of the joint in a controlled manner. They are most commonly used for fractures of the tibia or femur. Functional cast braces can be:
  - Simple, such as for the elbow
  - Complex, e.g. polyaxial at the knee.

Complications

Tight casts:

- Due to tight casting, ridges in the cast due to poor application or limb swelling. This may lead to vascular compression and compartment syndrome. Warn patients of the symptoms of compartment syndrome (see Notes, below) – if there is any suspicion that the cast is too tight, remove it
- Loosening of the cast leading to failure of fixation

Skin complications:

- On application – pressure sores can occur, particularly over bony prominences, and are best prevented by adequate padding
- On removal – abrasions and lacerations can occur, especially if an electric saw is used
- Foreign body – may fall into the cast, necessitating replacement
- Allergic reactions (rare).

Advantages of newer cast materials

- Lighter
- Stronger
- More radiolucent
- Waterproof
- Resistant to wear and tear
- Different colours available (for children and young-at-heart adults)
- Less untidy to apply (than plaster of Paris).

Disadvantages of newer cast materials

- Expense
- Skin irritation (gloves should be worn by the applicant)
- Less deformation after setting, therefore increased risk of neurovascular compromise if the limb swells
- More difficult to apply
- Can be very difficult to remove in an emergency situation without a proper plaster saw.

Plaster of paris – points of note

- Use first described by Antonius Mathijsen, a Flemish military surgeon, in 1854 for war injuries
- The name originates from the Montmartre region of Paris where it was first mined
- Consists of open-weave cloth or muslin strip impregnated with dehydrated calcium sulphate
- On addition of water, a latent heat of crystallisation reaction occurs; calcium sulphate becomes hydrated and then rapidly sets
- Cloth is made stiffer using dextrose or starch
- Hardening rates can be altered using accelerators or inhibitors.

Newer cast materials – points of note

- Knitted material of cloth or glass fibre impregnated with a monomer or polymer of polyurethane with substituted isocyanate terminal groups
- On addition of water, the compound polymerises and releases carbon dioxide
- Highly reactive material which is packaged in resistant containers.

Notes

- Compartment syndrome is defined as elevated compartment pressures within a soft-tissue envelope (either due to decreased space or increased pressure)
- Remember all the Ps for symptoms and signs
  - **P**ain out of **P**roportion to injury
  - **P**ain on **P**assive flexion
  - **P**alpate tense compartment
  - **P**allor, **P**aralysis, **P**araesthesia and **P**ulselessness (these are all seen late in the condition)
- The diagnosis is made clinically and can be confirmed with compartment pressure monitoring – with the latter, urgent treatment is needed if the absolute compartment pressure is greater than 30 mmHg or if the compartment pressure is within 30 mmHg of the diastolic blood pressure
- The treatment is emergency fasciotomy to decompress the involved compartments.

CASE 99 SIMULATED REDUCTION OF FRACTURES **

INSTRUCTION

You may be asked to demonstrate the reduction of a common fracture (e.g. fracture of the distal radius) on a patient model – your understanding of the principles of fracture reduction is being examined, e.g. 'This lady has presented to you in Accident and Emergency with a fracture of the right distal radius which you have confirmed on X-ray views. I would like you to demonstrate how you would reduce this fracture in A&E.' You may be shown an X-ray of the fracture at this point and there may be only one view, e.g. lateral only (Fig. 3.65).

APPROACH

Introduce yourself to the patient and begin by describing the fracture on the X-ray that you have been shown (the site of the fracture, any associated displacement, deviation or shortening, involvement of the ulna, etc.).

VITAL POINTS

Initiation

- Place yourself on the same side of the patient as the injury
- Explain the fracture to her and the need for reduction
- Explain that you will provide pain relief with a combination of inhaled nitrous oxide and local haematoma block with local anaesthetic (or your own preferred choice of analgesia).

Assistance

- Tell the examiner that you would use him as an assistant and position his hands proximal

to the fracture site in order to provide countertraction (usually just distal to the flexed elbow).

Traction

- Demonstrate the way that traction is performed, but do not pull with any force – do not harm the patient
- Explain that the first manoeuvre is linear traction from distal to the fracture site – traction serves to relax the musculature around the fracture site due to the inverse stretch reflex and needs to be maintained for several minutes before the reflex sets in.

Reduction

- The manoeuvres performed essentially serve to reverse the direction in which the fragment displaced at the time of injury and will depend upon the fracture itself, e.g. with dorsal displacement of the fragment, an opposing volar force is needed to effect the reduction. Sometimes it is necessary (while applying longitudinal traction) to increase the angulatory deformity in order to disimpact the fracture, and then to angle it back into the opposite direction.

Hold

- The fracture is held post-reduction, in this case by a below-elbow dorsal backslab (not a complete cast, as swelling may occur post-application)
- A broad arm sling provides additional comfort.

X-rays

- Anteroposterior and lateral X-rays are taken in order to check the reduction.

Follow-up

- A fracture clinic appointment is made in a few days time in order to check the reduction and complete the cast once the swelling has reduced

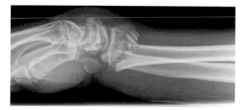

Figure 3.65 Lateral X-ray view of distal radius fracture of the wrist.

- It is particularly important to X-ray the wrist at 7–10 days as this is the most common time point for the fracture to re-displace
- Say that you would like to give the patient an information leaflet on

the care and complications of casts
- Explain that the fracture would normally take 4–6 weeks to heal, after which she may need physiotherapy for any resulting stiffness.

CASE 100 | LUMBAR DISC HERNIATION   ★★

INSTRUCTION

'This lady is complaining of pain in her lower back radiating down to her right leg. Ask her a few questions, examine her and tell me what you think the problem is.'

APPROACH

The ideal patient for this case would be one with a known lumbar disc prolapse in whom there are focal neurological signs to be elicited. Be as gentle as possible when examining the patient's back in order to minimise the chances of hurting her.

VITAL POINTS

Important features to extract are:

- Age
- Occupation
- Features of the pain, especially site, radiation, any history of injury and relieving and exacerbating factors
- Neurological symptoms (e.g. weakness, numbness and paraesthesia) and their distribution
- Sphincter disturbance – bladder and bowel symptoms (unlikely in patients used for examination purposes)
- Effect on patient's lifestyle, e.g. work, sleep
- Previous treatments, e.g. use of analgesia, physiotherapy, caudal epidurals, operative intervention
- Explore other causes of back pain, e.g. diseases of the pancreas, abdominal aortic aneurysm, loin pain from renal causes.

Examination

It is essential to examine the patient in her underwear so that the whole back and lower limbs are exposed. Start with the patient standing facing away from you and examine her gait first, then her back and finally, examine her lower limbs after asking her to lie down on the examination couch.

Gait

Half-shut knife position – patient leans forward with a painful, partially flexed back.

Look

- Skin – scars, sinuses
- From the side – loss of normal lumbar lordosis
- Posture – the 'sciatic list' is an involuntary attempt by the patient to reduce nerve root irritation by leaning to one side in an effort to open up the neural foramen.

Feel

- Muscle – erector spinae muscle spasm/ tenderness.

Move

- Forward flexion – ask the patient to touch her toes; normally her fingertips should be able to reach to within 5 cm of the floor (estimate distance from bony landmarks, e.g. ankle or knee)
- Extension – normally 30°
- Lateral flexion – ask the patient to slide hand down outside of leg; normally 30° to each side
- Rotation – ask the patient to sit down (to fix the pelvis) and fold her arms across her chest; normally 40° to each side.

Lie the patient supine

Straight-leg raising (SLR)

- Demonstrates lumbosacral nerve root irritation
- With the knee fully extended, gently flex the hip and record the angle at which there is onset of pain. This angle is normally 80° and Lasègue's sign is positive if pain is felt in the back, buttock and thigh at less than 60°
- A feeling of tightness in the hamstring is not significant
- Crossed SLR – if SLR on unaffected side produces pain on the affected side, this suggests L4/5 lumbar disc protrusion (this is the most specific sign for lumbar disc herniation).

Sciatic stretch test

- Having extended the hip as above, dorsiflexion of the foot should induce further pain
- Flexing the extended knee relieves the pain.

Neurological examination of the lower limbs

- Tone
- Power: test in particular for movements affected by the involved nerve roots
- Reflexes: knee/ankle/plantars
- Sensation: looking for specific dermatomal loss (see Table 3.1 and Fig. 3.66).

Finish your examination here

Completion

Say that you would like to:

- Examine the patient prone – in particular, perform a femoral stretch test to exclude an L2/3/4 root lesion
- Examine the peripheral pulses – to exclude a vascular cause
- Examine the abdomen – to exclude intra-abdominal pathology that may cause back pain
- Perform a digital rectal examination – to check anal tone, perianal sensation and the anal reflex to exclude cauda equina compression (not likely to be encountered in the clinical examination!).

Say you would record your findings.

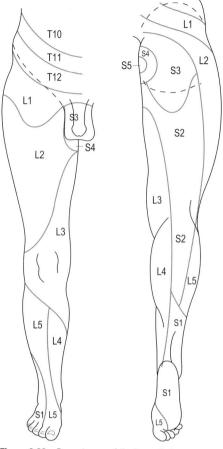

Figure 3.66   Dermatomes of the lower limb.

? QUESTIONS

(a) What factors increase the risk of developing symptomatic disc degeneration and herniation?

Physiological:

- Increasing age
- Poor posture
- Poor overall aerobic fitness
- Poor strength of spinal extensor and abdominal muscles
- Decreased spinal mobility

Environmental:

- Smoking

Occupational:

- Heavy physical work
- Frequent bending, lifting, pushing, pulling and twisting
- Repetitive work postures

- Static work postures
- Vibration
- Psychological and psychosocial work factors.

(b) How would you treat a lumbar disc herniation?

Non-surgical:

- Short period of bed rest (not more than 2 days) with appropriate analgesia (combination of muscle relaxant, non-steroidal anti-inflammatories and opioids) for acute attacks
- Physiotherapy ('back school') aimed at muscle strengthening and stabilisation, with emphasis usually on extension exercises, which strengthen back extensors and are less likely to increase intradiscal pressures

Epidural analgesia:

- Injection of a long-acting steroid with an epidural anaesthetic results in 60–85% short-term pain relief rate which falls to 30–40% at 6 months

Surgical: indicated with a herniated disc where there is a progressive neurological deficit and/or severe incapacitating pain (or failure of non-surgical treatment).

Options include:

- Chemonucleolysis of the disc with chymopapain – success rate ~70% but out of favour due to complications such as severe postoperative pain and spasms, and rarely, transverse myelitis and anaphylactic reactions
- Percutaneous discectomy – decompresses the nerve root by removing disc material from the centre of the disc space; ~50% success rate
- Endoscopic discectomy – success rates reported to be ~80%, but technique still in evolution
- Open hemilaminotomy and discectomy – gold standard with 85% success rate and

performed with the use of loupe magnification or operating microscope.

? ADVANCED QUESTIONS

(a) What is the difference between sciatica and referred pain?

- The term sciatica should only be used to refer to nerve root pain in a specific dermatomal distribution
- Referred pain is pain caused by any lesion in a spinal motion segment which radiates distally in a non-dermatomal pattern, e.g. to the buttocks, thighs, hips and occasionally the lower leg from the back. This pain is usually poorly localised, dull and less superficial than nerve root pain.

(b) What is the pathology of disc herniation?

- Pre-existing degeneration contributes to disc herniation
- A disc consists of an outer annulus fibrosus and an inner nucleus pulposus
- Herniation is the end process of progressive rupture of the nucleus pulposus through the posterior annulus and herniation of this material into the spinal canal
- The initial pathology is asymptomatic disc fissuring and fragmentation
- This is followed by progressive annular disruption from the inner to the outer layers
- In some patients, this finally results in a complete annular rupture with herniation of disc material into the canal.

FURTHER READING

Simon J, McAuliffe M, Shamim F, et al: Discogenic low back pain. *Phys Med Rehabil Clin N Am* 25(2):305–317, 2014.

www.arthritisresearchuk.org/arthritis-information/conditions/back-pain.aspx – information for patients.

CASE 101   EXAMINATION OF THE CERVICAL SPINE   *

INSTRUCTION

'This gentleman is complaining of pain in his neck and tingling in his right arm. Take a focused history and examine him, then tell me your differential diagnosis and plan.'

APPROACH

You may be presented with a patient who has a neck deformity and/or focal neurology. Ensure you are gentle when you examine him and explain what you are doing.

VITAL POINTS

Important features to extract are:

- Age
- Occupation
- Features of the pain, especially site, radiation, any history of injury, and relieving and exacerbating factors
- Neurological symptoms (e.g. weakness, numbness and paraesthesia) and their distribution
- Sphincter disturbance – bladder and bowel symptoms (unlikely in patients used for examination purposes)
- Effect on patient's lifestyle, e.g. work, sleep, clumsiness
- Previous treatments, e.g. use of analgesia, physiotherapy, operative intervention

EXAMINATION

It is essential to examine the patient with his neck and chest exposed to perform a full examination. Start with the patient standing facing away from you and examine his gait first; notice the position in which he holds his neck. Then ask the patient to sit in a chair in front of you and examine his neck and finally his upper limbs.

Look

- Skin – scars, sinuses, rashes, masses, stigmata of disease such as café-au-lait spots or neurofibromas (e.g. neurofibromatosis)
- From the side – loss of normal cervical lordosis or thoracic kyphosis
- Posture – torticollis can result from a contracture of sternocleidomastoid or lateral flexion from erosion of the lateral mass of the atlas in rheumatoid arthritis.

Feel

- Bone – the midline spinous processes from the occiput to T1, noting any tenderness or step deformities
- Muscle – the paraspinal, trapezius and interscapular muscles for muscle spasm/tenderness.

Move

- Forward flexion – ask the patient to bring his chin to his chest, normally 80° (state if reduced distance from chin to chest and estimate the magnitude)
- Extension – ask the patient to look up to the ceiling; normally 50°
- Lateral flexion – ask the patient to touch his ear to the ipsilateral shoulder; normally 45°
- Rotation – ask the patient to turn his neck to look at the wall behind him (in both directions); normally 80° to each side.

If any of these movements are restricted in active motion, perform gentle passive movements to note the resistance of the end of the range – is it limited by the pain the patient is experiencing or by a mechanical block?

Ask the patient to sit on the chair.

Spurling's test

This test can be useful in diagnosing nerve root pain (radiculopathy) in the cervical region.

With the patient sitting, warn him you will be performing a test that may reproduce his symptoms. Turn the patient's head to the affected side, then extend the neck and apply axial compression (push downward) – if pain or tingling radiates into the ipsilateral arm within 30 s, then the test is positive.

Neurological examination of the upper limbs

- Tone
- Power: test in particular for movements affected by the involved nerve roots
- Reflexes: biceps, triceps and supinator reflex
- Sensation: looking for specific dermatomal loss.

Finish your examination here

Completion

Say that you would like to:

- Examine the patient's whole spine if positive features are found in the cervical spine
- Examine the peripheral pulses – to exclude a vascular cause
- Examine the neck – to exclude other organic causes of neck pain, including malignancy or thoracic outlet syndrome
- If there are any concerns about cord compression, perform a full neurological examination, including the lower limbs and assess for red flags.

? QUESTIONS

(a) What factors increase the risk of developing symptomatic disc degeneration in the cervical spine?

Physiological:

- Peak age – between 40 and 50 years
- Poor posture
- Poor overall aerobic fitness
- Poor strength of spinal extensor and abdominal muscles
- Decreased spinal mobility

Sex:

- Men affected more than women

Environmental:

- Smoking

Occupational:

- Frequent bending or carrying heavy loads on the head
- Repetitive work postures
- Posture as a result of excessive driving
- Psychological and psychosocial work factors.

(b) How would you investigate this patient's neck pain with upper-limb paraesthesia?

- Plain X-ray: anteroposterior, lateral and oblique (shows foraminal stenosis). Flexion/extension views can demonstrate instability. This *must* cover C1–T1.

- CT: this is more commonly used for the cervical spine in a trauma setting to demonstrate acute bony injury. For this case, CT with the use of intrathecal dye (CT myelography) can demonstrate neural compression.
- MRI: this will demonstrate pathology in the spinal cord, disc degeneration and bony change. There is a high rate of false positives and so findings must be correlated clinically.
- Nerve conduction studies: this can help differentiate between peripheral nerve compression, neurological conditions and radiculopathy. There are high rates of false positives.

? ADVANCED QUESTION

(a) What radiographic findings would you expect in cervical spondylosis?

- Osteophyte formation
- Disc space narrowing
- Endplate sclerosis
- Reduced canal diameter (sagittal diameter)
- Degenerative changes of facet joints

FURTHER READING

Takagi I, Eliyas K, Stadlan N: Cervical spondylosis: an update on pathophysiology, clinical manifestation, and management strategies. *Dis Mon* 57:583–591, 2011.

CASE 102 | BRACHIAL PLEXUS LESIONS *

INSTRUCTION

'This gentleman suffered an injury to his right upper limb 5 years ago in a road traffic accident. Ask him a few questions first, then examine him and tell me what you think.'

APPROACH

Ensure both upper limbs are fully exposed – ask him to take off his shirt if he has not already undressed. Note that the patient may have a mixed picture of upper and lower brachial plexus injuries (Fig. 3.67).

VITAL POINTS

- Mechanism of injury:
  - If traction injury to the abducted arm, suspect lower brachial plexus lesion
  - If fall on to tip of shoulder, suspect upper brachial plexus lesion
- Clinical consequences – enquire about pain/sensory loss/paraesthesia/weakness
- Functional consequences – use of the limb for daily activities
- Previous treatments – ask about operative interventions, e.g. contracture release, nerve repair, tendon transfers
- Effect of the condition on the patient's quality of life and activities of daily living.

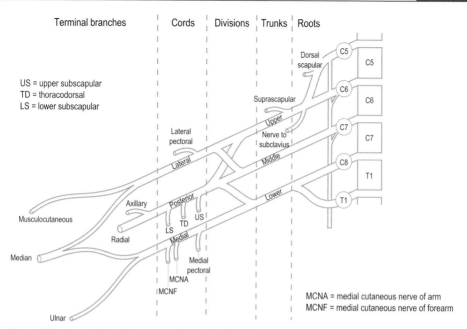

Figure 3.67 Organisation of the nerves within the brachial plexus.

Examination

You are essentially performing a neurological examination in order to distinguish between the various lesions.

INSPECT

- Limb position
  - 'Waiter's tip' position in Erb's palsy (Erb–Duchenne injury) – C5 and C6 involvement – adducted shoulder, extended elbow and forearm pronated and internally rotated
  - 'Claw hand' in Klumpke's palsy (Dejerine–Klumpke injury) – C8 and T1 involvement – paralysis of the small/intrinsic muscles of the hand
- Scars: traumatic/operative
- Muscle wasting/atrophy
- Fasciculations of involved muscles
- Inspect the face for evidence of ipsilateral Horner's syndrome (ptosis, anhidrosis, miosis and enophthalmos) (see Case 19).

Tone

- Flaccidity and hypotonia – lower motor neurone lesion.

Power

- Compare power of muscle groups in affected limb to contralateral limb – note that in C5/6 lesions, there is decreased shoulder abduction and elbow flexion, while in C8/T1 lesions, there is decreased wrist flexion, and finger abduction and adduction.

TOP TIP

NERVE ROOTS RESPONSIBLE FOR MOVEMENTS OF THE UPPER LIMB

Shoulder abduction: C5

Shoulder adduction: C5–C7

Elbow flexion: C5–C6

Elbow extension: C7

Wrist flexion: C7–C8

Wrist extension: C7

Finger flexion: C7–C8

Finger extension: C7–C8

Finger abduction: T1

TOP TIP

MEDICAL RESEARCH COUNCIL GRADING OF MUSCLE POWER

M0 – No contraction

M1 – Flicker or trace of contraction

M2 – Active movement with gravity eliminated

M3 – Active movement against gravity

M4 – Active movement against gravity and resistance

M5 – Normal power

REFLEXES

- Hyporeflexia or absent reflexes in involved roots, e.g. biceps and supinator reflexes affected in C5–6 lesions

✓

TOP TIP

✓ A way to remember limb reflexes (12345678!)

S1–2 – Ankle reflex

L3–4 – Knee reflex

C5–6 – Biceps and supinator reflexes

C7–8 – Triceps reflex

✓

Sensation

- Test light touch (cotton wool) and pain (orange stick) in all dermatomes compared with the unaffected side (Fig. 3.67) –
  - In C5–6 lesions, the outer aspect of the arm (over the insertion of deltoid) is affected
  - In C8–T1 lesions, the ulnar side of the hand and forearm are affected.

COMPLETION

Say that you would like to:

- Determine whether the level of injury is more proximal than C5 – test trapezius (C3–4 root value) by asking the patient to shrug his shoulder against resistance
- Examine the neck to exclude compression from thoracic outlet syndrome, especially if there is no history of trauma (see Case 128).

❓ QUESTIONS

(a) What are the branches of the brachial plexus? (Fig. 3.67)

- The brachial plexus is formed by the anterior rami of C5, 6, 7, 8 and T1 nerve roots (five roots)
- Three trunks: upper, middle and lower lying in the posterior triangle of the neck
- Six divisions: anterior and posterior division of each trunk at the level of the clavicle

- Three cords: lateral, medial and posterior formed as the six divisions enter the axilla (name of the cord denotes relationship to the axillary artery)
  - Lateral cord – anterior divisions of upper and middle trunks
  - Medial cord – anterior division of lower trunk
  - Posterior cord – all three posterior divisions
- Nerve branches: remember the $3:1:0:3:5:5$ rule (Table 3.4).

(b) How would you differentiate between pre-ganglionic and post-ganglionic injuries?

Pre-ganglionic injuries have a worse prognosis, as the nerve roots have been avulsed directly from the spinal cord and, as there is no proximal peripheral nerve tissue, surgical repair is difficult. The features of a pre-ganglionic injury are:

- Bruising in the posterior triangle of the neck
- Pain in an insensate hand
- Loss of sensation above the clavicle

Table 3.4

3 from root	Long thoracic nerve (C5, 6, 7)
	Nerve to subclavius (C5)
	Dorsal scapular nerve (C5, 6)
1 from upper trunk	Suprascapular nerve
0 from division	
3 from lateral cord	Lateral pectoral nerve
	Musculocutaneous nerve
	Lateral contribution to median nerve
5 from medial cord	Medial cutaneous nerve of arm
	Medial cutaneous nerve of forearm
	Medial pectoral nerve
	Medial contribution to median nerve
	Ulnar nerve
5 from posterior cord	Upper subscapular nerve
	Lower subscapular nerve
	Thoracodorsal nerve
	Axillary nerve
	Radial nerve

- Ipsilateral Horner's syndrome (avulsion of C8–T1 nerve roots)
- Loss of muscle function of branches direct from the roots of the brachial plexus, e.g. long thoracic nerve (C5–6–7 – winging of the scapula) and phrenic nerve (C3–4–5 – elevated hemidiaphragm seen on chest X-ray).

? ADVANCED QUESTIONS

(a) How would you assess the prognosis of a brachial plexus injury?

Three types of injury pattern have been described which provide a guide to prognosis:

- Root avulsion: direct avulsion of roots from spinal cord which is not amenable to surgical repair
- Rupture: of the plexus outside the vertebral column and, although the injury is unlikely to heal spontaneously, surgery may be of some benefit
- Nerve damage without rupture: improvement likely to occur spontaneously.

(b) What do you know of the staged management of brachial plexus injuries?

Staged management depends upon:

- Mechanism of injury, e.g. gunshot injuries – debride and treat as closed injury (see below)
- Whether the injury is open or closed – if open, primary epineural repair and if closed, staged management
- Staged management is as follows:
  - Stage I (3 months) – treat expectantly and assess clinically and electrophysiologically

(electromyographic and nerve conduction studies)
- Stage II (3–6 months) – if clinical or electrophysiological improvement, continue to treat expectantly; if not, nerve exploration
- Stage III – nerve exploration and/or repair
- Stage IV – from time of exploration and repair to 1–2 years later (involves active hand therapy)
- Stage V (at 2 years) – final assessment of recovery made and adjunct procedures considered, such as tendon transfers, arthrodesis and amputation.

Joseph Jules Dejerine (1849–1917). French neurologist and psychiatrist, and Professor of Neurology at the Salpêtrière Hospital, Paris.

Madame Dejerine-Klumpke née Auguste Klumpke (1859–1927). American-born neurologist married to Joseph Dejerine.

Guillaume Benjamin Amand Duchenne (1806–1875). French neurologist.

Wilhelm Erb (1840–1921). German neurologist and Professor of Medicine at Leipzig and Heidelberg.

Johann Friedrich Horner (1831–1886). Professor of Ophthalmology, Zurich, Switzerland.

FURTHER READING

http://patient.info/doctor/brachial-plexus-assessment-and-common-injuries – information for patients.

Limthongthang R, Bachoura A, Songcharoen P, et al: Adult brachial plexus injury: evaluation and management. *Orthop Clin North Am* 44(4):591–603, 2013.

CASE 103 | IVORY OSTEOMA *

INSTRUCTION

'Look at this gentleman's forehead and tell me the diagnosis.'

APPROACH

For the 'spot diagnosis'-type question, simply introduce yourself to the patient as the examiner wants a quick answer to the question. Ivory osteomas are commonly found on the vault of the skull and frequently the forehead.

VITAL POINTS

Examine as for any lump (see Case 1).

INSPECT

- Sessile, flat mounds.

PALPATE

- Smooth surface
- Bony hard in consistency

- Can move the superficial layers of the scalp across the top of the lump.

TOP TIP

LAYERS OF THE SCALP

☑ Remember the mnemonic that spells the word **SCALP**:

Skin

Connective tissue

Aponeurotic muscle

Loose areolar tissue

Periosteum.

? QUESTIONS

(a) What is an ivory osteoma?

Ivory osteomas are the most common benign tumours of the skull vault. They arise from cortical bone and radiologically may resemble sclerotic reaction produced by a meningioma (a CT scan may be needed to differentiate the two).

(b) How should they be managed?

They should not be resected unless they are symptomatic.

CASE 104 | CHONDROMA *

INSTRUCTION

'Examine this lump and tell me your diagnosis.'

APPROACH

Examine the relevant area – note that chondromas are usually found in the tubular bones of the hand or feet (e.g. phalanges).

VITAL POINTS

Examine as for lumps (see Case 1). Note that an enchondroma grows from the centre of the bone and an ecchondroma (periosteal chondroma) grows over the surface of the bone.

INSPECT

- Visible solitary or multiple swellings
- May be fusiform (enchondroma) or sessile lumps (ecchondroma).

PALPATE

- Smooth surface
- Hard consistency.

? QUESTIONS

(a) What is the differential diagnosis?

- Benign cysts (no calcification)
- Chondrosarcoma (older patients, especially in large bones).

(b) What is a chondroma?

- Benign cartilaginous tumour within or on the surface of long bones
- X-rays show well-defined lucent area in the medulla and characteristic specks of calcification.

? ADVANCED QUESTIONS

(a) What is the surgical treatment?

Surgical excision or curettage with bone grafting.

(b) What is Ollier's disease?

- Multiple chondromas – this is a sporadic disorder with equal sex distribution where pathological fractures and growth arrest occur
- The rare combination of enchondromas with cutaneous haemangiomas is known as Maffucci's syndrome
- Patients with Ollier's disease have a 30% chance of developing malignant transformation to chondrosarcomas, and also have an increased risk of visceral malignancies.

A. Marfucci (1847–1903). Professor of Pathology, Pisa, Italy.

L. Ollier (1830–1900). French surgeon who was senior surgeon at the Hôtel-Dieu in Lyons, France, in 1860.

CASE 105 | CHARCOT'S JOINTS *

INSTRUCTION

'Examine this gentleman's foot.' (Fig. 3.68)

APPROACH

Compare both feet, ideally by exposing the entire lower limbs, keeping the patient's underwear on.

VITAL POINTS

Look

- Look for swelling of the feet
- Colour of the overlying skin is usually normal, but can appear erythematous
- There may be ulceration (Fig. 3.68) – describe as in Case 2.

Feel

- Foot not tender or warm (although it may have been in the early stages)
- Crepitus may be felt
- The normal contours of the joints of the foot are lost and the joints may be hypertrophic or atrophic
- The joints may be subluxed or dislocated.

Move

- Instability of the joints may be demonstrated by abnormal movements and hypermobility.

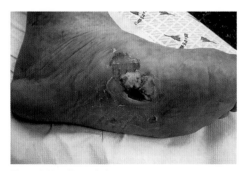

Figure 3.68   Charcot's foot.

Finish your examination here

Completion

Say that you would like to:

- Perform a neurological examination of the affected limb, particularly looking for loss of sensation and joint position sense
- Dip the urine for sugar (to exclude diabetes mellitus).

? QUESTIONS

(a) What is a Charcot's joint?

It is a progressive destructive joint arthropathy secondary to a disturbance of sensory innervation to a joint. The end result is a painless deformed joint resulting from repetitive minor trauma. It is thought that autonomic innervation is disrupted (neurogenic theory), causing hyperaemia in the foot (vascular theory), osteopenia and fragility fractures with joint dislocation and disordered architecture (vascular theory). Ulceration can develop under bony prominences.

(b) What are the causes of a Charcot's joint?

Peripheral:

- Diabetic neuropathy
- Peripheral nerve injuries
- Leprosy

Central:

- Syringomyelia
- Cauda equina syndrome, e.g. secondary to myelomeningocoele
- Tabes dorsalis.

Jean-Martin Charcot (1825–1893). French neurologist and son of a Paris coachbuilder. Professor of Pathological Anatomy, Salpêtrière Hospital, Paris, in 1872. Subsequently he became the Professor of Nervous Diseases in 1882. His pupils included Freud and Babinski.

FURTHER READING

Varma AK: Charcot neuroarthropathy of the foot and ankle: a review. *J Foot Ankle Surg* 52(6):740–749, 2013.

www.diabetes.usyd.edu.au/foot/Chartec1 .html – Charcot's arthropathy.

CASE 106 | WINGING OF THE SCAPULA *

INSTRUCTION

'Look at this gentleman's back and tell me your diagnosis.'

APPROACH

Expose fully to waist and ask the patient to turn around and face away from you.

VITAL POINTS

This case is essentially a spot diagnosis, and if asked to 'look at' the back, do not touch the back.

Look

- Asymmetry of the shoulders (this may not be obvious until the patient pushes against a wall – see below)
- Any obvious scapular winging
- Bilateral involvement.

Move

- Ask the patient to abduct his arm above the horizontal (there may be difficulty in performing this action)
- Ask him to stand up facing a wall and to push firmly with both hands against the wall (this makes winging more prominent and it is clinically easy to determine).

Finish your examination here

Completion

Say that you would like to:

- Examine the upper-limb musculature to exclude muscular dystrophy.

? QUESTIONS

(a) What is the most common cause of winging of the scapula?

Weakness of the serratus anterior muscle secondary to:

- Damage to the long thoracic nerve (anterior rami of C5, 6 and 7) which supplies serratus anterior, e.g. secondary to axillary surgery
- Upper brachial plexus injury
- Viral infections of C5, 6 and 7 nerve roots
- Certain types of muscular dystrophy, e.g. fascioscapulohumeral dystrophy (Dejerine–Landouzy syndrome).

? ADVANCED QUESTIONS

(a) What other causes are you aware of?

- Trapezius palsy secondary to injury to the spinal accessory nerve (at risk of iatrogenic injury in the posterior triangle of the neck)
- Post-glenohumeral fusion
- Abduction contracture of the deltoid.

(b) How would you treat this condition?

- Non-surgical – if disability minimal
- Surgical – tendon transfers or scapulothoracic fusion.

Sir Charles Bell (1774–1842). Scottish surgeon, physiologist and painter.

J. J. Dejerine (1849–1917). French neurologist

L. T. J. Landouzy (1845–1917). French physician.

FURTHER READING

Meininger AK, Figuerres BF, Goldberg BA: Scapular winging: an update. *J Am Acad Orthop Surg* 19(8):453–462, 2011.

CASE 107 | EXTERNAL FIXATORS *

INSTRUCTION

You may be shown an external fixator on a patient or on an X-ray and asked to comment (Fig. 3.69). The following is a guide to external fixators.

Principles

- Focus: this is the area of bone being supported, i.e. the fracture

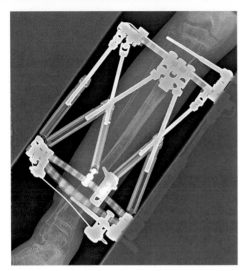

Figure 3.69 Circular Taylor spatial frame external fixator.

- Segment: this is the area of bone into which the external fixator is inserted in order to control the focus.

The external fixator device is made up of pins and frame (the former connect the frame to the bone).

Classification of pins

External fixators are inserted into bone by:

SCREW-THREADED HALF PINS

- Applied to one side of the bone
- Advantage is the low risk of neurovascular damage
- But there is a risk of loosening.

TRANSFIXING PINS

- Passes through the bone from one aspect of the limb to the other
- Provides better control of the fracture
- Disadvantages include possible damage to neurovascular structures as the pins pass through the bone, and risk of loosening
- Therefore transfixing pins are only used in very simple constructs such as joint fusions and temporary stabilisation of severely traumatised limbs.

TENSIONED FINE WIRES

- Also pass all the way through the limb
- This support is made of multiple small, thin wires placed into the bone at different orientations which are then tightened to support the bone

- Are less traumatic to the blood supply of the limb and tend not to loosen but are more expensive and complicated to apply.

Classification of frames

- Uniaxial: half-pin (frame is adjacent to one side of the limb only)
- Circular: Ilizarov frame (frame circles around the limb) or Taylor spatial frame (as in Fig. 3.69)
- Hybrid: supports one segment using rings and other segments using uniaxial constructs
- Pinless: metal clamps that tighten on to the bone and therefore avoid interfering with the medullary canal when later definitive internal fixation is being considered.

Indications

- Multiple trauma – there is evidence that adult respiratory distress syndrome may complicate intramedullary nailing when there has also been a concurrent chest injury, therefore external fixators are an alternative
- Periarticular fractures
- Intra-articular fractures
- Open fractures
- Pelvic fractures – to reduce life-threatening haemorrhage
- Bone transport (Ilizarov technique) – to encourage fracture union and replace lost bone.

Complications

- Pin-track infections
- Chronic pain
- Pin loosening and breakage
- Neurovascular damage
- Joint stiffness.

Professor Gabriel Abramovitch Ilizarov graduated from medical school in the Soviet Union in 1943, near the end of the Second World War. After graduation, he was assigned to practice in Kurgan, a small town in western Siberia. He was the only physician within hundreds of miles and had little in the way of supplies and medicine. Faced with numerous cases of bone deformities and trauma victims due to the war, Professor Ilizarov used the equipment at hand to treat his patients. Through trial and error, with handmade equipment, this self-taught orthopaedic surgeon created the Ilizarov technique of distraction osteogenesis. This refers to the formation of new bone between two bone surfaces that are pulled apart in a controlled and gradual manner.

CASE 108 | INTRAMEDULLARY NAILS *

INSTRUCTION

You may be shown an intramedullary nail, particularly one that has been removed from a patient (the nail is likely to be lying next to a patient or may be shown as a prop in between cases) or on an X-ray (Fig. 3.70). You should be able to recognise that it is an intramedullary nail and know some basic principles.

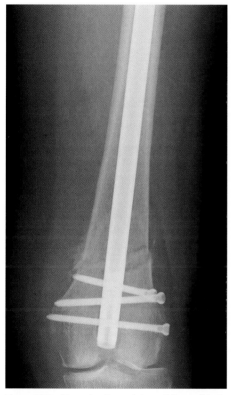

Figure 3.70 X-ray showing an intramedullary nail in the femur.

Material

- Most nails are made from stainless steel, titanium or titanium alloys (e.g. titanium–aluminium–vanadium)
- Titanium and its alloys are stronger, lighter, more resistant to infection and better osseointegrated than stainless steel.

Locking

Screws inserted proximally and distally:

- Provide longitudinal and rotational stability
- May be static or dynamic – in the former, the screws are inserted through round holes, thus forming a fixed construct, whereas in the latter, some element of movement at the fracture site is allowed by locking one end of the nail or placing one screw through an oblong hole
- Dynamisation – this is the process of removing one or more screws in order to allow collapse, which increases the loading of the fracture site and hastens union.

Controversies of reaming

- Enlarges medullary canal and therefore permits insertion of the stronger, wider nail – this may not be necessary with modern materials
- Weakness due to the loss of endosteal bone
- Disturbance of medullary blood supply may cause cortical necrosis
- Time-consuming
- May cause embolism of debris into medullary veins – this is implicated in the aetiology of adult respiratory distress syndrome in severe trauma.

CASE 109 | PAGET'S DISEASE OF BONE *

INSTRUCTION

'Have a look at this gentleman's legs.'

APPROACH

Expose the patient's legs but preserve his dignity by keeping his underwear on.

VITAL POINTS

Look

- Anterior bowing of the tibia (also known as sabre tibia)
- There may be lateral bowing of the femur.

Feel

- The affected bone for warmth.

Finish your examination here

Completion

Say that you would like to:

- Examine for the typical appearance of the skull – enlarged due to increased skull diameter (note that more than 55 cm is abnormal)
- Ask the patient if he has any hearing difficulties (either a conduction defect due to involvement of the ossicles or neural due to compression of the eighth nerve)
- Ask about osteoarthritic involvement of joints (e.g. limitation of hip abduction and fixed flexion deformity of the knees)
- Inspect the neck for a raised jugular venous pressure (cardiac failure secondary to a hyperdynamic circulation)
- Inspect the spine for kyphosis (and auscultate over the vertebral bodies for bruits – secondary to hyperdynamic circulation).

? QUESTIONS

(a) What is Paget's disease?

Paget's disease is a remodelling disease of isolated skeletal areas – there is increased bone turnover, increased numbers of osteoblasts and osteoclasts, and bone enlargement, deformity and weakness.

(b) What are the biochemical features of Paget's disease?

- Normal serum calcium and phosphate (occasionally hypercalcaemia)
- Markedly raised serum alkaline phosphatase (due to increased osteoblastic activity)
- Increased urinary hydroxyproline secretion (due to increased bone resorption).

(c) What are the complications of Paget's disease?

- Bone: increased risk of fractures, sarcomatous change (affects 1% of patients who have the disease for more than 10 years)
- Neurological: cranial nerve palsies, cord compression due to basilar invagination,

nerve root lesions due to vertebral damage, headache, fits
- Cardiac: high-output cardiac failure.

(d) How would you treat Paget's disease?

- Symptomatic: simple analgesics, progressing to bisphosphonates (e.g. alendronate), which inhibit osteoclast-mediated bone resorption. Calcitonins, which act by reducing osteoclastic activity, are less effective than bisphosphonates
- Surgical, e.g. hip arthroplasty for symptomatic osteoarthritis.

? ADVANCED QUESTIONS

(a) What are the radiological features of Paget's disease?

The hallmarks on plain X-rays are localised bony enlargement and patchy cortical thickening with sclerosis, osteolysis and deformity. More specific features include:

- Skull – 'honeycomb' and 'cotton wool' appearance with underlying osteoporosis circumscripta
- Vertebrae – 'picture frame' appearance due to sclerotic margins
- Pelvis – 'brim sign' due to thickening of the iliopectineal line, enlargement of the ischial and pubic bones
- Long bones – increased trabeculation (note that bone scans are more sensitive for assessing the extent of disease).

(b) What do you know about the aetiology of Paget's disease?

Several theories exist, including:

- Genetic: exact mechanisms unclear; may be linked to gene coding for the protein sequestosome 1 (SQSTM1)
- Infectious: may be due to slow viral infection, e.g. paramyxovirus, canine distemper virus, respiratory syncytial virus

(c) What changes can be seen on fundoscopy in patients with Paget's disease?

- Optic atrophy
- Angioid streaks – known as Terry syndrome.

Sir James Paget (1814–1899). English surgeon, St Bartholomew's Hospital, London and Professor of Surgery, Royal College of Surgeons. Described Paget's disease of bone as osteitis deformans.

Also described:

- Paget's disease of the nipple – intraepidermal, intraductal cancer involving the areola and/or the nipple characterised by large cells with a clear cytoplasm
- Paget's disease of the skin – skin cancer involving the apocrine glands characterised by large cells with a clear cytoplasm
- Paget–Schroetter syndrome – idiopathic axillary venous thrombosis
- Paget's sign (on testing whether a lump is fluctuant) – rest two fingers of one hand on opposite sides of the lump and press the middle of the lump with the index finger of your other hand – if the fingers are moved apart, the lump is fluctuant and you have demonstrated Paget's sign (see Case 1).

T. L. Terry (1899–1946). US ophthalmologist.

FURTHER READING

Al-Rashid M, Ramkumar DB, Raskin K, et al: Paget disease of bone. *Orthop Clin N Am* 46(4):577–585, 2015.

http://www.arthritisresearchuk.org/arthritis-information/conditions/pagets.aspx – information for patients.

CASE 110 | ACHONDROPLASIA *

INSTRUCTION

'Have a look at this gentleman and describe what you see.'

APPROACH

Introduce yourself, step back and talk systemically through the physical appearance of the patient. Remember not to lay a hand on the patient unless the examiner prompts you to.

VITAL POINTS

Height

- Reduced (dwarfism, but avoid use of this word in the exam – you can use the term 'disproportionate short stature' instead)
- Normal trunk size
- Shortened extremities.

Hands

- Short and broad
- Wedge-shaped gap between middle and ring fingers (trident hands).

Skull

- Macrocephaly
- Frontal bossing (prominent forehead)
- Saddle nose (depression of the root of the nose)

- Maxillary hypoplasia
- Mandibular prognathism (protrusion of the jaw).

Spine

- Thoracolumbar kyphosis
- Excessive lumbar lordosis.

Knees

- Genu varum.

Finish your examination here

Completion

Say that you would like to:

- Take a family history (see below)
- Assess the effect of the symptoms on the patient's quality of life.

? QUESTIONS

(a) What is achondroplasia?

- Commonest form of disproportionate short stature with proximal shortening of long bones
- Equally common in males and females
- Prevalence is between 0.5 and 1.5 in 10 000 live births.

(b) What treatment options are available for the problems associated with achondroplasia?

Non-surgical:

- Subcutaneous human growth hormone to increase height

Surgical:

- Limb lengthening using distraction devices
  - Correct body proportion and axial deviation
  - Improve appearance, body-image and self-esteem
- Region-specific surgery, e.g.
  - Spinal surgery – correction of thoracolumbar kyphosis, decompression for spinal stenosis
  - Correction of genu varum (by guided growth arrest or osteotomy).

? ADVANCED QUESTIONS

(a) Do you know of any conditions resembling achondroplasia?

- Hypochondroplasia – similar to mild achondroplasia

- Pseudochondroplasia – similar to achondroplasia but normal head and face.

(b) What do you know about the genetics of achondroplasia?

- Autosomal dominant with complete penetrance
- Around 80% of cases represent new mutations
- Mutations in transmembrane domain of fibroblast growth factor receptor 3 mapped to chromosome 4p16.3.

FURTHER READING

Bouali H, Latrech H: Achondroplasia: current options and future perspective. *Pediatr Endocrinol Rev* 12(4):388–395, 2015.

http://www.littlepeopleuk.org/information-about-dwarfism-conditions/types-of-dwarfism/achondroplasia – information for patients.

CASE 111 | VARICOSE VEINS ***

INSTRUCTION

'Examine this lady's varicose veins.' (Fig. 4.1)

APPROACH

There is limited reliance on the Trendelenburg's / tourniquet tests described below in current clinical practice due to the widespread availability / superiority of venous duplex scanning. However, such patients remain widely available for inclusion in examinations, so you should remain familiar with clinical evaluation.

Expose the patient up to the groin, maintaining her dignity by keeping her genitalia covered.

VITAL POINTS

TOP TIP

☑ When performing vascular examinations it is useful to remember that there are three objectives to be completed for both inspection and palpation. This also applies to examination of arterial supply (see Case 113). When assessing the venous system of the lower limbs these are as follows:

☑ Inspection for the three **S**s:

- **S**ite and size of varicosities, including the presence of a saphena varix

- **S**kin for changes and scars

- **S**welling of the ankle

☑ Palpation for the three **S**s:

- **S**tate of the skin/subcutaneous tissues

- **S**ites of fascia defects

- **S**ite of incompetence (including the Trendelenburg and tourniquet tests)

Inspect

Ask the patient to stand (veins are collapsed when the patient is supine) and while kneeling in front of the patient, look for the three **S**s:

- **S**ite and size of varicosities, including the presence of a saphena varix:
  - Establish that any visible veins are varicosities (dilated *and* tortuous) as opposed to physiological (dilated only, e.g. as in athletes)

- Inspect for varicosities in the distribution of the long saphenous vein (LSV) (Figs 4.1 and 4.2)
- Ask the patient to turn around and inspect for varicosities in the distribution of the short saphenous vein (SSV) (Fig. 4.2)
- Try to decide whether the varicosities are long or short saphenous in origin, commenting that the distinction may be difficult below the knee
- Examine the groins for the presence of a saphena varix. This will be located at the saphenofemoral junction (SFJ) (see below)

- **S**kin for changes and scars
  - Look for scars indicating previous surgery, especially hidden in the groin creases
  - Determine whether there are signs of chronic venous insufficiency (see below) (see Case 121)
  - If there is evidence of ulceration, describe its characteristics fully (see Case 112)

- **S**welling of the ankle
  - Look for asymmetry between the lower limbs and establish the height and severity of the swelling.

TOP TIP

☑ Use the acronym **LEGS** to help you remember the signs of chronic venous insufficiency (see Case 121):

- **L**ipodermatosclerosis

- **E**czema

- **G**aps in the skin (i.e. ulceration) – active and healed (the latter causing a white patch called *atrophie blanche*)

- **S**welling (pedal oedema)

☑ Inspect specifically around the medial malleolus (the 'gaiter' area) for evidence of these changes

Palpate

- **S**tate of the skin/subcutaneous tissues
  - Palpate the skin for the presence of pitting oedema
  - Feel along the course of the long and short saphenous veins, determining whether there is induration of the subcutaneous tissues

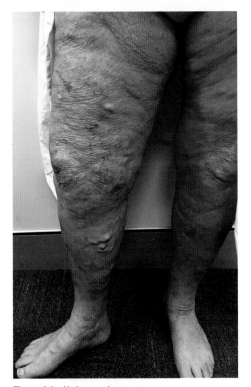

Figure 4.1 Varicose veins.

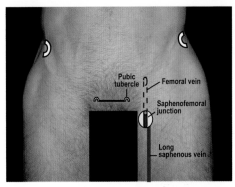

Figure 4.3 Anatomy of the saphenofemoral junction.

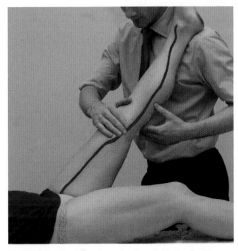

Figure 4.4 Emptying the veins in preparation for the Trendelenburg test.

Figure 4.2 Anatomy of the superficial venous system of the leg.

- Sites of fascia defects
  - Feel along the medial aspect of the leg for tenderness in the fascial defects at the site of perforator veins

- Site of incompetence
  - Ask the patient to turn to face you again and palpate the SFJ, which is located 3.5 cm (approximately two finger breadths) below and lateral to the pubic tubercle (Fig. 4.3)
  - Feel for the smooth swelling and palpable thrill of a saphena varix. If present, the cough test may be positive (Cruveilhier's sign)
  - The Trendelenburg test is performed with the patient first lying down. Elevate the leg gently to empty the veins (Fig. 4.4). Palpate the SFJ and ask the patient to stand while maintaining direct pressure over the SFJ with one finger (Fig. 4.5). If the veins do not refill then the SFJ is incompetent. Should the veins fill, then the SFJ may or may not be competent, but there are certainly distal incompetent perforators

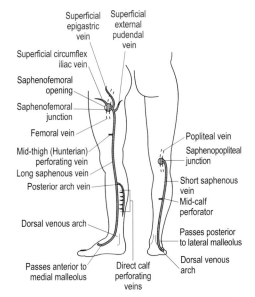

Superficial epigastric vein
Superficial external pudendal vein
Superficial circumflex iliac vein
Saphenofemoral opening
Saphenofemoral junction
Femoral vein
Mid-thigh (Hunterian) perforating vein
Long saphenous vein
Posterior arch vein
Dorsal venous arch
Passes anterior to medial malleolus
Direct calf perforating veins
Popliteal vein
Saphenopopliteal junction
Short saphenous vein
Mid-calf perforator
Passes posterior to lateral malleolus
Dorsal venous arch

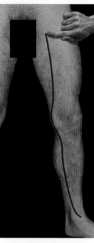

Figure 4.5 The Trendelenburg test with direct pressure over the saphenofemoral junction with one finger.

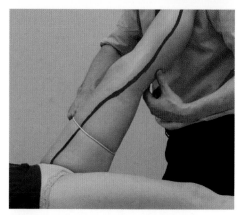

Figure 4.7 The tourniquet test in the mid-thigh.

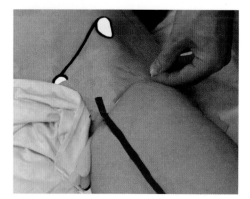

Figure 4.6 The tourniquet test in the upper thigh.

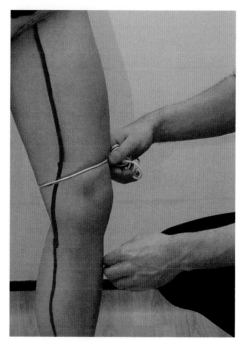

Figure 4.8 The above-knee tourniquet test.

- The tourniquet test employs a similar principle but uses a tourniquet to control the junction rather than fingers. Again, empty the leg in the supine position and apply the tourniquet (in the interests of infection control, a single-use examination glove is frequently employed for this purpose) (Fig. 4.6). Then ask the patient to stand and inspect for filling and collapse above and below the position of the tourniquet (see Top Tip, below). The tourniquet test has the advantage that perforators can be examined below the groin. To do this, this tourniquet should be positioned in the mid-thigh (Fig. 4.7), above- (Fig. 4.8) and below-knee regions (Fig. 4.9)
- A hand-held Doppler (if provided) may be used to allow identification of SFJ/

popliteal fossa reflux by squeezing the muscle of the thigh or calf, listening proximally as blood flows up the leg (normal) and then for a second 'swoosh' in incompetent veins as blood refluxes down the leg when the probe is positioned over the junction. (Note: this has largely been superseded by Duplex scanning in clinical practice and is not relied upon for patient assessment.)

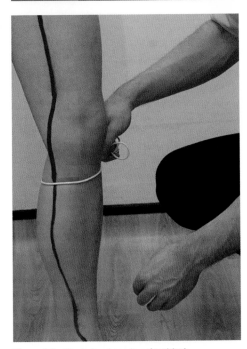

Figure 4.9 The below-knee tourniquet test.

☑ The tourniquet test is designed to reveal the presence and site of incompetent veins, especially at the sites of connection between the superficial and deep venous systems (Fig. 4.2). The test is interpreted by examining the condition of the veins below the level of the tourniquet as follows:

- Collapsed veins below the tourniquet indicate that the incompetent vein is at/above the level of the tourniquet
- Rapid filling of veins below the tourniquet indicate that the incompetent veins is below the level of the tourniquet.

Finish your examination here

Completion

Say that you would like to:
- Perform a tap test (Chevrier's tap sign)
- Auscultate the vein for bruits (indicating the presence of arteriovenous fistulae)
- Examine the abdomen for masses (including a digital rectal examination) to ascertain whether the varicose veins are primary or secondary.

? QUESTIONS

(a) What are the advantages of preoperative Duplex ultrasound scanning?

Over the last few years, routine preoperative duplex imaging has come to be considered mandatory prior to intervention. This imaging modality can accurately identify the presence of reflux or occlusion in deep and superficial venous systems.

Advantages include:
- Accurate characterisation of pattern of superficial reflux / incompetent perforators
- Identification of deep venous disease
- Assessment of suitability of superficial veins for endovenous intervention
- Accurate evaluation of recurrent varicose veins
- Identification of anatomical variants.

(b) How would you treat varicose veins?

Conservative:
- Graduated elastic compression stockings (grade II compression)
- Encourage weight loss and regular exercise

Ultrasound-guided foam sclerotherapy:
- The aim of sclerotherapy is to induce chemical ablation and fibrosis by injecting a sclerosant (e.g. 1% sodium tetradecyl sulphate) into an empty vein
- In recent years, the conversion of liquid sclerosant into foam by mixing it with air or carbon dioxide (Tessari method) has become popular as it makes it echogenic and easier to identify on ultrasound

Surgical:
- Traditional surgery
  - Ligation of the incompetent SFJ or saphenopopliteal junction with stripping of the LSV / SSV (reduced risk of recurrent varicosities) and stab avulsion of varicosities
  - Ligation of incompetent perforating vessels (with site of incompetence preoperatively marked with duplex)
- Endovenous thermal ablation – laser and radiofrequency ablation
  - Avoid general anaesthetic / outpatient procedures
  - Improved early morbidity with faster return to normal activities / work
  - Lower risk of nerve injury

A recently published multicentre randomised trial comparing the clinical effectiveness of endovenous laser ablation, foam sclerotherapy and surgery for the treatment of varicose veins showed no clinically substantial differences in quality of life between the treatment groups. All treatments had similar clinical efficacy, but there were fewer complications after laser treatment, and ablation rates were lower after treatment with foam (see Further reading).

(c) Assuming this patient is to undergo traditional surgery, what would you tell her about the procedure?

- Procedure usually performed as day case
- Need to wear tight-fitting (compression) stockings for 6 weeks postoperatively
- No driving for 1 week
- Does not alter the skin changes, including skin flares
- May not improve symptoms such as aching
- Bruising is very common after surgery, but more severe bleeding, requiring return to theatre, is rare
- There is a risk of deep vein thrombosis (DVT) in the order of 0.5–5%, although small, below-knee DVTs of questionable clinical significance
- There is a risk of nerve damage, with some numbness in up to 40% of patients
- Risk of recurrent veins (20–80% at 5–20 years).

? ADVANCED QUESTIONS

(a) What do you know about the pathophysiology of varicose veins?

Fibrous tissue invades the tunica intima and media of the vein and breaks up the smooth muscle, preventing the maintenance of adequate vascular tone. These changes are patchy and may not affect adjacent segments of vein.

(b) What syndromes are associated with varicose veins?

- Klippel–Trenaunay–Weber syndrome consists of a triad of varicose veins, port-wine stains and bony and soft-tissue hypertrophy of the limbs. This may present with varicose veins in an unusual position, classically over the lateral aspect of the thigh. Peripheral oedema is often significant, as the deep venous system may be abnormal
- Parkes–Weber syndrome is characterised by multiple arteriovenous fistulae, with limb hypertrophy. The arteriovenous fistulae may be so severe as to cause high-output cardiac failure.

M. Klippel (1858–1942). French psychiatrist and neurologist.

P. Trenaunay. French neurologist.

Professor F. Trendelenburg (1844–1924). German surgeon, Leipzig.

F. P. Weber (1863–1962). British physician.

FURTHER READING

Brittenden J, Cotton SC, Elders A, et al: A randomized trial comparing treatments for varicose veins. *N Engl J Med* 371:1218–1227, 2014.

Critchley G, Handa A, Maw A, et al: Complications of varicose vein surgery. *Ann R Coll Surg Engl* 79(2):105–110, 1997.

Houghton AD, Panayiotopoulos Y, Taylor PR: Practical management of primary varicose veins. *Br J Clin Pract* 50(2):103–105, 1996.

CASE 112 | VENOUS ULCER ***

INSTRUCTION

'Examine this patient's ankle and tell me the diagnosis.' (Fig. 4.10)

APPROACH

The patient should be exposed from the groin to the toes, preserving her dignity.

VITAL POINTS

Look

Observe the following characteristic features of a venous ulcer (see Case 1).

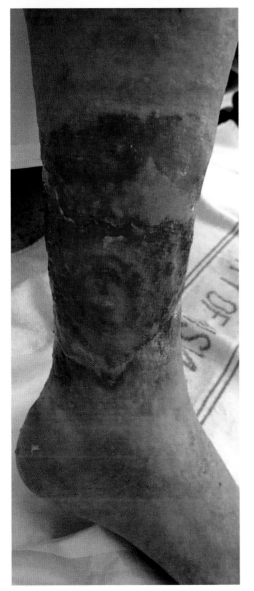

Figure 4.10 Venous ulceration.

Edge and base

- The edge is sloping and pale purple/brown in colour
- The base is usually covered with pink-coloured granulation tissue, but there may also be some white fibrous tissue
- They are usually rather shallow and often have a seropurulent discharge.

Surrounding skin

- Look for signs of primary varicose veins
- The signs of chronic venous disease are usually present: induration, pigmentation and brown discoloration of lipodermatosclerosis (see also Case 121)
- Oedema, spider veins and telangiectasia may be present.

Feel

- Feel the adjacent skin for temperature – it may be warmer than the rest of the leg (compared with the ischaemic ulcer, where the surrounding skin will be cold).

Finish your examination here

Completion

Say that you would like to:
- Examine the limb properly for varicose veins (see Case 111)
- Perform an ankle brachial pressure index measurement (see Case 113) as this must be >0.8 before compression bandaging can be used.

? QUESTIONS

(a) What are the causes of venous ulcers?

Any cause of deep venous insufficiency can lead to ulceration:
- Valvular disease:
  - Varicose veins
  - Deep vein reflux (such as post deep vein thrombosis [DVT])
  - Communicating vein reflux (post-thrombotic or non-thrombotic) – controversial (unusual)

Site

- The venous ulcer is most commonly found over the lower third of the medial aspect of the leg, immediately above the medial malleolus ('gaiter area').

Shape

- The size varies enormously, and venous ulcers can be extremely large.

- Outflow tract obstruction:
  - Often post-DVT
- Muscle pump failure:
  - Primary – stroke, neuromuscular disease
  - Secondary – due to musculoskeletal pathology/injury of the ankle.

(b) How are venous ulcers treated?

Non-surgical:

- High success – 50–70% will heal at 3 months, 80–90% at 12 months
- The patient should be warned to avoid trauma to the affected area
- Four-layer compression bandaging comprising:
  1. Non-adherent dressing over ulcer plus wool bandage
  2. Crêpe bandage
  3. Blue-line bandage
  4. Adhesive bandage to prevent the other layers from slipping
- Encourage rest and elevation of leg
- Once healed, grade II compression stockings should be fitted and continued for life

Surgical:

- If the ulcer fails to heal, careful consideration should be given to excluding other causes (such as a malignant Marjolin ulcer) and the area may need to be biopsied (2% of chronic leg ulcers are malignant)
- Otherwise, a split-skin graft should be considered with excision of the dead skin and the graft attached to healthy granulation tissue
- If ulceration is due to primary varicose veins, surgery to the superficial veins is required.

Rene Marjolin (1812–1895). Surgeon in Paris who described the formation of a carcinoma in a chronic, non-healing ulcer.

FURTHER READING

Fletcher A, Cullum N: A systematic review of compression treatment for venous leg ulcers. *BMJ* 315:376–380, 1997.

London NJ, Donnelly R: ABC of arterial and venous disease. Ulcerated lower limb. *BMJ* 320:1589–1591, 2000.

CASE 113 | PERIPHERAL ARTERIAL SYSTEM – EXAMINATION ***

INSTRUCTION

'Examine this gentleman's legs, focusing on the arterial system.' (Fig. 4.11)

APPROACH

Expose the patient's legs from the groin to the toes, preserving his dignity by keeping his underwear on.

VITAL POINTS

TOP TIP

☑ As with the assessment of the venous system (see Case 111), examination of arterial supply requires that three objectives be completed for both inspection and palpation. These are as follows:

☑ Inspection for:

- Colour changes
- Trophic changes
- Vascular angle

☑ Palpation for:

- Temperature
- Capillary refill
- Peripheral pulses

☑

Inspect

Most of the pathology will be around the feet and toes. However, be certain to examine the groin (and abdomen) for the presence of surgical scars from previous bypass or endovascular procedures. Typically, scars from arterial procedures are vertical, whereas those for venous / groin (e.g. open hernia repair) tend to be horizontal / placed in skin creases. Begin by looking carefully at the feet. Observe the following features (Fig. 4.11):

- Colour changes:
  - The skin of the lower limb may be red (vasodilatation of the microcirculation due to tissue ischaemia), white (advanced

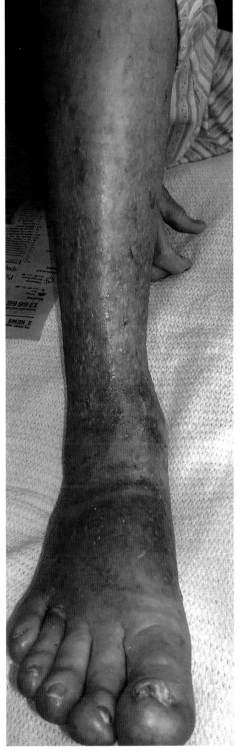

Figure 4.11 Chronic lower-limb ischaemia.

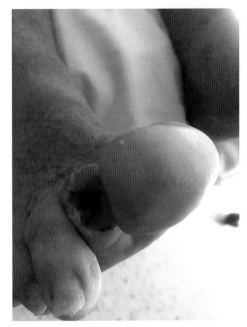

Figure 4.12 Ischaemia resulting in loss of toes.

ischaemia) or purple/blue (excess deoxygenated blood in the tissues)

- Trophic changes:
  - Loss of hair and small non-healing sores may be evident on the lower limbs/feet
  - Gangrene (especially between and at the tips of the toes) (see Case 122)
  - Loss of digits, due to previous gangrene/ amputation (Fig. 4.12)
  - Arterial (ischaemic) ulcers are found typically in the least well-perfused areas and over the pressure points, such as lateral aspect of foot and malleoli (see Case 120)
    - The lesions are punched out (because there is limited healing from the edges due to poor arterial inflow) and well circumscribed. They may be very tender, and the surrounding skin is cold
    - They may vary considerably in size but are usually smaller than venous ulcers
    - There is no / minimal granulation tissue, but there may be a thin layer of slough at the base, which is otherwise flat and pale
    - They may be very deep and penetrate surrounding tissue (e.g. bone / tendon)
    - The commonest differential is with a neuropathic ulcer. If there is any doubt, limb neurology should be examined

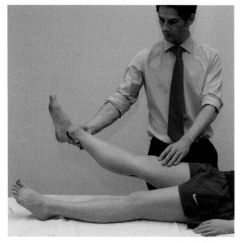

Figure 4.13 Examining for the vascular (Buerger's) angle.

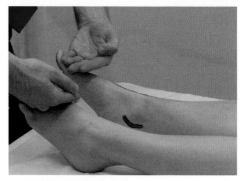

Figure 4.14 Palpation to assess and compare limb skin temperature.

- Be sure to look between each of the toes on both feet
- Ask the patient for permission, then lift the foot up to observe the heel for ulcers (neuropathic ulcers are commonest here) and the sole of the foot for ulceration of the metatarsal heads
- Vascular (Buerger's) angle:
  - Lift the leg until it becomes white as the perfusion drops
  - The angle between the horizontal and the leg when it becomes white is Buerger's angle (Fig. 4.13)
  - Venous guttering can also be observed
  - A normal leg can be raised to 90° and still remain perfused; if the angle is less than 20°, this indicates severe ischaemia
  - Assisting the patient to drop the leg over the side of the bed causes the diseased leg to become purple-red in colour due to reactive hyperaemia – this is the second part of Buerger's test. It represents dysfunction of the microcirculation (perhaps secondary to sympathetic dysfunction and loss of vasoconstrictive tone) due to chronic ischaemia.

Palpate

- Temperature
  - Feel for skin temperature, staying at the end of the bed next to the patient's feet – use the back of the hand, comparing both sides simultaneously for any difference (Fig. 4.14)

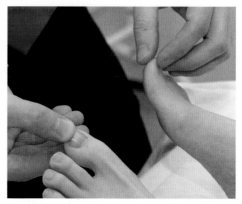

Figure 4.15 Palpation to assess the capillary refill time.

- Capillary refill
  - Examine the toes for capillary refill – use the thumb to push hard over the pulp of the big toe on both sides (Fig. 4.15). Normally the toe blanches but then returns to the normal colour within 2 s; any longer than this is abnormal
- Palpation of the peripheral pulses.

It is imperative that you know the surface anatomy of all the named peripheral arteries. Not only is this a favourite question of examiners, but such knowledge will allow you to expose such vessels surgically with confidence!

You should say that you wish to examine *all* peripheral pulses. However, if you have been asked to examine just the lower limbs, as in this case, it is sufficient to examine the radial pulse (to check its rate and rhythm), before concentrating on the lower limbs. The anatomy of the arteries of the lower limb is shown in Fig. 4.16.

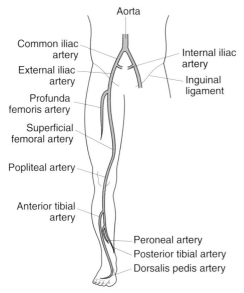

Figure 4.16 Anatomy of the arteries in the leg.

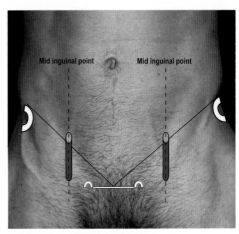

Figure 4.17 Surface anatomy of the femoral pulses.

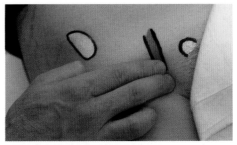

Figure 4.18 Palpation of the femoral pulse with the fingers parallel to the direction of the artery.

TOP TIP

☑ Vascular surgeons palpate the peripheral pulses using the following technique:

- Use more than one finger to palpate the pulse if the artery is big enough
- Position your fingers in the direction of the artery to optimise your chances of feeling it
- Palpate both sides simultaneously to detect subtle differences

If you cannot palpate the pulse having employed all of these measures, then it is (almost certainly!) *absent*. For the purposes of exams, peripheral pulses should be *specifically and confidently* reported to your examiner as: (1) present; (2) reduced; or (3) absent. Nothing annoys examiners more than hearing, 'I don't think that I can feel the pulse'.

Femorals:

- The femoral pulse lies at the mid inguinal point, halfway between the anterior superior iliac spine and the pubic symphysis (Fig. 4.17). It should be palpated with the fingers parallel to the direction of the artery (Fig. 4.18)

Popliteals:

- Next, move down to palpate the popliteal pulse, which is often quite difficult to palpate. Consequently, if it is easily palpable it should raise the suspicion of aneurysmal dilatation

- The pulse is most easily palpated by compressing it against the posterior aspect of the tibia
- Ask the patient to bend the knee slightly, and hold the knee between your hands. Use the pulps of your four fingers of both hands held alongside each other to feel the two heads of the gastrocnemius as they join (marking the lower borders of the popliteal fossa). The pulse lies between these two heads (Fig. 4.19)
- It is not possible to compare both sides simultaneously, so palpate each side in turn before moving on to the foot pulses

Foot pulses:

- Go to the bottom end of the examination couch to palpate the foot pulses
- Do not be tempted to palpate the dorsalis pedis artery (DPA) and posterior tibial artery (PTA) pulses simultaneously. Instead, examine each pulse in turn using two or

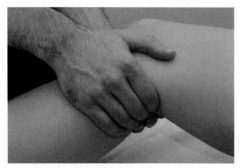

Figure 4.19 Palpation of the popliteal pulse.

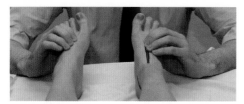

Figure 4.20 Palpation of both dorsalis pedis pulses simultaneously.

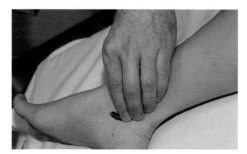

Figure 4.21 Palpation of the posterior tibial pulse in the line of the artery.

three fingers, while simultaneously comparing it with the contralateral side
- To examine the DPA, ask the patient to bring the big toe towards the ceiling (thus demonstrating the tendon of extensor hallucis longus). The artery lies immediately lateral to this tendon. Examine both DPAs simultaneously. It is easier to do this crouching down (Fig. 4.20)
- The PTA lies one finger's breadth below and behind the medial malleolus. Position your fingers in line with the artery as it curves forwards towards the dorsum of the foot (Fig. 4.21). Examine both PTAs simultaneously
- Remember that the foot pulses may be absent in 2% of normal subjects!

Listen

- Check for a bruit over the femoral artery and in the subsartorial canal (in the mid-thigh).

Finish your examination here

Completion

Say that you would like to:
- Examine the rest of the peripheral arterial system
- Examine the abdomen for aneurysmal dilatation of the aorta (see Case 117)
- Measure the ankle brachial pressure indices (ABPIs) on each side.

? QUESTIONS

(a) How would you demonstrate this patient's ABPI?

- The pressure cuff is inflated over the upper arm and the systolic pressure measured at the brachial artery using a Doppler probe
- The cuff is then placed over the calf
- When the dorsalis pedis pulse has been located with the Doppler, the cuff is inflated until the pressure is high enough to occlude the artery and thus the Doppler sound disappears
- Slowly lower the cuff pressure until the Doppler sound restarts; this is the ankle pressure
- The index is the ankle pressure divided by the brachial pressure.

(b) What is the significance of the ABPI?

- The normal index is 1
- As the perfusion of the leg begins to decrease in a patient with peripheral vascular disease, the ratio begins to fall
- Patients with intermittent claudication have an index of approximately 0.5–0.8
- Patients with rest pain tend to have an index <0.5
- An absolute pressure of less than 50 mmHg at the ankle is used in some definitions of critical ischaemia
- It is important to note that ABPIs are unreliable in patients with diabetes mellitus, who have erroneously elevated indices on account of calcification of the vessel. Indeed, this may lead to an ABPI >1.0.

Leo Buerger (1879–1943). Austrian who lived in the USA all his life. Surgeon and urologist who became Professor of Urology in New York and subsequently Los Angeles. Also named Buerger's disease (thromboangiitis obliterans) (see Case 129).

CASE 114 VASCULAR EFFECTS OF THE DIABETIC FOOT ***

INSTRUCTION

'This gentleman has diabetes. Examine his foot and describe your findings.' (Fig. 4.22)

APPROACH

Expose the patient's legs from the groin to the toes, preserving his dignity.

VITAL POINTS

Look

Inspect the foot as for any vascular case (see Case 113). Diabetic peripheral vascular disease is usually evident below the knee. Note especially:

- Presence of bilateral disease
- Any previous surgical scars, including excision of metatarsal heads or digits for gangrene

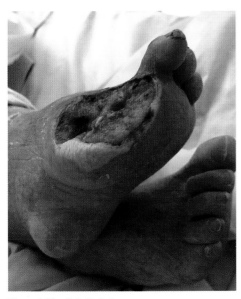

Figure 4.22 Diabetic foot.

- Charcot's joints are more common in diabetics with neuropathy (see Case 105)
- Signs of damage to the foot if the patient has a sensory neuropathy and cannot feel injuries such as hot bath water or nails digging into the feet
- Evidence of ulceration.

Feel

- The pulses may be preserved until very late in the disease and may in fact feel quite prominent due to calcification of arteries
- Take care when palpating the joints of the foot as they may be painful
- Test for sensation over the foot, and if any abnormality is detected, work proximally to find the level at which sensation returns to normal.

Finish your examination here

Completion

Say that you would like to:

- Examine the neurological system. Diabetic neuropathy is much commoner in type 1 diabetics and can form a glove-and-stocking-type sensory or mixed neuropathy. Isolated peripheral nerve lesions and autonomic neuropathy may also be present
- Examine the abdomen and the rest of the peripheral arterial system. In addition, say that you would like to perform fundoscopy and urinalysis for proteinuria (microalbuminuria is an early marker of renal impairment).

? QUESTIONS

(a) Why are diabetics particularly prone to foot pathology?

The 'diabetic foot syndrome' encompasses a number of pathologies, including: diabetic neuropathy, peripheral occlusive arterial disease, Charcot neuroarthropathy, osteomyelitis, foot ulceration and the potentially preventable end point of amputation.

Diabetic neuropathy and peripheral occlusive arterial disease are the major aetiological factors for the development of ulceration and may act alone, together or in combination with other factors such as microvascular disease, biomechanical abnormalities, limited joint mobility and increased susceptibility to infection.

(b) What is the aetiology of diabetic foot ulcers?

- Neuropathic (45–60% of ulcers)
- Ischaemic due to peripheral occlusive arterial disease (10% of ulcers)
- Mixed neuroischaemic (25–45% of ulcers).

Opinion is divided as to whether diabetic neuropathy occurs due to (1) microvascular disease leading to nerve hypoxia or (2) direct effects of hyperglycaemia on neuronal metabolism.

Atherosclerotic occlusive arterial disease is present (albeit in subclinical form in some) in virtually all long-term diabetics. Vascular disease is responsible for 70% of diabetic deaths. The distribution of peripheral occlusive arterial disease is different in diabetics, predominantly affecting below-knee vessels.

(c) It is known that the pulses are preserved in the diabetic – why is this?

Calcification of the walls of the vessels preserves the pulses until late in the natural history of disease, and prevents the sphygmomanometer from compressing the vessels. This tends to lead to an abnormally (and reassuringly) high ABPI measurement. A similar effect is seen in peripheral vascular disease caused by chronic renal failure.

? ADVANCED QUESTIONS

(a) What differences in management are there in diabetics?

Patients with diabetes often exhibit multiple complications of their diabetes, including retinopathy, nephropathy and ischaemic heart disease. Consequently, patients require a multidisciplinary team of physicians, surgeons and allied health professionals. The abnormal ABPI, plus the fact that patients often have occlusions at multiple levels, means that earlier recourse to intra-arterial digital subtraction angiography is indicated. Any infections should be treated aggressively with bed rest and intravenous antibiotics, together with meticulous foot care. Sepsis should be treated with surgical debridement. All diabetics should be seen regularly by the chiropodist with a view to preventing complications.

(b) Are there any problems with diabetics undergoing angiography?

They may have a degree of renal impairment which can be dramatically worsened following a dose of intra-arterial contrast. Patients should be kept well hydrated with intravenous fluids peri-procedure. If they are on metformin, this has to be stopped prior to the procedure, as lactic acidosis has been reported.

FURTHER READING

Caputo GM, Cavanagh PR, Ulbrecht JS, et al: Assessment and management of foot disease in patients with diabetes. *N Engl J Med* 331(13):854–860, 1994.

Frykberg RG, Armstrong DG, Giurini J, et al: Diabetic foot disorders: a clinical practice guideline. American College of Foot and Ankle Surgeons. *J Foot Ankle Surg* 39(5 Suppl):S1–S60, 2000.

CASE 115 | AMPUTATIONS ***

INSTRUCTION

'Examine this patient's lower limbs.'
(Fig. 4.23)

APPROACH

- Expose the patient's legs from the groin to the toes, keeping his underwear or a gown in place

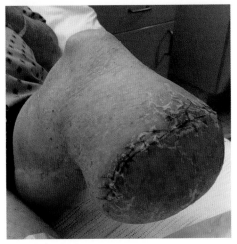

Figure 4.23 Below-knee amputation.

- The patient may be presented on a chair – if it is clear the examiner only wants you to look at the amputation, then the other leg should not be exposed.

VITAL POINTS

Look

- Examine the amputation stump first
- Describe the anatomical level of the amputation, usually above-knee (transfemoral) or below-knee (transtibial) (Fig. 4.23)
- Very occasionally, you may be presented with a knee disarticulation or Gritti–Stokes amputation, which is a modification of the traditional transfemoral amputation, with resection of the bone at a supracondylar femoral level and fixation of the patella to the distal part of the femur as an end cap. These amputations are usually reserved for patients who are unlikely to walk postoperatively
- If the patient has a partial foot amputation, then describe the level of amputation (Ray, transmetatarsal, Syme's)
- Comment on the stump – healthy stumps are cylindrical and the skin wound has healed completely
- Amputations are traditionally formed 12 cm above the knee or 14 cm below the knee
- Below-knee (transtibial) amputations can be performed in two ways:
  - Long posterior flap of Burgess – posterior calf muscles are used to cover the transected bone, but the muscle should

be debrided carefully so the flap is not too bulky to fit within the skin
  - Skew flap of Kingsley Robinson – the suture line runs obliquely (anterior–posterior)
- In above-knee (transfemoral) amputations, equal anterior and posterior semicircular flaps are formed – the vastus lateralis is sutured to the adductors, and the other quadriceps muscles to the hamstrings.

Feel

The soft tissue under the skin should move freely over the bone beneath.

Move

- Ask the patient actively to flex and extend the knee joint immediately above the amputation to demonstrate the fixed flexion deformity that often follows a below-knee amputation if good physiotherapy has not prevented it
- Manipulate the joint passively if the patient cannot move it at all
- If the patient's prosthesis is available, ask to look at it, and then ask the patient to fit the appliance and walk with it in place.

Finish your examination here

Completion

Say that you would like to:

- Examine the rest of the limb and the other limb for signs of peripheral vascular disease.

❓ QUESTIONS

(a) What are the indications for amputation?

Indications for amputation can be remembered as the four **D**s:

- **D**ead (ischaemic):
  - Peripheral vascular disease (80–90% of all cases)
  - Thromboangiitis obliterans (see Case 129)
  - Arteriovenous fistulae (see Case 133)
- **D**amaged (trauma):
  - Unsalvageable limbs
  - Burns
  - Frostbite

- **D**angerous (malignancy)
  - Bone
  - Soft tissue
- **D**amn nuisance (infection/neuropathy)
  - Osteomyelitis
  - Necrotising fasciitis
  - Charcot neuroarthropathy.

(b) How is the level of amputation selected?

- In general terms, the level depends on the healing and rehabilitation potential of the patient and prosthetic considerations
- More proximal amputations make it more difficult for the patient to achieve independent walking subsequently. Indeed, only 40–50% of transfemoral amputees achieve mobility
- More distal amputations preserve more joints and more control of prosthesis and offer better rehabilitation potential – up to 60–80% of patients achieve independent mobility. However, suboptimal below-knee perfusion can compromise stump healing / viability.

(c) What are the complications of amputations?

- Complications should be divided into specific to the amputation and general for any operation, and also into immediate (within 24 h), early (up to 1 month) and late (beyond 1 month)
- Mention at the beginning that these patients often have other medical problems, especially cardiovascular disease, putting them at particularly high risk
- Operative mortality is 20% and 1-year survival is 50%.

Specific early complications:

- Psychological and social implications
- Haematoma and wound infection, including gas gangrene (rare)

- Deep vein thrombosis and pulmonary embolus
- Phantom-limb pain – due to the sensory cortex 'believing' the limb is still present
- Skin necrosis (caused by poor perfusion of the stump) requires refashioning, usually at a higher level

Specific late complications:

- Osteomyelitis – infection transmitted to the bone through the stump
- Stump ulceration – can be caused by pressure from the prosthesis
- Stump neuroma – swelling of the distal nerve as it tries to regrow following division; during the initial procedure the nerve should be cut back far enough to prevent a neuroma from forming
- Fixed flexion deformity of the knee, especially with long-term disease
- Difficulty in mobilising
- Spurs and osteophytes in the underlying bone.

James Syme (1799–1870). Professor of Surgery, Edinburgh and University College Hospital, London, and father-in-law to Joseph Lister.

FURTHER READING

Dormandy J, Heeck L, Vig S: Major amputations: clinical patterns and predictors. *Semin Vasc Surg* 12(2):154–161, 1999.

Robinson KP, Hoile R, Coddington T: Skew flap myoplastic below-knee amputation: a preliminary report. *Br J Surg* 69(9):554–557, 1982.

CASE 116 | PERIPHERAL ARTERIAL SYSTEM – HISTORY ***

INSTRUCTION

'This lady has had previous surgery but still describes some pain in the calf on walking. Ask her some questions to help you define the cause.' (Fig. 4.24)

APPROACH

Within a short case or OSCE, you may be asked to take a history from a patient, and vascular long cases are extremely common in the final MB examination. The clue in this particular patient (Fig. 4.25) is that she has a vertical scar over the femoral artery, suggestive of arterial bypass surgery.

VITAL POINTS

The history should be structured to answer three basic questions, summarised in Table 4.1.

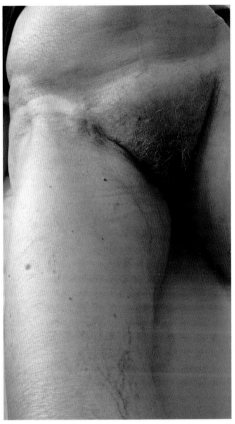

Figure 4.24 Groin scar from previous arterial bypass surgery.

Introduction

- Ask the patient's age
- Ask her occupation.

Pain of intermittent claudication

Site:

- Stenosis of the lower aorta and common iliac artery causes buttock claudication (and may be associated with impotence, which in association with absent femoral pulses is termed Leriche's syndrome)
- External iliac artery stenosis causes thigh claudication
- Superficial femoral artery stenosis leads to calf claudication

Intensity:

- The pain is always felt in the muscles, as it is due to increased oxygen demand from actively contracting muscle

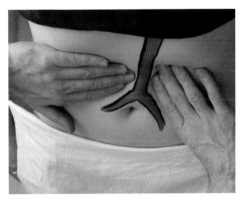

Figure 4.25 Examination of the aorta in the abdomen.

Table 4.1

Vascular symptoms	Risk factors for arterial disease	Fitness for surgery
Intermittent claudication	Smoking	Previous medical history
Rest pain	Diabetes	Anaesthetic history
Critical ischaemia	Hypertension Cholesterol Previous history (especially heart disease or stroke) Family history (Renal failure) (Hypothyroidism) (Gout)	Drug history and allergies Social history (related to postoperative rehabilitation)

- When the demand is not met due to ischaemia in the afferent arterioles, anaerobic metabolism ensues, leading to lactic acidosis
- The pain is due to anoxia, acidosis and the build-up of metabolites

Precipitating and relieving factors:

- The pain comes on during exercise and typically after a fixed distance
- It comes on more rapidly after walking up a hill rather than on the flat
- The pain is relieved after a few minutes of resting.

Rest pain

Site:

- Rest pain often begins in the least well-perfused (i.e. most distal) part of the leg, over the toes and forefoot. Thus, calf pain at night in the absence of foot pain is *unlikely* to be ischaemic in origin

Intensity:

- The pain is very severe, aching in nature and typically wakes the patient from sleep

Precipitating and relieving factors:

- The pain comes on at night when the patient is lying flat in bed
- It is relieved by getting up (assistance from gravity / hydrostatic pressure) and walking on a cold floor and sometimes patients describe that they have to sleep sitting up to prevent the pain from coming on
- Characteristically, the pain is also relieved by hanging the foot over the edge of the bed.

Critical ischaemia

It is important to immediately identify whether there is any feature in the history which suggests more severe (limb-threatening) disease. Ask specifically about the presence of ulcers or gangrene ('trophic changes').

Critical limb ischaemia is defined by the European consensus as:

1. Presence of arterial ulcers or gangrene, *or*
2. Rest pain that lasts for 2 weeks or more and is only relieved by opiate analgesia, *and*
3. An absolute ankle pressure (see Case 113) of <50 mmHg.

Function

As for the orthopaedic history:

- Impact on patient's life, e.g. work, sleep
- Going to the shops
- Walking aids
- Limp.

? QUESTIONS

(a) What is the differential diagnosis of intermittent claudication?

The causes of pain in the leg can be divided into:

- Musculoskeletal: pathologies of the knee, ankle or hip (such as osteoarthritis)
- Neurological: spinal stenosis (leading to spinal claudication)
- Vascular: intermittent claudication, deep vein thrombosis.

(b) Why do patients with rest pain typically get more severe pain at night?

The pain is caused by a reduced blood supply to the distal aspects of the limb. The pain gets worse at night because the perfusion of the limb is further reduced when the patient is lying down. This is due to:

- Decreased cardiac output at night
- Reduced effect of gravity, which normally acts to increase relative blood supply to the legs
- Relative dilatation of the skin vessels due to the warmth of the bedclothes.

(c) How can the severity of peripheral arterial disease be classified in clinical practice?

There are several classification systems but the simplest for use in clinical practice is the Fontaine classification:

Fontaine stage	Description
I Asymptomatic	Peripheral arterial disease present but no symptoms
II Intermittent claudication	Pain in muscles precipitated by walking/relieved by rest
III Rest pain	Constant pain in feet (often worse at night)
IV Tissue loss	Ischaemic ulceration or gangrene

René Leriche (1879–1955) was a famous French surgeon who was Professor of Surgery at the University of Strasbourg. He also named Sudek-Leriche syndrome – aseptic necrosis of the bone following injury (more commonly shortened to Sudek atrophy).

CASE 117 | ABDOMINAL AORTIC ANEURYSM ★★★

INSTRUCTION

'Examine this gentleman's abdomen.'

APPROACH

Expose the patient as for the abdominal examination (see Case 43).

VITAL POINTS

Inspect

- A midline pulsating mass may be visible, especially in deep inspiration – this is easier to identify in thin patients
- Note the presence of any abdominal scars.

Palpate

- Hand examination is likely to be normal, and the examiner will probably move you on immediately to palpation of the abdomen
- Gentle palpation of the nine abdominal areas may be normal
- A pulsatile mass may be identified on deeper palpation in the epigastric region
- The mass should be measured by bringing the lateral sides of the index fingers of both hands together to identify the borders of the aneurysm and estimating the distance between your fingers (in centimetres)
- An expansile mass moves your fingers laterally with each pulse; aneurysms are expansile as well as pulsatile (a transmitted pulsation is not expansile; see Case 2)
- Take care not to palpate too firmly
- Palpate over the course of the common iliac arteries
- Continue the examination by palpating the femoral arteries in the groin and the popliteal arteries (which may also be aneurysmal in nature).

Auscultate

- For aortic and iliac bruits.

Finish your examination here

Completion

Say that you would like to examine the heart, carotid vessels and legs for concurrent cardiac, carotid or peripheral vascular disease.

? QUESTIONS

(a) In which patients are abdominal aortic aneurysms (AAAs) most common?

Aneurysms are most common in:

- Men
- Aged >60 years
- Smokers
- Hypertensive patients
- Often strong family history.

(b) Which patients should have their aneurysms repaired?

- The reason for repairing AAAs is to prevent rupture
- The following aneurysms should be repaired:
  - Symptomatic aneurysms (back pain, tenderness over the aneurysm on palpation, distal embolic events, ruptured/ leaked aneurysms)
  - Asymptomatic aneurysms (≥5.5 cm diameter; increase of diameter of ≥1 cm per year, suggesting rapidly expanding aneurysm)
- The UK Small Aneurysm Trial suggests that if the aneurysm is between 4.0 and 5.5 cm in diameter, open surgical repair is not recommended, and for those greater than 5.5 cm in diameter, the patient will benefit from surgery

- The risk of rupture of a >5.5 cm aneurysm is 10% per year, increasing with the size of the aneurysm.

(c) What is the operative mortality of AAA repair?

- The elective 30-day mortality from open AAA repair is 5%, but this figure may be lower in specialist centres
- If the patient suffers a ruptured aneurysm and reaches the hospital, operative mortality rises to 50%, but only 50% of patients reach hospital alive
- Mortality is usually from haemorrhage, subsequent myocardial infarction or renal failure.

? ADVANCED QUESTIONS

(a) Are there any other options other than open AAA repair?

- Laparoscopic (minimally invasive open) repair of abdominal aneurysms is claimed to be associated with less surgical trauma, with benefits in terms of lower operative mortality and morbidity rates and more rapid recovery of the patients. However, reliable comparative data are lacking
- Endovascular repair (EVAR), using grafts placed into the abdominal aorta from the femoral artery by a vascular surgeon and/or a radiologist, is increasingly performed
- The goal of EVAR is sustained aneurysm exclusion from the systemic circulation by means of a stent graft, preventing further aneurysm expansion and thus eliminating rupture risk
- Although the operative mortality is lower, there are no long-term data to suggest that outcome is better from this procedure. There is a significant failure rate (approximately 25%) and medium-term complications like endoleaks are of increasing concern.

(b) Should we be screening for AAA?

- A UK screening programme has never been agreed, and opinions differ as to the value of screening on a population basis

- The Multicentre Aneurysm Screening Study (MASS) trial revealed a significantly reduced prevalence of aneurysm-related death in the screened male population between 65 and 74 years of age, with a 53% reduction in those who attended for screening. Analysis of the 10-year MASS data shows that the NHS AAA Screening Programme will prevent significant numbers of AAA ruptures and AAA deaths. Over 10 years, for every 10 000 men scanned, 65 AAA ruptures will be prevented, saving 52 lives. However, there will also be six post-elective surgery deaths involving men whose aneurysm is detected under the screening programme.

(c) Do you know of any infectious agents associated with AAA?

- *Salmonella typhi* is the most common infective organism
- Mycotic aneurysms sometimes occur as a result of staphylococcal infection
- Syphilitic aneurysms have been consigned to history, although recent increasing rates of infection may cause a resurgence in the future.

FURTHER READING

Ashton HA, Buxton MJ, Day NE, et al: The Multicentre Aneurysm Screening Study (MASS) into the effect of abdominal aortic aneurysm screening on mortality in men: a randomised controlled trial. *Lancet* 360(9345):1531–1539, 2002.

Thompson SG, Ashton HA, Gao L, et al: Screening men for abdominal aortic aneurysm: 10 year mortality and cost effectiveness results from the randomised Multicentre Aneurysm Screening Study. *Br Med J* 338:b2307, 2009.

UK Small Aneurysm Trial Participants: Mortality results for randomised controlled trial of early elective surgery or ultrasonographic surveillance for small abdominal aortic aneurysms. *Lancet* 352(9141):1649–1655, 1998.

Note

The actor George C. Scott died from a ruptured abdominal aortic aneurysm in September 1999, as did Sir John Hunter (see Case 119).

CASE 118 | CAROTID ARTERY DISEASE ***

INSTRUCTION

'Listen to this gentleman's neck.'

APPROACH

Expose the patient's neck as for the neck exam (see Case 6).

VITAL POINTS

This is a direct instruction and you should proceed immediately to auscultation.

Auscultate

- Notice the bruit over one or both carotid arteries
- The bruit is best heard over the course of the common carotid artery, which runs behind and medial to the sternocleidomastoid in the anterior triangle of the neck
- The bruit is best heard in expiration
- Tell the examiner that you would listen over the precordium to ensure this is not a transmitted aortic stenosis murmur (heard as an ejection systolic murmur in the aortic area – second intercostal space immediately to the right of the sternum).

Finish your examination here

TOP TIP

- The subject of carotid bruits and cerebrovascular events may also be brought up by asking you to question the patient with regards to his bruit
- In this case, you should ask about previous transient ischaemic attacks or strokes, asking about temporary or resolving neurological symptoms such as weakness or paraesthesia
- Also ask about amaurosis fugax, the visual sensation of a curtain being drawn down slowly in front of one eye
- Neurological symptoms occur on the contralateral side but transient monocular blindness (amaurosis fugax) is ipsilateral to the side of the carotid stenosis

Completion

Say you would perform a neurological examination to look for signs of a previous cerebrovascular event, and would also check for signs of atherosclerosis elsewhere (heart, abdominal aorta and peripheral vascular system).

? QUESTIONS

(a) How would you investigate a patient who was referred with a carotid bruit?

The patient should have a full work-up for atherosclerosis:

General investigations:

- Urinalysis for proteinuria, marker of atherosclerotic renal disease
- Blood tests
  - Haematology: full blood count for anaemia, which might precipitate symptoms
  - Biochemistry: renal function for possible undetected renal disease
  - Glucose: exclude diabetes
  - Cholesterol: to identify hypercholesterolaemia
- Electrocardiogram: To look for evidence of atrial fibrillation, cardiac disease, previous infarction, ischaemia or left ventricular dysfunction

Special investigations:

- An echocardiogram would also be an option, especially if the patient had a precordial bruit
- In most UK centres, carotid duplex scanning is the investigation of choice for detecting and evaluating the severity of carotid artery disease
- Computed tomography angiography (CTA) and magnetic resonance angiography (MRA) are increasingly used to assess disease and have replaced elective catheter angiography, which incurs a stroke/death risk of 1.5% and thus is no longer part of the routine work-up of patients
- In a systematic review on the performance of non-invasive imaging modalities in the assessment of a 70–99% carotid stenosis, CTA had the highest specificity (0.94), followed by MRA (0.93), then ultrasound (0.84) (see Further reading).
- The National Clinical Guideline for Stroke 2004 (see Further reading) recommends that duplex findings be confirmed by MRA (or second duplex). If a second duplex approach

is taken, it is good practice to ensure that this is performed by a second practitioner.

(b) What is the consequence of carotid stenosis?

- Stroke is the third leading cause of death in the West, 80% of strokes are ischaemic (the remainder are haemorrhagic) and 80% of these affect the carotid territory. Thromboembolism of the internal carotid or middle cerebral arteries is the principal cause
- Atherosclerosis affects the intracranial circulation, particularly the circle of Willis and the vertebrobasilar system
- Transient ischaemic attacks (neurological symptoms resolving completely within 24 h) and transient monocular blindness (amaurosis fugax) are usually caused by repeated microemboli from the plaque, consisting of clusters of platelets and cholesterol
- The same symptoms can be caused by microemboli from the heart and aortic arch.

? ADVANCED QUESTIONS

(a) Which patients might be considered for carotid endarterectomy (Fig. 4.26)?

- The North American (North American Symptomatic Carotid Endarterectomy Trial: NASCET) and European (European Carotid Surgery Trial: ECST) trials were set up to investigate evidence-based indications for carotid endarterectomy
  - The Carotid Endarterectomy Trialists Collaboration combined data from ECST, NASCET and the Veterans Affairs trials, and includes 5-year outcomes in >6000 patients
  - Carotid endarterectomy confers maximum benefit in the recently symptomatic (<6 months), with a 70–99% NASCET stenosis
  - Carotid endarterectomy confers modest (but significant) benefit in the recently symptomatic (<6 months), with a 50–69% NASCET stenosis (ECST 70–85%)
  - Carotid endarterectomy is not indicated in symptomatic patients with a 0–50% NASCET stenosis
- These trials demonstrated that, for patients with severe stenosis (over 70%), surgery reduced the relative risk of disabling stroke or death by 48%.

(b) What would you warn the patient of when you ask him to give consent for an endarterectomy?

- The advantages of having surgery are a sixfold reduction in the rate of stroke at 3 years
- The 30-day stroke / mortality risk is 6%
- Specific risks of haematoma, hypoglossal nerve injury and numbness of the ipsilateral earlobe should also be mentioned.

> *Thomas Willis (1621–1675).* English physician and anatomist who described the sweet taste of diabetic urine, myasthenia gravis, general paralysis of the insane and whooping cough and identified the intercostal, spinal and spinal accessory nerves. He gave names to 'reflex' and 'neurology' and was buried in Westminster Abbey.

FURTHER READING

Cina CS, Clase CM, Haynes RB: Carotid endarterectomy for symptomatic carotid stenosis. *Cochrane Database Syst Rev* 2:CD001081, 2000.

European Carotid Surgery Trial (ECST): Randomised trial of endarterectomy for recently symptomatic carotid stenosis – final results of the MRC ECST. *Lancet* 351(9113):1379–1387, 1998.

Intercollegiate Stroke Working Party: *National Clinical Guidelines for Stroke*, 2nd edn. London: Clinical Effectiveness & Evaluation Unit, 2004.

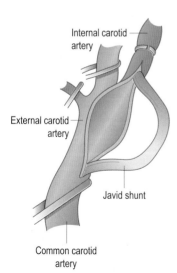

Internal carotid artery

External carotid artery

Javid shunt

Common carotid artery

Figure 4.26   Carotid endarterectomy.

North American Symptomatic Carotid Endarterectomy Trial (NASCET) investigators: National Institute of Neurological Disorders and Stroke and Trauma Division: Clinical alert: benefit of carotid endarterectomy for patients with high-grade stenosis of the internal carotid artery. *N Engl J Med* 22(6):816–817, 1991.

CASE 119 | POPLITEAL ANEURYSM **

INSTRUCTION

'Examine the pulses in this gentleman's legs.'

APPROACH

Expose the patient's legs from the groin to the toes, preserving his dignity. If asked to examine the pulses, rather than the limb, be sure to begin by palpating the femoral pulse – you have not been asked to examine the feet for signs of peripheral arterial disease.

VITAL POINTS

Palpate the leg pulses

- Begin with the femoral pulses, comparing one side with another (see Case 113)
- Comment on whether the pulses are present or absent and whether the character of the pulse is normal
- Move down to the popliteal pulses
- Note the expansile pulsation behind the knee
- The aneurysmal pulse is relatively easy to find and the artery does not need to be compressed against the tibia
- Slide the fingers of your two hands apart and comment on the diameter of the vessel. A popliteal aneurysm is 2 cm or greater in diameter
- The pulsating mass does not alter with change in position of the knee
- The ankle and foot pulses may not be palpable if the aneurysm is thrombosed
- 50% are bilateral – don't forget to examine the other knee.

Finish your examination here

Completion

Say that you would like to:

- Examine the rest of the limb and the other limb for signs of peripheral vascular disease

- Examine the abdomen, as 50% will also have an abdominal aortic aneurysm.

? QUESTIONS

(a) How might a patient with a popliteal aneurysm present?

- Popliteal aneurysms represent 80% of all peripheral (non-aortic) aneurysms
- The patient may have presented with a lump behind the knee if the aneurysm has grown to such a size that it has expanded beyond the popliteal fossa
- 50% present with distal-limb ischaemia caused by thrombosis or embolism
- Patients may present with an acutely ischaemic leg
- Less than 10% rupture.

(b) Under what circumstances would they be treated?

Surgery is indicated for:

- Symptomatic aneurysms
- Those containing thrombus
- Those greater than 2 cm.

The aneurysm is surgically repaired by either an excision bypass, where the popliteal artery is ligated above and below the diseased segment and a graft interposed, or a simple resection and anastomosis without the use of a graft (Hunter's ligation).

Acute ischaemia caused by thrombus can be treated with thrombolysis.

Sir John Hunter (1728–1793). Scottish surgeon and anatomist. Also described Hunter's canal (subsartorial adductor canal) and Hunterian chancre (syphilitic chancre). Interestingly, he died of a ruptured abdominal aortic aneurysm and was buried in Westminster Abbey.

FURTHER READING

Thompson MM, Bell PR: ABC of arterial and venous disease. Arterial aneurysms. *BMJ* 320(7243):1193–1196, 2000.

CASE 120 | ISCHAEMIC ULCER **

INSTRUCTION

'Examine this patient's feet.' (Fig. 4.27).

APPROACH

Again, ideally expose the whole of the legs from the groin, maintaining the patient's dignity, but if the patient is in an environment where other patients are present, this would be inappropriate and you should just comment on the feet.

VITAL POINTS

Begin examining the legs as for the peripheral arterial system examination (see Case 113).

Look

Observe the following characteristic features of an ischaemic ulcer.

Site:

- Characteristically over the tips of the toes and over the pressure areas

Shape:

- The size of the ulcer varies from a few millimetres on the tips of the toes to several centimetres over the lower leg

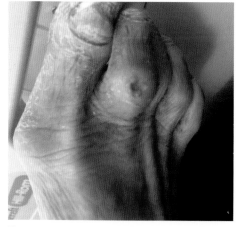

Figure 4.27 Ischaemic ulceration.

Edge and base:

- The edge is punched out and clean cut because there has been no partial healing of the wound
- The base may contain slough and may be infected, but there is no healthy red granulation tissue as the blood supply is too poor
- The ulcer may be very deep and penetrate down to bone and the underlying joints – the bone may be exposed at the base

Surrounding skin:

- The skin around the ulcer is a grey/blue colour.

Feel

- Palpate for temperature using the back of the hands – note the surrounding skin is cold compared with the proximal limb and the contralateral foot
- Check the peripheral pulses, noting the most distal pulse that is still palpable
- Check the pulses of the other leg.

Finish your examination here

TOP TIP

☑ Almost all of the examination is 'Look' and you should spend as much time as possible commenting on the features without progressing to 'Feel', as this will score marks very quickly.

? QUESTIONS

(a) What are the causes of ischaemic ulcers?

These can be divided into large- and small-vessel arterial disease:

- Large-vessel
  - Atherosclerosis
  - Thromboangiitis obliterans (see Case 129)
- Small-vessel
  - Diabetes mellitus
  - Polyarteritis nodosa
  - Rheumatoid arthritis.

Alternatively, an anatomical classification.

Luminal causes:

- Emboli (atherosclerotic / cholesterol)
- Thrombotic / hypercoagulable states (antiphospholipid syndrome, etc.)

Arterial wall – the acronym **SAD** is useful as an *aide-mémoire*:

- **S**pasm – Raynaud's phenomenon
- **A**therosclerosis / **A**rteritis
  - Takayasu's
  - Buerger's disease
  - Giant cell
  - Polyarteritis nodosa
  - Small-vessel vasculitides – connective tissue diseases, Behçet's, etc.
- **D**iabetes mellitus / **D**ilatation (aneurysm)

Outside the artery:

- Trauma
- Compression.

(b) What kinds of analgesia would be appropriate for this patient?

- Ischaemic ulcers can be extremely painful and even removing the bandages from around the ulcer can cause pain that lasts for several hours
- Consider the analgesic ladder (Table 4.2), remembering that combinations of drugs administered regularly in a variety of different formulations (oral, intramuscular, etc.) can be more effective.

(c) What other non-surgical treatments are available?

Risk-factor modification:

- Stopping smoking
- Good diabetic and hypertensive control
- Optimised serum lipid levels

Symptom modification:

- Avoidance of drugs which might worsen symptoms, such as beta-blockers
- Commencement of low-dose aspirin (75 mg/day), which reduces the incidence of cardiac and cerebrovascular events in high-risk patients
- Intravenous prostaglandins act by inhibiting platelet aggregation, stabilising leukocytes and endothelial cells, and are vasodilators. They can have some effect in healing ulcers, relieving rest pain and reducing the risk of amputation
- Lumbar sympathectomy reduces sympathetic-mediated vasoconstriction and improves perfusion by allowing for unopposed vasodilatation of the skin vessels. This is often unsuccessful in diabetics who may have autonomic neuropathy causing 'autosympathectomy'.

(d) What is the differential diagnosis of leg ulcers?

TIN CANS

- **T**rauma
- **I**nfection / **I**mmunological (tuberculosis; syphilis; rheumatoid arthritis) (see Case 124)
- **N**eoplasia squamous cell carcinoma (see Case 14) / basal cell carcinoma (see Case 16)
- **C**hronic venous insufficiency (see Case 112)
- **A**rterial insufficiency
- **N**europathic (see Case 124)
- **S**kin conditions – e.g. pyoderma gangrenosum (see Case 40)

Different types of leg ulcers

See Table 4.3.

Table 4.2 The analgesic ladder

Stage	Analgesia
I	Simple, oral agents such as paracetamol or non-steroidal anti-inflammatory drugs (NSAIDs) like ibuprofen – taking great care in the elderly and patients with renal impairment. Selective cyclooxygenase-2 inhibitors such as rofecoxib are also available, which reduce the incidence of gastrointestinal bleeding
II	Stronger oral agents, such as a mixture of orally acting opioids like codeine and paracetamol
	Stronger NSAIDs such as diclofenac
III	Intramuscular, stronger oral or intravenous opioids such as morphine, diamorphine

Table 4.3 Comparison of different types of leg ulcer

	Venous	Ischaemic	Neuropathic
Site	Gaiter region over medial malleolus of ankle	Tips of toes and pressure areas	Heel, underneath metatarsal heads (pressure-bearing areas)
Shape	Variable, usually irregular	Regular outline	Regular outline, follows skin contour
Size	Can be very large	Varying size, few mm to several cm	Several cm
Edge	Usually sloping pale purple/brown	Punched out, clean	Clean
Base	Pink granulation tissue or white fibrous tissue characteristic	Bone may be exposed, no granulation tissue	Often exposing bone
Surrounding skin	Chronic venous signs, e.g. lipodermatosclerosis	Grey/blue	Normal
Skin temperature	May be warmer	Cold	Normal
Pulses	Present	Absent	Present

FURTHER READING

London NJ, Donnelly R: ABC of arterial and venous disease. Ulcerated lower limb. *BMJ* 320(7249):1589–1591, 2000.

Sarkar PK, Ballantyne S: Management of leg ulcers. *Postgrad Med J* 76(901):674–682, 2000.

Note

About 400 years BC, Hippocrates wrote, 'In case of an ulcer, it is not expedient to stand, especially if the ulcer be situated on the leg'. Hippocrates himself had a leg ulcer.

CASE 121 | POST-THROMBOTIC LIMB **

INSTRUCTION

'Examine this gentleman's legs.' (Fig. 4.28).

APPROACH

Expose the patient's legs, maintaining his dignity and keeping his underwear on. Ensure that you can see his feet and position him lying comfortably on the couch.

VITAL POINTS

Look

Note the features of chronic venous insufficiency (Fig. 4.28), comparing one side with the other:

- Swelling
- Dilated superficial veins (as blood cannot return to the inferior vena cava through the deep veins)

- Skin pigmentation, possibly restricted to the medial malleolus ('ankle flare')
- Venous eczema
- Lipodermatosclerosis
- Venous ulceration or evidence of previous ulceration.

Feel

- Compare the temperature of both legs
- Check for pitting oedema (watching the patient's face at all times).

Finish your examination here

Completion

Say that you would like to:

- Test for deep venous occlusion – Perthes test – place a high tourniquet around

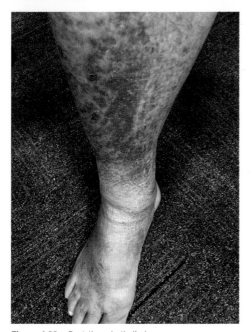

Figure 4.28   Post-thrombotic limb.

the top of the patient's thigh and ask him to walk. If the deep venous system is occluded, the leg will become swollen and blue with dilated superficial veins distal to the tourniquet.

? ADVANCED QUESTIONS

(a) What is venous gangrene?

Venous gangrene is a rare complication of deep vein thrombosis in the iliofemoral segment and presents in three phases:

1. Phlegmasia alba dolens (white leg)
2. Phlegmasia cerulea dolens (blue leg)
3. Gangrene – occurs as a consequence of acute ischaemia and may be restricted to the foot or spread up the leg.

(b) What investigations are appropriate for deep venous disease?

- Duplex – shows areas of reflux and deep venous occlusion
- Venography:
  - Ascending – identifies deep venous patency and perforator incompetence
  - Descending – identifies areas of reflux
- Varicography: shows sites of communication
- Ambulatory venous pressures.

(c) What are the surgical options available for deep venous occlusion/reflux?

Reflux:

- Trahere transplantation – use a segment of axillary vein with valve and insert it into the deep venous system of the leg, wrapping it in a polytetrafluoroethylene cuff
- Kistner's operation – valvuloplasty of damaged valves

Obstruction:

- Palma operation – use contralateral long saphenous vein (LSV) and anastomose to the femoral vein to bypass iliofemoral obstruction
- Warren bypass – use LSV to bypass deep venous blockage – no longer used.

Notes

Post-thrombotic limbs:

- 90% are due to reflux following deep vein thrombosis
- 10% are due to obstruction following deep vein thrombosis.

FURTHER READING

Hopkins NF, Wolfe JH: ABC of vascular diseases: deep venous insufficiency. *BMJ* 304:107, 1992.

CASE 122 | GANGRENE   ✱✱

INSTRUCTION

'Examine this patient's foot' (Fig. 4.29).

APPROACH

Expose the patient and examine the legs (see Case 113).

VITAL POINTS

Look

- Note the appearance of gangrene, which often begins between the toes
- Comment on whether the gangrene is wet (Fig. 4.29) or dry

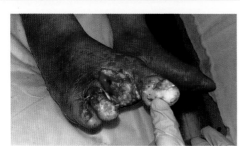

Figure 4.29   Wet gangrene in a patient with toe amputation.

- Wet gangrene is due to either acute ischaemia or local trauma, and may be complicated by infection
- Wet gangrene usually has an ill-defined, spreading edge (Fig. 4.29)
- Skin blistering may occur
- A line of demarcation gradually appears between the viable and dead tissue – if this has occurred, the gangrene is 'dry' and the dead tissue may eventually fall off (autoamputation)
- Continue to comment on the other features of peripheral vascular disease (see Case 113).

Feel

Palpate the peripheral pulses and check for temperature differences between the legs (see Case 113).

Finish your examination here

? QUESTION

(a) What are the causes of gangrene?

Gangrene is the result of irreversible tissue necrosis and has a number of causes:

- Diabetes (the commonest cause)
- Embolus and thrombosis – both leading to acute limb ischaemia, mesenteric infarction, critical limb ischaemia, 'trashing' of feet

- Raynaud's syndrome – see Case 123
- Thromboangiitis obliterans (Buerger's disease) – see Case 129
- Ergot poisoning
- Vessel injury secondary to extreme cold, heat, trauma or pressure
- Drug-induced, e.g. warfarin.

? ADVANCED QUESTION

(a) What is Fournier's gangrene?

- Rare necrotising subcutaneous infection involving the scrotum, penis and perineum
- Scrotum is red and swollen with crepitus on palpation due to dermal gangrene
- Multiple organisms are responsible, usually coliforms and anaerobes.

Jean Alfred Fournier (1832–1914). French dermatologist who specialised in the study of venereal diseases. Fournier's gangrene was actually first described by Baurienne in 1764 but was named after Fournier following five cases he presented in clinical lectures in 1883. His name is associated with two other medical terms:
- Fournier's sign: scars on the mouth following the healing of lesions in congenital syphilis
- Fournier's tibia: fusiform thickening and anterior bowing of the tibia in congenital syphilis.

CASE 123 | RAYNAUD'S PHENOMENON **

INSTRUCTION

'Look at this lady's hands and ask her a few questions.'

APPROACH

The examiner will often use a leading question like this in order to stimulate a spot diagnosis and lead to some supplemental questions. In this situation, the key is to ascertain the presence of the central clinical features (in this case, of Raynaud's) and then to try to identify any precipitating features.

TOP TIP

☑ Be clear about terminology:

- Raynaud's phenomenon: characteristic cold-induced changes associated with vasospasm
- Raynaud's disease: primary disease occurring in isolation
- Raynaud's syndrome: secondary Raynaud's phenomenon associated with other diseases (see below)

VITAL POINTS

Ask questions at the same time as looking at the hands:

- What is the main problem you have with your hands?
- When does this symptom occur?
- Is it precipitated by any specific weather conditions?
- Can you describe the colour changes your fingers go through during these episodes?

Look

- Note that the pathology is usually bilateral
- In between acute attacks, the skin may be dry and red, especially around the tips of the fingers, and the nails brittle
- Also note any ulcers or gangrene on the pulps.

Feel

- The radial pulse is normal.

TOP TIP

☑ The acronym **WBC** may help you recall the order of the skin colour changes of the fingers seen in Raynaud's:

- **W**hite – blanching of digits
- **B**lue – cyanosis and pain
- **C**rimson – reactive hyperaemia – fingers turn red in colour

Finish your examination here

Completion

Say that you would like to:

- Ask about symptoms and look for signs of the secondary causes of Raynaud's.

? QUESTIONS

(a) What is the pathogenesis of Raynaud's phenomenon?

- If the vessels are normal in calibre, the clinical features may be caused by relatively overactive alpha receptors in the wall, leading to abnormal smooth-muscle contraction or changes in elasticity
- Alternatively, there may be a fixed obstruction in the vessel wall, which reduces the distal flow and thus renders the digits susceptible to the effects of cold.

(b) What are the predisposing factors?

The causes can be divided into primary and secondary:

- Primary Raynaud's (Raynaud's disease) is due to vasomotor malformation
- Secondary Raynaud's occurs as a consequence of pathology affecting the vessel wall.

In general the secondary causes, especially when related to connective tissue diseases, cause more severe problems with necrosis and gangrene.

TOP TIP

☑ The secondary causes can be remembered using the acronym **BADCaT**:

- **B**lood disorders, e.g. polycythaemia
- **A**rterial, e.g. atherosclerosis, thromboangiitis obliterans
- **D**rugs, e.g. beta-blockers, oral contraceptive pill
- **C**onnective tissues disorders, e.g. rheumatoid arthritis, systemic lupus erythematosus, scleroderma, polyarteritis nodosa
- **T**rauma, e.g. vibration injury

(a) What are the treatment options for Raynaud's?

Non-surgical:

- Use of gloves and discontinuing any predisposing drugs, e.g. beta-blockers
- Using warm pads in gloves and socks in the winter
- Encourage patients to stop smoking

Medical (used with variable success):

- Calcium channel blockers, e.g. nifedipine
- Naftidrofuryl oxalate (Praxilene)
- Prostacyclin analogues (e.g. iloprost)

Surgical:

- Cervical sympathectomy and amputation of the affected phalanges

- Cervical sympathectomy may not be a permanent solution and may only relieve symptoms for 2 years or less
- Amputate only if digits are threatened with gangrene.

Maurice Raynaud (1834–1881) was a physician in Paris. He described the differences between primary Raynaud's disease and secondary Raynaud's phenomenon in his MD thesis at the age of 28.

FURTHER READING

Block JA, Sequeira W: Raynaud's phenomenon. *Lancet* 357(9273):2042–2048, 2001.

www.nhlbi.nih.gov/health/public/blood/other/raynaud.htm – information for patients.

CASE 124 | NEUROPATHIC ULCER **

INSTRUCTION

'Examine this lady's foot.' (Fig. 4.30)

APPROACH

As previously (see Case 112).

VITAL POINTS

Look

Observe the characteristic features of a neuropathic ulcer.

Site:

- They are usually found over the pressure areas, over the metatarsal heads on the sole of the foot and the balls of the toes; they can also occur on the heel

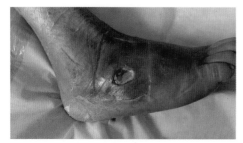

Figure 4.30 Neuropathic ulcer.

Shape:

- Irregular, corresponding to the shape of the pressure point that has become exposed

Edge and base:

- Clean edge
- Base may be deep, with exposure of bone and tendon

Surrounding skin:

- The surrounding skin has a normal blood supply and therefore looks normal.

Feel

- Feel the temperature of the surrounding skin, which is expected to be normal
- The peripheral pulses are usually normal
- Test the sensation over the dermatomes using light touch and pinprick; note the absence of sensation around the ulcer and describe the extent of the sensory abnormality.

Finish your examination here

Completion

Say that you would like to:

- Perform a complete neurological examination, including cranial and peripheral nerves.

TOP TIP

☑ It can be difficult to distinguish between an ischaemic and neuropathic ulcer; however, neuropathic ulcers are:

- Painless
- Associated with normal appearance of the surrounding skin
- Associated with local sensory loss

✔

? QUESTIONS

(a) What are the causes of neuropathic ulcers?

They can be caused by any disease that leads to a peripheral sensory neuropathy, or by causes of spinal cord disease. Causes of peripheral neuropathy include:

- Systemic diseases:
  - Diabetes – by far the most relevant cause in clinical practice
  - Vasculitis (systemic lupus erythematosus)
  - Hypothyroidism
  - Vitamin B$_{12}$ deficiency
- Drugs and toxins:
  - Prescribed drugs (amiodarone/metronidazole, etc.)
  - Alcohol
  - Toxins
- Infections:
  - Tuberculosis, leprosy
  - HIV
- Carcinomas, especially lung cancer and polycythaemia rubra vera
- Idiopathic (50–60%).

(b) Why do these ulcers form?

Peripheral neuropathy has several effects:

- Slowly progressive sensory loss, with numbness and tingling of the feet and sometimes also hands. The sensory loss is often 'glove-and-stocking' in distribution and may also be associated with motor impairment. Due to the sensory loss, damage over the pressure areas is not noticed by the patient
- Motor neuropathy may result in wasting of the intrinsic foot muscle and an altered foot shape, with claw toes and prominent metatarsal heads

- Autonomic neuropathy reduces sweating, leading to a dry foot susceptible to cracking.

Therefore, the insensitive, mechanically abnormal, dry foot is at risk from unperceived external trauma (e.g. from shoes) and from repetitive (and often relatively minor) painless injury (e.g. foreign body in shoe). Progressive skin loss and ulceration may occur.

FURTHER READING

Phillips TJ: Successful methods of treating leg ulcers. The tried and true, plus the novel and new. *Postgrad Med* 105(5):159–174, 1999.

www.skinwound.com/online_training_manual/neuropathic_wounds.htm – guide to neuropathic ulcers.

Note: Rarer causes of leg ulceration

The following causes of leg ulcers may also be encountered in the clinical examination. A couple of characteristics are listed for each type:

Tuberculosis:

- Undermined edge
- Shallow ulcer

Pyoderma gangrenosum:

- Undermined edge
- Violaceous
- Necrotic ulcer with hypertrophic margins

Syphilis:

- Gumma of tertiary syphilis has a typical punched-out ulcer, over the anterior surface of the lower leg, and has a yellow-coloured 'wash leather' base
- 'Scalloped' border

Arteriovenous fistulae:

- Ulcer is distal to the fistula
- Shallow indolent ulcers

Rheumatoid arthritis:

- Necrotising vasculitis
- Purpuric, haemorrhagic bullae

Squamous cell carcinoma:

- Rolled or raised edge
- Often on sun-damaged skin

Sickle cell disease:

- Small, punched-out ulcers
- Often over medial aspect of lower leg.

CASE 125 | LYMPHOEDEMA **

INSTRUCTION

'Examine this patient's legs.' (Fig. 4.31)

APPROACH

Expose the patient's legs, preserving the patient's dignity.

VITAL POINTS

Look

- The legs may be grossly swollen, with no particular distribution
- Tends to be bilateral
- Note the loss of contour at the ankle, which causes a 'buffalo hump' appearance on the dorsum of the foot
- There may be lichenified fronds on the toes and the skin looks thick and indurated (hyperkeratosis, lichenification and *peau d'orange*)
- Yellow discoloration of nails.

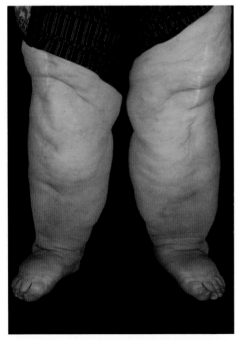

Figure 4.31 Lymphoedema (from Beard JD: Vascular and Endovascular Surgery: A Companion to Specialist Surgical Practice, 5th edn. London: Saunders, 2013).

Palpate

- Determine whether or not the oedema is pitting in nature
- Initially the oedema is characteristically pitting but later it stops pitting as tissue resistance increases
- Palpate the groin for inguinal lymphadenopathy (which may be present).

Finish your examination here

Completion

Say that you would like to:

- Examine the jugular venous pulse, heart and lungs to exclude right-sided cardiac failure
- Palpate the liver to identify hepatomegaly
- Ask the patient some questions to determine any hereditary conditions that predispose to lymphoedema

TOP TIP

☑ The commonest cause of unilateral ankle oedema is venous disease; lymphoedema is much more commonly bilateral

? QUESTION

(a) What is the differential diagnosis of swollen legs?

Lymphoedema can be similar in appearance to any other cause of swollen legs, but tends to be bilateral:

- Central causes include right heart failure, hypoalbuminaemia, nephrotic syndrome and hypothyroidism
- Peripheral (local) causes are usually venous, disease such as deep vein thrombosis, Klippel–Trenaunay syndrome, chronic venous insufficiency or post-phlebitic limb (see Cases 111, 112 and 121)
- Rare causes are angio-oedema, arteriovenous malformations (Parkes–Weber syndrome, multiple arteriorvenous fistulae) and hemi-hypertrophy.

❓ ADVANCED QUESTIONS

(a) What is the difference between primary and secondary lymphoedema?

Primary lymphoedema refers to congenital disease or primary lymphatic failure. It is three times more common in women and the pathology originates from within the lymphatics. It is also known as Milroy's disease.

Secondary lymphoedema can be classified according to the cause:

- Malignancy: infiltration of nodes; may also cause a chylothorax or chylous ascites when this occurs in nodes in the thorax and abdomen
- Infections, e.g. filiaris (infection by the *Wuchereria bancrofti* worm), tuberculosis
- Post surgery or radiotherapy, such as axillary dissection in breast surgery and inguinal irradiation.

(b) What are the treatment options?

Non-surgical:

- Advise patient to elevate the leg as much as possible and stress the importance of cleanliness and careful chiropody
- Manual lymphatic drainage / massage
- Grade III compression stockings to apply 40 mmHg pressure at the ankles
- Intermittent pneumatic compression device
- Complex decongestive physiotherapy
- Cellulitis should be treated
- Benzopyrones, although a Cochrane review failed to reach firm conclusions about their effectiveness (see Further reading)

Limb elevation reduces intravascular hydrostatic pressure and the stockings increase extracellular hydrostatic pressure, together reducing the level of tissue oedema. These measures can be very successful, but patient motivation is key and it may take some time for the results to become apparent.

Surgical:

- Used rarely: the results tend overall to be poor
- More likely to be successful where there is discrete occlusion of the lymphatics

- Options include debulking or bypass procedures:
  - Direct lymphovenous anastomosis
  - Stripping a piece of small-intestine mucosa, exposing the rich submucosal plexus – this can then be used to replace a leg lymph node, which then forms new connections with distal lymphatics in order to drain the leg
  - Debulking to reduce the volume of the leg – Homans' procedure is an example of such an operation. Flaps are raised above and below the knee (beginning on the medial side and then returning to surgery later if required to complete the lateral flap) and strips of subcutaneous tissue are removed before the flap is sutured. If the skin is in poor condition, a different operation, which excises the skin in addition to the soft tissues, can be performed and the skin covered with a split-skin graft (Charles' procedure).

Joseph Bancroft (1836–1894). Surgeon to the General Hospital, Brisbane, Australia.

John Homans (1877–1954). Professor of Clinical Surgery, Harvard Medical School, Boston. He also described Homans' sign, which occurs when passive dorsiflexion of the foot gives pain in the calf in the presence of a deep vein thrombosis.

W. F. Milroy (1855–1942). North American physician.

FURTHER READING

Badger C, Preston N, Seers K, et al: Benzo-pyrones for reducing and controlling lymphoedema of the limbs. *Cochrane Database Syst Rev* 2, 2004,

Cohen SR, Payne DK, Tunkel RS: Lymphedema: strategies for management. *Cancer* 92(4 Suppl):980–987, 2001.

Rockson SG: Lymphedema. *Am J Med* 110(4):288–295, 2001.

www.cancerbacup.org.uk/info/lymphoedema.htm – online booklet from CancerBACUP about lymphoedema.

www.lymphoedema.org/lsn/ – information and support network for patients.

CASE 126   HYPERHIDROSIS   ✱✱

INSTRUCTION

'Examine this patient's hands.'
(Fig. 4.32)

APPROACH

Expose to the elbows and ask the patient to place the hands palm upwards on a pillow (if available).

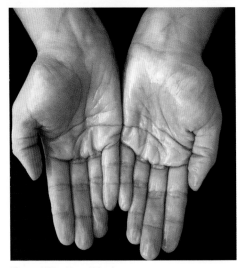

Figure 4.32 Hyperhidrosis.

VITAL POINTS

Describe the presence of excessive sweat on the palmar surface of both hands, confirming this by palpation.

Finish your examination here

Completion

Say that you would like to:

- Examine the axillae, groins and soles of the feet for excessive sweating
- Enquire about the social effects of the symptoms
- Exclude underlying causes (see below).

? QUESTIONS

(a) What is the differential diagnosis?

- Anxiety
- Hyperthyroidism
- Hyperhidrosis erythematosus traumatica – rare occupational form where a vibratory surface (e.g. capstan lathe) produces excessive sweating of the skin on contact
- Phaeochromocytoma.

(b) How do you treat this condition?

- Reassurance: if symptoms are not distressing to the patient
- Medical: aluminium hexachloride solution painting for axillary hyperhidrosis
- Surgical:
  - Axillary – excise hair-bearing skin/intradermal Botulinum A neurotoxin (Botox) – this has a 62% cure rate
  - Palmar – cervical sympathectomy (T2–T4) via thoracoscopic approach – this has a 98% cure rate
  - Plantar – lumbar sympathectomy.

(c) What side-effects would you warn this patient about if considering cervical sympathectomy?

- Excessive dryness of skin
- Compensatory sweating around trunk (in up to 50% of patients)
- Horner's syndrome (a consequence of damage to the stellate ganglion) – 0.1%
- Pneumothorax/haemothorax
- Important to warn of the risks of a general anaesthetic for what may be largely a cosmetic problem.

? ADVANCED QUESTIONS

(a) What other part of the body can be affected by hyperhidrosis?

The face can be affected in patients with:

- Syringomyelia
- Frey's syndrome (see Case 21).

FURTHER READING

Chiou TS, Chen SC: Intermediate-term results of endoscopic transaxillary T2 sympathectomy for primary palmar hyperhidrosis. *Br J Surg* 86(1):45–47, 1999.

Glogau RG: Botulinum A neurotoxin for axillary hyperhidrosis. No sweat Botox. *Dermatol Surg* 24(8):817–819, 1998.

CASE 127 | FALSE ANEURYSM **

INSTRUCTION

'Examine this patient's groin.'
(Fig. 4.33)

APPROACH

Expose the patient's groin and begin your examination (see Case 42).

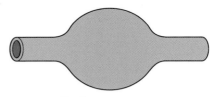

Fusiform aneurysm

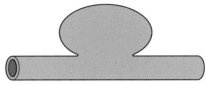

Saccular aneurysm

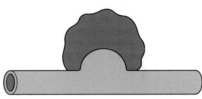

False aneurysm

A cavity in a haematoma
which connects with the
lumen of the artery

Figure 4.34 The types of aneurysm.

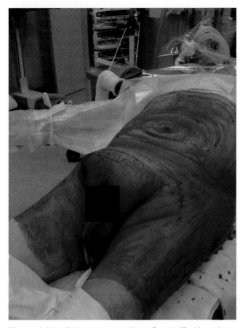

Figure 4.33 False aneurysm (from Beard JD: *Vascular and Endovascular Surgery: A Companion to Specialist Surgical Practice*, 5th edn. London: Saunders, 2013).

VITAL POINTS

TOP TIP

☑ Most false aneurysms in exams affect the common femoral artery, occurring following radiological puncture during arteriography.

Inspection

- Note the presence of a mass in the groin. It is usually obvious that it is pulsatile from inspection alone
- Note the presence of any surgical scars or (much more subtly) puncture sites in the groin and accurately describe their position. Scars will usually be longitudinal, indicating previous exposure of the common femoral artery.

Palpate

- Describe the pulsatile swelling underneath one of the scars
- Fully describe all the characteristics of the swelling
- Define the anatomical position of the swelling, which is usually located at the mid-

inguinal point, as it should be closely associated with the transition from external iliac artery to common femoral artery as at passes under the inguinal ligament
- Continue to palpate the distal peripheral pulses.

Auscultate

There may be a bruit over the swelling.

Finish your examination here

❓ QUESTIONS

(a) What is the difference between a false and a true aneurysm?

- An aneurysm (see Case 117) is an abnormal dilatation of a blood vessel (Fig. 4.34)
- A true aneurysm involves all layers of the arterial wall
- A false aneurysm follows a partial laceration of the vessel wall, causing blood to leak out of the vessel into the surrounding tissues

- A false aneurysm is the same as a pulsating haematoma and is most common in the common femoral artery
- Fibrous tissue forms around the haematoma and then contracts, producing a false sac which contains thrombus but remains connected to the lumen of the damaged vessel
- Pulsation transmitted from the artery tends to increase the size of the cavity with time.

(b) What are the causes of a false aneurysm?

- Traumatic
- Iatrogenic
  - Following angiography, blood continues to leak from the

puncture site (easy to repair with suture to arterial wall)

- Following bypass, e.g. femoropopliteal, is often associated with infection (more complex and often needs vein patch to reconstruct).
- Complicates approximately 1% of transfemoral interventions.

(c) What are the treatment options?

- Compression therapy (direct /ultrasound-guided) of the false aneurysm
- Thrombin injection
- Surgical repair
- Observation and review.

CASE 128 | THORACIC OUTLET OBSTRUCTION *

INSTRUCTION

'Examine this lady's right arm.'

APPROACH

Expose the patient's arm and shoulder, also taking care to expose the contralateral arm.

VITAL POINTS

Look

- Inspect the arm from the anterior and posterior aspects
- Note the presence of oedema, cyanosis or pallor due to *reduced venous outflow* from the arm – the patient may describe the appearance or worsening of these symptoms on exercise
- Inspect the hand especially carefully, with the hand resting on a white pillow, noting the possible *arterial complications* of thoracic outlet syndrome:
  - Patchy gangrene of the tips of the fingers and palm
  - Fingertip necrosis
- Continue by examining for wasting of the small muscles of the hand (T1 distribution), a feature caused by the *neurological deficit* from the obstruction.

Palpation

- Palpate the neck, in thin people – there may be a bony swelling of the cervical rib above the clavicle in the supraclavicular fossa

- A pulsatile mass might be present (due to post-stenotic dilatation)
- If there is any evidence of oedema, palpate this and note that it is characteristically pitting in nature
- The radial pulse is usually present and normal.

Auscultation

- There might be a bruit over the subclavian artery (Fig. 4.35).

Sensation

- Test sensation in the dermatomes of the arm specifically – there may be sensory loss over the T1 region, along the medial aspect of the arm around the elbow joint.

Finish your examination here

? QUESTIONS

(a) What is the differential diagnosis of thoracic outlet obstruction?

This is often a difficult diagnosis to make because the clinical signs are the result of a mix of arterial, venous and neurological complications of the obstruction.

Arterial symptoms (fingertip gangrene, necrosis) are more commonly due to:

- Raynaud's phenomenon (see Case 123)
- Thromboangiitis obliterans (see Case 129)
- Takayasu's arteritis

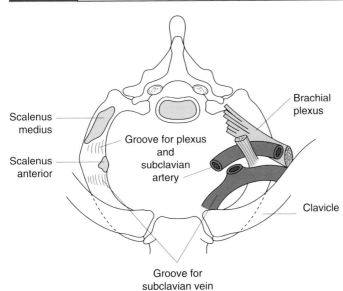

Figure 4.35 Anatomy of the first rib.

Brachial plexus

Scalenus medius

Groove for plexus and subclavian artery

Scalenus anterior

Clavicle

Groove for subclavian vein

Venous symptoms (oedema, cyanosis or pallor of the arm) may be caused by:

- Axillary vein thrombosis
- Damage to axillary drainage following surgery (such as axillary dissection in breast surgery)

Neurological symptoms may be due to:

- Cervical spondylosis
- Pancoast's tumour
- Cervical disc protrusions
- Ulnar nerve neuropathy.

(b) What investigations may help to confirm the diagnosis?

- There may be a cervical rib or prominent transverse process on the chest X-ray or thoracic outlet views
- Duplex examination may be useful in quantifying the postural changes and post-stenotic dilatation
- CT / MR arteriograms of the subclavian artery may show a marked kink in the artery or even the vein, and sometimes there is a localised aneurysm at the site of the narrowing.

(c) What is the pathogenesis of thoracic outlet obstruction?

Congenital:

- Usually due to a cervical rib (arising from the seventh cervical vertebra) and the subclavian artery is compressed between the rib and either the scalenus anterior muscle or the clavicle

Acquired:

- The obstruction may also follow a fractured clavicle, hypertrophy of the scalene muscles or occasionally a pathological enlargement of the first rib.

Henry Khunrath Pancoast (1875–1939). Professor of Roentgenology, University of Pennsylvania, Philadelphia, USA.

Mikito Takayasu (1860–1938). Japanese surgeon who described an obliterative arteritis affecting the subclavian and carotid arteries of young Asian women.

FURTHER READING

Parziale JR, Akelman E, Weiss AP, et al: Thoracic outlet syndrome. *Am J Orthop* 29(5):353–360, 2000.

CASE 129   THROMBOANGIITIS OBLITERANS (BUERGER'S DISEASE)   *

INSTRUCTION

'Look at this man's feet and ask him some questions.' (Fig. 4.36)

APPROACH

Expose the patient and examine the legs as for any peripheral arterial case (see Case 113).

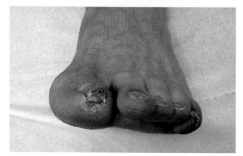

Figure 4.36 Thromboangiitis obliterans (Buerger's disease). (from Puechal X, Fiessinger J-N 2007 Thromboangiitis obliterans or Buerger's disease: challenges for the rheumatologist. *Rheumatology*, 2007. 46 (2): 192-199, with permission).

VITAL POINTS

Look

- Nicotine staining of the fingers
- The patient may complain of chronic paronychia and early ulcers that heal poorly
- There may be a history of intermittent claudication
- Note the presence of distal gangrene and other appearances of chronic ischaemia in the feet, and of erythema nodosum
- Patients often have multiple amputations.

Feel

When examining the pulses, the typical pattern is that the femoral and popliteal pulses are present and the foot pulses are absent.

Finish your examination here

? QUESTIONS

(a) What is the pathogenesis of thromboangiitis obliterans?

- It is a collagen vascular disease, caused by infiltration of plasma cells into the arterial wall
- This leads to luminal thrombosis and affects small and medium-sized arteries of the lower limb
- Eventually, collagen is deposited and forms a thick fibrous coat
- Heavy smoking is very strongly associated with this condition.

(b) What specific investigations would you perform?

- Collagen antibodies are present in 45% of patients
- There is an association with HLA-B5
- Angiography has typical appearances of normal proximal vessels with distal occlusion and 'corkscrew' collaterals.

Leo Buerger (1879–1943). North American urologist.

FURTHER READING

Olin JW: Thromboangiitis obliterans (Buerger's disease). *N Engl J Med* 343(12):864–869, 2000.

CASE 130 | SUPERIOR VENA CAVA OBSTRUCTION *

INSTRUCTION

'Look at this patient's thorax and tell me what the problem is.' (Fig. 4.37)

VITAL POINTS

Look

- Note the tortuous, visible, dilated veins overlying the chest wall and neck – these veins would not be expected to be compressible
- The face may be plethoric and swollen

- Comment if the patient is dyspnoeic at rest.

Finish your examination here

Completion

Tell the examiner you would examine the patient further to find a cause for the obstruction, including looking for peripheral stigmata of lung carcinoma (e.g. nicotine stains, digital clubbing and Horner's syndrome), lymphadenopathy and examining the chest.

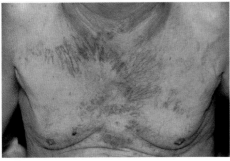

Figure 4.37 Superior vena cava obstruction. (from Wieser S, Kohler M 2010 An early sign of superior vena cava syndrome. *QJM* 103(9): 707, with permission).

? QUESTIONS

(a) What are the causes of superior vena cava (SVC) obstruction?

Causes can be divided into pathology within and outside the SVC. Within the SVC obstruction tends to be as a consequence of thrombosis within intravenous jugular or subclavian lines (central venous pressure lines), especially when hyperosmolar solutions are infused for feeding.

Outside the SVC (compression from pathologies in adjacent structures):

- Carcinoma of the lung
- Lymphoma
- Carcinoma of the thyroid
- Aortic aneurysm
- Mediastinal goitre
- Mediastinal fibrosis
- Constrictive pericarditis.

? ADVANCED QUESTIONS

(a) How can the extent of the obstruction be determined?

- An intravenous injection of contrast into the veins in the arm can illustrate the degree of obstruction
- Increasingly, CT / MR angiography is used in clinical practice

- Cross-sectional imaging of the thorax may demonstrate the cause of the obstruction and the length of SVC affected.

William Harvey (1578–1657). Physician at St Bartholomew's Hospital, London and President of the Royal College of Physicians. He gave the first account of the circulation of blood in his book *De Motu Cordis* in 1628, although he first spoke of its existence in 1616.

Johann Friedrich Horner (1831–1886). Professor of Ophthalmology in Zurich who described Horner's syndrome – ipsilateral ptosis, miosis, hypohidrosis and enophthalmos due to damage to the cervical sympathetic chain.

FURTHER READING

Markman M: Diagnosis and management of superior vena cava syndrome. *Cleve Clin J Med* 66(1):59–61, 1999.

Notes

There are two other conditions where dilated veins can be observed across the trunk:

- Inferior vena cava obstruction, where the dilated veins occur across the lower abdomen; the commonest cause is intra-abdominal malignancy
- Caput medusae – dilated veins around a portosystemic anastomosis in the umbilical veins.

The three causes of dilated abdominal wall veins can be distinguished by the direction of flow within the dilated veins. This is detected by placing two fingers on the vein, sliding one finger along the vein to empty it and then releasing one finger, watching to see which direction the empty segment fills (Harvey's test).

In relation to the umbilicus:

- In SVC obstruction the direction of flow above the umbilicus is downwards
- In inferior vena cava obstruction the direction of flow below the umbilicus is upwards
- In caput medusae the direction of flow is away from the umbilicus (both below and above).

CASE 131 | CAROTID ARTERY ANEURYSM AND DILATED COMMON CAROTID ARTERY *

INSTRUCTION

'Examine this patient's neck.'

APPROACH

Expose the patient and proceed as for the neck exam (see Case 6).

VITAL POINTS

Inspect

- A pulsatile swelling can be noted in the line of the carotid artery at the base of the neck
- It is normally unilateral.

Palpate

- The aneurysm is firm and expansile.

Auscultate

- A bruit may be heard.

Finish your examination here

Completion

Say that you would like to:

- Look for neurological associations (ipsilateral Horner's syndrome and focal neurological signs caused by embolisation of the aneurysm)

- Examine for other cardiovascular associations (measuring the blood pressure, examining the peripheral pulses and heart).

? QUESTIONS

(a) How would the patient be investigated?

Other risk factors and cardiovascular disease elsewhere would be excluded and the neck imaged with a duplex scan or occasionally an intravenous digital subtraction angiogram.

(b) What is the cause of these aneurysms?

- True aneurysms are uncommon and are generally caused by atherosclerosis, and occasionally by dissection, trauma, previous carotid surgery or infection
- When a true aneurysm has been excluded, the patient can be reassured and discharged
- Dilated, tortuous common carotid arteries are much more common – the artery is kinked or coiled and there is a prominent carotid bifurcation.

CASE 132 | LYMPHANGIOMA *

INSTRUCTION

'Examine this patient's neck.'

APPROACH

Begin to examine the neck as described in Case 6. Lymphangiomas are usually found in childhood and rarely present in younger adults; they are extremely rare in older adults.

VITAL POINTS

Look

- There is a swelling above the clavicle in the posterior triangle of the neck.

Feel

- The swelling feels soft and smooth
- More solid areas may be palpable within the mass
- Characteristically brilliantly transilluminable (because it is full of lymph)
- The skin overlying the lump is normal.

Finish your examination here

? QUESTIONS

(a) What is the origin of lymphangiomas?

Some 50% are present at birth and they are thought to represent a congenital abnormality during the evolution of embryonic lymph nodes into the adult type.

(b) How are they classified?

Lymphangiomas can be:

- Cystic (cystic hygroma, as in this case – for further information, see Case 37)

- Solid or diffuse – may involve any part of the body, usually present at birth; local overgrowth of tissues and bone may occur, which can render surgical correction extremely difficult
- Cutaneous (lymphangioma circumscriptum) – present as groups of multiple small transparent blisters lying close to each other. They are usually not present at birth but develop later. They tend to be cosmetically more disfiguring and also ooze fluid or bleed frequently; early surgical treatment is therefore warranted. An ellipse of skin and underlying subcutaneous tissue should be excised.

FURTHER READING

Orvidas LJ, Kasperbauer JL: Pediatric lymphangiomas of the head and neck. *Ann Otol Rhinol Laryngol* 109(4):411–421, 2000.

CASE 133 | ARTERIOVENOUS FISTULA   *

INSTRUCTION

'Examine this patient's forearm and tell me the diagnosis.' (Fig. 4.38)

APPROACH

- Expose the patient's arms and place them palm upward on a white pillow if available
- Check that both hands and forearms are exposed to compare one side with the other.

VITAL POINTS

Inspect

- There is a swelling over the mid forearm
- Describe this swelling as for any other lump (see Case 2)
- The arteriovenous (AV) fistula may have been surgically created, i.e. a Cimino–Brescia fistula for haemodialysis in patients with chronic renal failure (in which case there

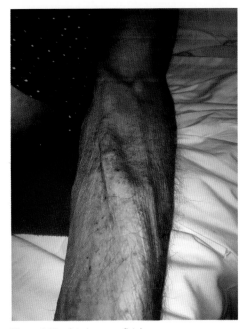

Figure 4.38 Arteriovenous fistula.

should be a precise scar over the skin) or it could be traumatic, or occasionally congenital

- The lump may be pulsatile.

Palpate

- Check that the patient does not have any pain and then palpate the mass
- There is also a thrill palpable.

Auscultate

- The lump has a machinery murmur in systole.

Finish your examination here

Completion

Say that you would like to:

- Examine the rest of the patient to try to determine why the fistula had been formed in the first place.

? ADVANCED QUESTIONS

(a) How is a Cimino–Brescia AV fistula fashioned?

- The procedure can be performed under a regional (brachial plexus), local or general anaesthesia
- A longitudinal incision 3–4 cm in length is made to access the radial artery and the cephalic vein
- The cephalic vein is mobilised and tributaries divided
- The radial artery is also identified and dissected and a longitudinal venotomy and parallel longitudinal arteriotomy performed
- Fine non-absorbable sutures are used to join the two
- The distal cephalic vein is ligated altogether.

(b) What are the specific complications of a Cimino–Brescia fistula?

- Thrombosis during or just after haemodialysis, which may be due to relative hypotension and damage to the intima of the vein
- Venous hypertension in the hand causes swelling and ischaemia of the fingertips. This

should be avoided by ligating the distal vein segment

- High-output cardiac failure secondary to massive run-off through the fistula
- Pseudoaneurysm formation.

(c) How would you determine clinically the degree of shunt caused by a large fistula?

- The Branham–Nicoladoni sign indicates the degree of shunting and cardiac impairment resulting from a large AV fistula
- The carotid pulse is palpated and then a tourniquet placed around the proximal affected limb and inflated above systolic pressure
- The pulse during the period when the tourniquet is inflated is compared with the pulse beforehand
- Normally an AV fistula causes a hyperdynamic circulation – sinus tachycardia may be present
- When the fistula is cut off from the circulation, this is corrected and so the pulse will slow during the test
- This indicates the presence of a left-to-right shunt.

H. H. Branham. Nineteenth-century North American surgeon.

M. J. Brescia. Contemporary renal physician, VA Hospital, New York.

J. E. Cimino. Contemporary renal physician, VA Hospital, New York.

Other types of arteriovenous fistula – these are all rare

? CONGENITAL

- Most commonly occur in the head, neck and limbs
- They can lead to AV aneurysms
- In the head, they most commonly involve the superficial temporal artery
- If the overlying mucous membrane or skin ulcerates, the fistula may haemorrhage
- Small asymptomatic fistulae may be treated expectantly or occasionally with therapeutic embolisation
- Surgical options include occlusion of the feeding vessel and excision of the fistula and

surrounding aneurysm if present, or radiological embolisation.

? MULTIPLE ARTERIOVENOUS FISTULAE (PARKES–WEBER SYNDROME)

- These are almost always in the limbs and present with an overall increase in the size of the affected limb
- The limb has the appearance of extensive varicose veins
- These are very often complicated by severe lipodermatosclerosis and ulceration
- Bruits and thrills may be present
- The Branham–Nicoladoni sign is normally positive (see above)

- Usually it is impossible to excise or embolise each individual fistula unless they are all derived from a single peripheral artery.

? TRAUMATIC

- May follow a simultaneous partial laceration through a vein and artery lying in apposition
- Occur several days after the injury
- More common after open injuries
- The patient may notice a thrill or buzzing
- The other situation where this may occur is following cannulation of vessels by radiologists or cardiologists
- These fistulae normally need to be explored, the vessels separated and the defect closed.

CASE 134 | COARCTATION OF THE AORTA *

INSTRUCTION

'Examine this lady's back and describe the abnormalities you see.'

APPROACH

Expose the patient to the waist, and ask her to stand or sit forward on the side of the bed so that you can examine the back adequately (see Case 101).

VITAL POINTS

Look

- Note the large, prominent, tortuous blood vessels running over the left scapula
- Palpate the vessels to demonstrate that they are arteries
- Listen to the vessels and confirm the presence of a systolic murmur.

Finish your examination here

Completion

Say that you would like to:

- Compare the pulses in the arms and legs – the upper-limb pulses are much stronger than the leg pulses. The patient is usually hypertensive

- Examine for radiofemoral delay and examine the precordium for an ejection systolic murmur heard over the left sternal edge.

? QUESTIONS

(a) What is the pathophysiology of coarctation?

- The aorta is narrowed below the origin of the left subclavian artery and therefore blood flow to the abdomen and legs is reduced
- The prominent vessels over the back are large collaterals that have developed to bypass the obstruction and supply the legs
- The collaterals form between branches of the subclavian artery, especially the internal mammary and scapular vessels, which feed the intercostals from the third rib down.

(b) What investigations would be helpful in confirming the diagnosis?

- Notching on the underside of the ribs may be seen on a chest X-ray (CXR) – this sign is caused by erosion by the intercostal collateral vessels
- On the CXR the aorta may be abnormal – it contains two bulges – the 'three sign'
- A barium swallow shows the opposite – the 'reverse three sign' in the oesophagus
- An echocardiogram shows the site of the coarctation and may demonstrate concurrent aortic stenosis.

(a) What associations of coarctation are you aware of?

Coarctation may be associated with:

- Bicuspid aortic valves
- Aortic stenosis
- Aneurysms in the circle of Willis.

(b) What are the treatment options?

Non-surgical:

- Investigation and treatment of concurrent abnormalities (present in 50%)
- Management of hypertension

Surgical:

- End-to-end anastomosis, patching and the use of the left subclavian artery as a flap are all surgical options.

FURTHER READING

McCrindle BW: Coarctation of the aorta. *Curr Opin Cardiol* 14(5):448–452, 1999.

CASE 135 | ATRIAL FIBRILLATION *

INSTRUCTION

'Take this lady's pulse and comment on it.'

VITAL POINTS

- Ask for permission, and then take the patient's right radial pulse and then a central (carotid) pulse
- Rate and rhythm (Table 4.4) should be ascertained from the radial pulse
- Character and volume are determined from the carotid pulse
- It is often easier to use the thumb to palpate the carotid pulse, but be careful to avoid giving the sensation of strangling the patient by using the right thumb to take the pulse in the left side of the neck.

Finish your examination here

Completion

Say that you would like to:

- Continue to examine the rest of the cardiovascular system and look especially for complications of atrial fibrillation (see below).

(a) What are the causes of atrial fibrillation?

Cardiac disease:

- Hypertension
- Myocardial infarction, ischaemia
- Mitral valve disease
- Cardiomyopathy
- Endocarditis

Respiratory disease:

- Pneumonia
- Lung cancer
- Sarcoidosis

Other:

- Hyperthyroidism
- Idiopathic (lone atrial fibrillation), where it is not due to any of the causes listed above.

(b) What are the complications of atrial fibrillation?

- The major risk is of embolic stroke, which results from thrombus accumulating in an inefficiently contracting left atrium
- Several risk assessment calculators are available. The commonest is the **CHADS2** score, which includes:

•	**C**ongestive heart failure	1 point
•	**H**ypertension	1 point
•	**A**ge >75 years	1 point
•	**D**iabetes mellitus	1 point
•	**S**troke/transient ischemic attack	2 points (Table 4.5)

- Emboli can also lodge in the mesenteric vessels, causing intestinal ischaemia
- Patients are also at risk from acute limb ischaemia if emboli lodge in the arteries of the leg.

Table 4.4 Assessment of rate, rhythm, character and volume of pulse

Rate	Expressed in beats/min
	Count for 15 s and multiply beats by 4
Rhythm	Regular or irregular
	If irregular, can be regularly or irregularly irregular
	Regularly irregular:
	Extrasystoles
	Sinus arrhythmias (faster in inspiration)
	Pulsus paradoxus (weaker in inspiration)
	Pulsus alternans (alternating weak and strong beats)
	Irregularly irregular:
	Atrial fibrillation
Character	Rate of increase and decrease of the pressure within the wave of the pulse
	Collapsing pulse ('waterhammer pulse') – steep rise then rapid fall is characteristic of aortic regurgitation
	Anacrotic pulse – a slow rise and a slow fall in aortic stenosis, as the normal dicrotic notch is lost
Volume	The expansion of the artery with each beat is palpated in the carotid artery
	High cardiac output leads to a strong pulse
	A patient with severe blood loss and shock has a thready pulse

Table 4.5

CHADS2 score	Annual stroke risk (%)	Recommendation
0	1.9	Daily low-dose aspirin (LDA)
1	2.8	LDA or warfarin
2	4	Warfarin unless contraindicated
3	5.9	Warfarin unless contraindicated
4	8.5	Warfarin unless contraindicated
5	12.5	Warfarin unless contraindicated
6	18.2	Warfarin unless contraindicated

- Patients with controlled atrial fibrillation may decompensate following the stress of surgery and, in the most severe cases, this can lead to hypotension
- Finally, the underlying cause for the atrial fibrillation, such as ischaemic heart disease, is still present and may contribute further to anaesthetic risk.

FURTHER READING

Falk RH: Atrial fibrillation. *N Engl J Med* 344(14):1067–1078, 2001.

(c) What are the surgical problems associated with atrial fibrillation?

- Anaesthesia is more complicated because of the increased risk of stroke
- In addition, patients with atrial fibrillation may be anticoagulated and, if on warfarin, this medication needs to be discontinued prior to elective surgery

COMMUNICATION SKILLS WITH THOMAS CROMPTON AND ROSHANA MEHDIAN

SECTION 5

CASE 136 | INTRODUCTION TO COMMUNICATION SKILLS ***

INTRODUCTION

To communicate effectively you must:

- Listen to, ask for and respect patients' views about their health and respond to their ideas, concerns and expectations
- Share with patients, in a way they can understand, the information they want or need to know about their condition, its likely progression and the treatment options available to them, including risks and uncertainties
- Answer questions and keep patients informed about the progress of their care
- Make sure that patients are informed about how information is shared with other professionals involved in their care.

Although communication skills are examined at all levels in surgery, we have included a section here on what is expected of the candidate in the MRCS examination.

FORMAT OF MRCS EXAM

Communication skills will be formally assessed at four of the 18 OSCE stations in the MRCS part B examination. Two manned stations examine history-taking skills; these may be from the patient or from a relative, carer or colleague. One station will focus on delivering information to a patient or relative, such as explaining the need for an operation. A final station will require you to deliver information to a colleague or other professional, such as handing over a patient or making a telephone call to a consultant.

- Usually actors replace patients and are generally briefed thoroughly and carefully – they will know the scenario much better than you will!
- One examiner may be a trained lay examiner who is paired with a surgical examiner
- Of the six domains being assessed in the MRCS, the communication skills stations will award marks in the following three domains:
  - Communication with colleagues – 20
  - Talking with relatives and carers – 20
  - History taking – 40

Clinical knowledge will not be specifically examined but beware as obvious errors or giving the wrong clinical information may result in a fail.

Specific stations may require the candidate to:

1. Communicate with a patient or relative in typical clinical situations. For example:
   - Explaining a diagnosis
   - Explaining investigations
   - Conveying bad news
   - Obtaining informed consent
   - Explaining the uncertainties of diagnosis, outcome or prognosis
2. Take a focused medical history in a variety of clinical situations, for example outpatients or Accident and Emergency (A&E)
3. Demonstrate an ability to convey information to colleagues and other healthcare professionals in an appropriate manner, to a satisfactory standard and using a variety of methods. These might include:
   - Verbal communication such as case presentations to colleagues
   - Written communications such as referral or patient transfer letters
   - Investigation request forms
   - Telephone communication.

PREPARATION

Read the case through carefully and make sure you know how long you have to prepare. Paper and pens will be provided to make notes when required.

Some general points on the cases:

1. Do you know the patient/relative, e.g. is it someone you see every day on the ward round or a new patient in clinic?
2. Classify the problems into medical and psychosocial
3. Deal with each problem separately
4. What is the patient's frame of mind likely to be (e.g. angry/anxious/bereaved)? This is best assessed by asking yourself the question, 'how would I feel if I was the patient?'
5. Plan your conversation.

THE CONSULTATION

Points are awarded for the approach to the actor or patient and you should either introduce yourself formally, if you have never met the patient before, or remind the patient who you are if you have met frequently.

- Ensure a seating plan with no objects between you and your patient; consider your environment
- Diagrams often help patient understanding
- Avoid any medical jargon (like 'neck of femur fracture')

- When delivering information, 'chunk and check' with your patient – give a small amount of information and ensure it is understood before moving on
- Finally, the actor usually has an input into the marks you are awarded for the case – so make sure you establish a good rapport with him or her.

CASE 137 | INFORMATION GATHERING – BACK PAIN ***

SCENARIO

You are an orthopaedic core trainee on call at a district general hospital. Your registrar has asked you to see a referral from a general practitioner – a 43-year-old male mechanic with a long history of lower-back pain and a recent exacerbation. On this occasion, he felt as if he pulled a muscle in his back when lifting a heavy car part at work and he now has lower-back pain radiating down both legs. He has not passed more than a dribble of urine, despite feeling the need to go. Take a history from him and formulate a plan.

KEY POINTS

Medical

Take a full history as you normally would in any medical consultation, beginning with age and occupation. You need to confirm your suspicion of cauda equina syndrome (CES) by taking a complete pain history, enquiring about urinary symptoms, bowel symptoms and altered sensation in the perineum (e.g. you can ask if toilet paper feels different on wiping).

Although the history is not typical, you must screen for the rarer causes of CES or other sinister causes of back pain. This will show your knowledge to the examiner. Enquire about weight loss, lethargy, fevers, night sweats, appetite, etc. to screen for spinal tumours, metastases or spinal infections leading to compression of the cauda equina.

Complete the medical history focusing on surgically relevant information such as past surgical history, medical conditions affecting fitness for surgery and medications that may affect or contraindicate surgery (e.g. anticoagulants).

At the end, the examiners will most likely ask you for a plan. You suspect CES. You would carry out a full neurological examination, record the results clearly and act on the outcome. If your examination findings could not rule out a cauda equina, the patient requires radiological investigation. MRI scanning is the gold standard following standard radiography and discussion with your local neurosurgical centre urgently is indicated. Don't forget to escalate to your senior colleagues as early as possible and document all of the above.

Psychological

You need to keep the patient informed. The diagnosis you suspect will probably be a shock to him. There is an element of the 'giving a difficult diagnosis' scenario that may also come up in this consultation. The patient may well ask what you think the diagnosis is and to tell him the possible outcomes. Remember that it is fine to employ silence; this often allows your patient to express concerns and questions. You may also need to enquire as to the support, e.g. family members, that the patient has access to, and to involve any allied health professionals, e.g. senior nursing staff, as early as possible.

CASE 138 | INFORMATION GATHERING – TRAUMA CALL ***

SCENARIO

You are an orthopaedic core trainee in a large district general hospital. It is 7 p.m. and a 14-year-old boy has been brought in by the ambulance service having been hit by a car. He was a pedestrian and had bulls-eyed the windscreen. He was combative at the scene and so was intubated and ventilated. He has an obvious head injury and an open tibial fracture. The primary and secondary surveys have been completed and no further injuries have been found. He is awaiting a CT scan of his head, cervical spine, chest and pelvis. The registrar is running the trauma call with the only nurse available and asks you to speak to the mother who witnessed the event. The mother is obviously distressed and is sitting in the relatives' room attached to A&E.

Speak to the mother giving her any information you can about her son while obtaining the important information necessary for the boy's care. Once you have the information, you will present the key points back to your registrar.

KEY POINTS

As you have been told in the scenario, the mother is going to be distressed having witnessed the accident. You will have to comfort and reassure her as much as possible while getting the information you need.

Firstly ensure you plan for an appropriate environment. Take her to a quiet room and suggest a nurse be available. Ensure your seating plan has no objects between you and the patient.

Find out what she already knows about her son's injuries from the ambulance crew or nurses. Comment that he is now in a safe area with a team of doctors and nurses looking after him.

Give her the facts without any emotional comments. He has a head injury and is awaiting a CT scan of his head, neck, chest, abdomen and pelvis. Explain this is needed to rule out other life-threatening injuries and to define the head injury further. He has badly broken his leg (with the bone exposed) and will require an operation tonight to prevent infection and for stabilisation.

For his treatment you need to take a focused trauma history and *not* a full medical history from birth to the present day. The **AMPLE** history described as part of the Advanced Trauma Life Support protocol is a useful guide.

A – **A**llergies

M – **M**edications

P – **P**ast medical history

L – **L**ast meal

E – **E**vents/**E**nvironment related to injury.

Once you have the information, you need to tell the mother that you will be back to update her after the scan results are available. You will then be able to give her much more information about his injuries.

Check her understanding and ask if she has any questions before presenting your information to the examiner/registrar. It may be worth asking if she wants someone to stay with her, e.g. a nurse, so that she is not left alone in the room. It is also useful to give her an idea of when she can see her son.

CASE 139 | INFORMATION GATHERING – VASCULAR REFERRAL ***

SCENARIO

You are a general surgical core trainee in a busy clinic. The consultant has just seen a patient with bilateral leg pain, referred by a GP. With further questioning it has become obvious that the pain is vascular in nature. The consultant has asked you to take a history and

then write a referral letter to the local vascular consultant. In the first station you will take the history from the patient, using notepaper as necessary, and then in the second station you will write the referral letter to the vascular surgeon. You change jobs in one week and will be working for the vascular surgeon to whom you are referring.

PART 1 – HISTORY TAKING

Key points

- Name, age, sex and occupation
- Initial symptoms, time of first presentation and subsequent progression or regression of symptoms are important
- The exact site of pain, walking distance at which it develops, maximum walking distance and time for pain to resolve on resting need to be noted
- Direct questioning must exclude rest pain in the limbs and other cardiovascular disease
- The effects of the symptoms on the patient's work, life and hobbies need to be addressed
- Take a full medical history to try to glean the aetiology of the peripheral vascular disease, include smoking, ischaemic heart disease, diabetes or any family history of vascular disease.

PART 2 – REFERRAL LETTER

This is a formal letter, which must include the name and address of referring hospital, preferably on headed paper, with details of the referring consultant clinic, the name and address of the receiving consultant and the date of referral.

- Other details include the patient's contact details, including address and telephone, and the GP name, address and telephone
- A concise letter detailing all relevant information from your history should follow the above

- Finish with a polite request to review the patient in clinic
- Finally your details and contact information should be included, and remember to copy the letter to the GP and the patient.

> General Surgical Consultant
> General Surgical Clinic
> St Elsewhere Hospital
> London E1
> 25th December 2016

Vascular Consultant
Another Hospital
London
E2

Dear Mr Vascular

RE:	Mr SMITH	GP:	Dr GP
	Acacia Avenue		Another Road
	London		Anytown
	K1		Z1
	NHS no. 987 654 3421		
	Tel: 01234 567891		Tel: 01234 987654

This 64-year-old retired teacher presented to Mr Abdomen's clinic this morning having been referred from his GP with bilateral leg pain … etc. etc.

Yours sincerely

Mr Newly Qualified Surgeon

cc. GP
cc. Patient

CASE 140   INFORMATION GIVING – OBTAINING INFORMED CONSENT   ***

SCENARIO

You are a registrar in general surgery and the consultant has asked you to consent Mrs Smith, a 40-year-old singer, for a total thyroidectomy, as you have assisted with the operation on several occasions recently. The patient is aware of the diagnosis of thyroid cancer and the need for an operation.

You have examined Mrs Smith and taken a full history. Examination is otherwise unremarkable but she states that her voice has changed in recent weeks.

Obtain informed consent from this patient for a total thyroidectomy. A generic consent form is provided and you have a 5-min preparation station to fill in the form, including all the patient's details.

KEY POINTS

Remember you have not met this patient before so you must review her understanding of the diagnosis first and explain the indications for operation.

- Explain the process of consent to the patient: to discuss the need for the operation, the alternatives, the benefits and the risks in order to ensure she understands the information fully before proceeding

- Explain the procedure at an appropriate level for this patient, including where the incision will be made. Use diagrams if necessary to ensure understanding
- Mention the specific complications and the more general risks of surgery and ask about previous anaesthetic problems. Any complication of greater than 1% must be mentioned and don't forget to get Mrs Smith to sign a consent form after you have answered all her questions
- If you are unsure of any points, you may need to defer to your consultant – say that you will speak to him and get back to her. Remember that your consultant is ultimately responsible for the care of this patient.

TOP TIP

☑ COMPLICATIONS

- Complications from any surgical procedure can be divided into *early* (days or weeks) and *late* (months)
- Complications are also divided into *general* to any operative procedure and *specific* to the operation in question. This gives a framework on which to base your discussion of complications from any procedure

✓

COMPLICATIONS OF THYROIDECTOMY

General

- Early
  - Bleeding/haematoma
  - Infection
  - Scar
  - Anaesthetic risk
- Late
  - Hypertrophic scarring.

Specific

- Respiratory obstruction: oedema, bleeding or recurrent laryngeal nerve palsy
- Recurrent and superior laryngeal nerve damage: voice change characterised by an inability to create a high-pitched sound (crucial given the patient's occupation!) – preoperative cord inspection is essential
- Hypocalcaemia due to deliberate or inadvertent removal of all parathyroid tissue
- Hypothyroidism and need for medication.

CASE 141 | INFORMATION GIVING – BREAST CARCINOMA ***

SCENARIO

You are a general surgery registrar in a breast clinic. A 52-year-old housewife is attending following a routine mammography showing calcification consistent with ductal carcinoma in situ in the right breast. You have taken a history and performed both a general examination and clinical examination of the breasts, which are unremarkable. Explain the results to the patient and inform her of the plan.

KEY POINTS

Introduce yourself formally, as you have not met the patient before.

Medical

Explain the mammography and clinical examination findings to the patient in appropriate non-medical language. Explain carcinoma in situ and the difference to breast carcinoma/cancer (abnormal cells in ducts but no invasion outside ducts as yet) – it is essentially a pre-malignant condition in which a proportion, if left untreated, will go on to develop invasive cancer.

- Explore her understanding of the diagnosis and explain in simple terms what will happen next
- Knowledge of triple assessment is necessary
- Make sure the patient understands the need for biopsy and explain that the options for surgery will depend on the biopsy results. She will probably require wide local excision and radiotherapy but this will depend on the histology
- If asked about prognosis, you must not give specific information until you have the necessary results. You need to wait for biopsy results and also the surgical histology results with clearance margins and lymph node involvement before an accurate prognosis can be given.

Psychosocial

Allow time for active listening to the patient's concerns, especially the shock of the suspected diagnosis and the degree of uncertainty at this stage.

- There will be worries about treatment, as patients have preconceived ideas about breast removal, chemotherapy and/or radiotherapy. She may know of other patients who have gone through similar experiences

- Give her the opportunity to return with her family to discuss treatment and prognosis and offer her support and continuity of care. Let your consultant know, in case she returns when you are not in clinic
- It is often best to get allied health professionals such as senior nurses involved in the patient's support network as early as possible. Give her any information leaflets available and hand over to the Macmillan nurse, if available, in clinic for further discussion about the diagnosis.

CASE 142   INFORMATION GIVING – TESTICULAR TUMOUR   ***

SCENARIO

You are a urology core trainee in clinic. You have just received a phone call from the radiologist about a patient you sent for an urgent testicular ultrasound scan. He is 30 years old and newly married with no children. He presented, after much persuasion from his wife, with a painless swelling of the testicle. The radiologist confirms the results are consistent with a tumour, as you suspected from your clinical assessment. The scan has not been discussed with the patient, who is coming straight to clinic. He is anxious and suspecting bad news. You are due to assist in theatre in 10 minutes time.

KEY POINTS

- No need for a formal introduction as you sent him for the scan
- Remember to phone the surgeon you are due to assist to avoid interruptions during your consultation when theatres try to contact you if your consultation is prolonged
- Remember to give a 'warning shot' early in the consultation
- Give adequate time to explore the patient's concerns and answer his questions.

Medical

Explain that the ultrasound results and clinical examination suggest that cancer is the diagnosis. Give the news early in the

consultation and use the term 'cancer' – not lesion or lump, as this leads to confusion. Explore the patient's understanding of the diagnosis and explain in simple terms what will happen next.

Make sure the patient understands the need for early surgery and also that surgery is partly diagnostic. He will need to have urgent blood tests and a staging CT scan to assess prognosis. Sperm banking should also be discussed at this stage.

Psychosocial

Ensure you will not be interrupted for your consultation by turning your pager off and informing the clinic nurse.

- Allow time for active listening to the patient's concerns and consider the shock of the suspected diagnosis but also a degree of uncertainty at this stage. He will have worries about treatment. Depending on surgical results, he may require chemotherapy or, less likely, radiotherapy
- It is difficult to give any useful prognosis at this stage, as it will depend on the staging scan and histology following surgery
- You must offer the chance to return with his wife to discuss treatment and prognosis. Offer support, continuity of care and any information leaflets you have available
- If you have to rush away at the end, ensure that another health professional, e.g. clinic nurse, stays with him to explore any further issues.

CASE 143 | INFORMATION GIVING – LOSS OF FUNCTION ***

SCENARIO

You are a vascular surgery registrar. A week ago, the team admitted a 55-year-old policeman with an ischaemic right limb. He smokes 15 cigarettes per day and has insulin-dependent diabetes. An angiogram revealed an occluded right superficial femoral artery, with reasonable collaterals. An electrocardiogram, echocardiogram and carotid duplex scan were all within normal limits. He underwent a bypass procedure 7 days previously, at which you assisted. Unfortunately, the clinical scenario has deteriorated and, there is now gangrene affecting the ankle and foot, the lower limb is insensate distal to the calf and he is unable to move his right ankle.

You have to explain that he needs a below-knee amputation (BKA).

KEY POINTS

- You have met the patient before and therefore you should establish early on what he already understands about his leg and what he has had done already. This case is about loss of function
- Find out what sort of work he does as a policeman, as he may have to modify or change his job
- He may already expect the worst, as he has not been able to move his leg since the operation.

Medical

You must be clear in your own mind about the necessity for amputation here. His foot is unviable and he has a fixed ankle, indicating irreversible loss of function.

- Use a diagram if necessary to explain what has happened to his leg
- You must be able to explain how a BKA is performed and the reasons why this is a much better option for him than an above-knee amputation
- You must be able to list the complications of BKA if he asks
- You must also be prepared to discuss ways in which his life afterwards can be normalised.

Psychosocial

- He is initially going to need a wheelchair at home, so an occupational therapy assessment is required
- He lives with his wife, so does have someone at home with him and you should ask if he would like you to get his wife in to discuss all of this with both of them together
- Empathy is key to the success of your approach with this scenario and you should try to understand the psychological consequences to this active man of losing his leg
- The use of a prosthetic limb will be crucial to his rehabilitation and this should be mentioned. He will be able to drive a car and walk eventually, although he will initially need assistance
- Remember to enlist the assistance of allied health professionals such as prosthetists and senior nursing staff.

CASE 144 | INFORMATION GIVING – THE ANGRY PATIENT ***

SCENARIO

You are an orthopaedic registrar in a large trauma centre. At the end of a 12-hour on-call shift, you go to the bedside of a 28-year-old barrister with a closed ankle fracture whose operation has been cancelled for the third day running. The patient was admitted on Saturday morning and it is now Monday of a bank holiday weekend.

She was seen by one of your colleagues this morning, who, she states, 'promised the operation would definitely be today'. Since then there have been two major trauma calls, both requiring emergency surgery. The nurses have been busy, so she has not had analgesia for 6 hours and she has spent much of the day off the ward with her leg not elevated to use her mobile phone. She has missed crucial meetings with her clients and wants to make a complaint.

You have to explain the reasons for cancellation (more urgent trauma cases and only limited capacity at the weekend), while advising her about elevation of the leg.

KEY POINTS

Reading the case, it is clear that the communication scenario is to 'deal with' the angry patient. This is difficult and must be planned carefully.

Medical

If possible, find somewhere private to talk, with a nursing colleague present, and ensure you are not interrupted.

- Begin by introducing yourself – she has met a lot of different doctors and it is important she knows your role as the on-call surgeon
- Apologise early for the cancellation and explain the reasons of clinical priority. Explain how the operations are prioritised, as this may calm the situation. All patients will get their operation as soon as space is available on the list and it will not change her long-term outcome from the operation

- Avoid blaming anyone for what has happened, as this undermines professionalism
- Offer analgesia immediately, as being comfortable may change her perception of the situation
- Give her a chance to vent her anger before trying to interject. You could apologise on behalf of your colleague but explain he had good intentions trying to allay her anxiety and could not predict the arrival of major traumas
- Try to move the discussion on to focus on her treatment and offer advice regarding elevation of her leg to reduce swelling and prevent wound problems postoperatively.

Psychological

- Be understanding by trying to put yourself into this patient's shoes
- Expect that she will be angry, even unreasonable, but that your reaction would be similar
- Enlist the help of allied health professionals such as senior nursing staff, as she may need someone to talk to following your departure from the ward.
- Do not mirror any potentially aggressive movements, e.g. a patient standing up; if this happens, allow her some time to get things off her chest and then invite her to sit down so that you can discuss it in more detail.

INDEX

Page numbers followed by "*f*" indicate figures, "*t*" indicate tables, and "*b*" indicate boxes.